AF693062

Oxygen Variations, 2nd Edition

Oxygen Variations, 2nd Edition

Guest Editors

Costantino Balestra
Simona Mrakic-Sposta
Gerardo Bosco

MDPI

Basel • Beijing • Wuhan • Barcelona • Belgrade • Novi Sad • Cluj • Manchester

Guest Editors
Costantino Balestra
Environmental, Occupational & Ageing Physiology Laboratory
Haute Ecole Bruxelles-Brabant (HE2B)
Brussels
Belgium

Simona Mrakic-Sposta
National Research Council
Institute of Clinical Physiology
Milan
Italy

Gerardo Bosco
Department of Biomedical Sciences
University of Padova
Padova
Italy

Editorial Office
MDPI AG
Grosspeteranlage 5
4052 Basel, Switzerland

This is a reprint of the Special Issue, published open access by the journal *International Journal of Molecular Sciences* (ISSN 1422-0067), freely accessible at: https://www.mdpi.com/journal/ijms/special_issues/8PU70RA6UC.

For citation purposes, cite each article independently as indicated on the article page online and as indicated below:

Lastname, A.A.; Lastname, B.B. Article Title. *Journal Name* **Year**, *Volume Number*, Page Range.

ISBN 978-3-7258-7536-8 (Hbk)
ISBN 978-3-7258-7537-5 (PDF)
https://doi.org/10.3390/books978-3-7258-7537-5

© 2026 by the authors. Articles in this reprint are Open Access and distributed under the Creative Commons Attribution (CC BY) license. The reprint as a whole is distributed by MDPI under the terms and conditions of the Creative Commons Attribution-NonCommercial-NoDerivs (CC BY-NC-ND) license (https://creativecommons.org/licenses/by-nc-nd/4.0/).

Contents

About the Editors vii

Costantino Balestra, Gerardo Bosco and Simona Mrakic-Sposta
Oxygen Variations, 2nd Edition: Integrative Insights from Cellular Models to Clinical Physiology
Reprinted from: *Int. J. Mol. Sci.* **2026**, *27*, 1863, https://doi.org/10.3390/ijms27041863 . . . . . . **1**

Yuliya Sidorova, Nikita Petrov, Nadezhda Biryulina, Ilya Sokolov, Anastasiya Balakina, Nikita Trusov and Alla Kochetkova
The Study of Approaches to Modeling Oxidative Stress in Male Wistar Rats: The Comparative Analysis of Diet-Induced, Chemically Induced, and Physiologically Induced Models
Reprinted from: *Int. J. Mol. Sci.* **2025**, *26*, 6872, https://doi.org/10.3390/ijms26146872 . . . . . . **7**

Dominika Orzoł, Martyna Kępska and Magdalena Zyzak
Orientin Reverses Premature Senescence in Equine Adipose Stromal Cells Affected by Equine Metabolic Syndrome Through Oxidative Stress Modulation
Reprinted from: *Int. J. Mol. Sci.* **2025**, *26*, 6867, https://doi.org/10.3390/ijms26146867 . . . . . . **28**

Federico Pierro, Manlio Fazio, Giuseppe Murdaca, Fabio Stagno, Sebastiano Gangemi and Alessandro Allegra
Oxidative Stress and Mitochondrial Dysfunction in Myelodysplastic Syndrome: Roles in Development, Diagnosis, Prognosis, and Treatment
Reprinted from: *Int. J. Mol. Sci.* **2025**, *26*, 6415, https://doi.org/10.3390/ijms26136415 . . . . . . **48**

Michele Salvagno, Elda Diletta Sterchele, Mario Zaccarelli, Simona Mrakic-Sposta, Ian James Welsby, Costantino Balestra and Fabio Silvio Taccone
Oxidative Stress and Cerebral Vascular Tone: The Role of Reactive Oxygen and Nitrogen Species
Reprinted from: *Int. J. Mol. Sci.* **2024**, *25*, 3007, https://doi.org/10.3390/ijms25053007 . . . . . . **71**

Franziska Münz, Thomas Datzmann, Andrea Hoffmann, Michael Gröger, René Mathieu, Simon Mayer, et al.
The Effect of Targeted Hyperoxemia on Brain Immunohistochemistry after Long-Term, Resuscitated Porcine Acute Subdural Hematoma and Hemorrhagic Shock
Reprinted from: *Int. J. Mol. Sci.* **2024**, *25*, 6574, https://doi.org/10.3390/ijms25126574 . . . . . . **96**

Elizabeth G. Damato, Joseph S. Piktel, Seunghee P. Margevicius, Seth J. Fillioe, Lily K. Norton, Alireza Abdollahifar, et al.
Exposure to Non-Steady-State Oxygen Is Reflected in Changes to Arterial Blood Gas Values, Prefrontal Cortical Activity, and Systemic Cytokine Levels
Reprinted from: *Int. J. Mol. Sci.* **2024**, *25*, 3279, https://doi.org/10.3390/ijms25063279 . . . . . . **111**

Alessandra Vezzoli, Simona Mrakic-Sposta, Andrea Brizzolari, Costantino Balestra, Enrico Maria Camporesi and Gerardo Bosco
Oxy-Inflammation in Humans during Underwater Activities
Reprinted from: *Int. J. Mol. Sci.* **2024**, *25*, 3060, https://doi.org/10.3390/ijms25053060 . . . . . . **130**

Mariana Cannellotto, Ali Yasells García and María Silvina Landa
Hyperoxia: Effective Mechanism of Hyperbaric Treatment at Mild-Pressure
Reprinted from: *Int. J. Mol. Sci.* **2024**, *25*, 777, https://doi.org/10.3390/ijms25020777 . . . . **149**

Jelena Nesovic Ostojic, Sanjin Kovacevic, Milan Ivanov, Predrag Brkic, Maja Zivotic, Nevena Mihailovic-Stanojevic, et al.
Hyperbaric Oxygen Reduces Oxidative Stress Impairment and DNA Damage and Simultaneously Increases HIF-1α in Ischemia–Reperfusion Acute Kidney Injury
Reprinted from: *Int. J. Mol. Sci.* **2024**, *25*, 3870, https://doi.org/10.3390/ijms25073870 . . . . . . **161**

About the Editors

Costantino Balestra

Costantino Balestra is the Director of the Integrative Physiology Laboratory and a full-time Professor at the Haute École Bruxelles-Brabant (HE2B) in Brussels, where he teaches physiology, biostatistics, and research methodology, while also holding academic affiliations with the Université Libre de Bruxelles (ULB) and the Vrije Universiteit Brussel (VUB). His expertise lies in environmental and occupational physiology, with a specific focus on diving medicine, hyperbaric medicine, and integrative physiology, and he is particularly interested in the neurophysiology of fatigue and the application of intermittent oxygen doses. His clinical work focuses on translating performance-enhancing oxygen protocols for sportsmen into therapeutic applications to trigger beneficial healing reactions, specifically in oncologic patients. An internationally recognized authority in his field, he serves as Vice President of DAN Europe for Research and Education, is a former President of the European Underwater and Baromedical Society (EUBS), a former Vice President of the Undersea and Hyperbaric Medical Society (UHMS), and Vice President of The Belgian Society of Hyperbaric and Diving Medicine (SBMHS).

Simona Mrakic-Sposta

Simona Mrakic-Sposta is a molecular researcher at the Istituto di Fisiologia Clinica, part of the Consiglio Nazionale delle Ricerche (CNR) in Milan, and also serves as an adjunct professor of anatomy at Università Telematica San Raffaele (UNIROMA 5). Her research focuses on biomarkers of oxidative stress, inflammation, organ damage, and neuroplasticity, as she studies the physiological adaptation of the whole organism to extreme environmental conditions. Her work encompasses investigations into physiological adaptations in extreme environments, including high altitudes (hypobaric and normobaric hypoxia), saturation diving, breath-hold diving, and space environments. Since October 2017, she has been a member the Società Italiana di Medicina di Montagna (SIMeM), where she now serves as the Secretary.

Gerardo Bosco

Gerardo Bosco is currently a Full Professor at the University of Chieti-Pescara in the Department of Medicine and Aging Sciences, and until 2025 he served as Associate Professor at the University of Padua, where he was also Director of the Second-Level Master's Program in Underwater and Hyperbaric Medicine. His research focuses on respiratory mechanics, cardiovascular adaptations during exercise, metabolic disorders, and oxygen toxicity under environmental stress, in addition to his interest in human performance and safety in extreme environments and perioperative care. His work has highlighted the preventive role of pre-oxygenation and the ketogenic diet in diving, and he explores hypoxia modulation and the mechanisms of hyperbaric oxygen therapy; in 2016, his group validated femoral head osteonecrosis as a new indication for hyperbaric oxygen therapy. A specialist in Underwater and Hyperbaric Medicine and Nutrition Sciences, he has held significant leadership roles in academic medical programs, including directing the Master's Program in Underwater and Hyperbaric Medicine at the University of Padua.

International Journal of
Molecular Sciences

MDPI

Editorial

Oxygen Variations, 2nd Edition: Integrative Insights from Cellular Models to Clinical Physiology

Costantino Balestra [1,2,3,4,*], Gerardo Bosco [5] and Simona Mrakic-Sposta [6]

1 Environmental, Occupational, Aging (Integrative) Physiology Laboratory, Haute Ecole Bruxelles-Brabant (HE2B), 1160 Brussels, Belgium
2 Anatomical Research and Clinical Studies, Vrije Universiteit Brussels (VUB), 1090 Brussels, Belgium
3 DAN Europe Research Division (Roseto-Brussels), 1160 Brussels, Belgium
4 Physical Activity Teaching Unit, Motor Sciences Department, Université Libre de Bruxelles (ULB), 1050 Brussels, Belgium
5 Department of Medicine and Sciences of Aging, G. d'Annunzio University of Chieti-Pescara, 66100 Chieti, Italy; gerardo.bosco@unich.it
6 Institute of Clinical Physiology, National Research Council (CNR), 20162 Milan, Italy; simona.mrakicsposta@cnr.it
* Correspondence: cbalestra@he2b.be or Costantino.Balestra@ulb.be or costantinobalestra@gmail.com

Introduction

As we have been studying oxygen for 250 years [1], we may think that we know it all. Admittedly, we have learned a considerable amount since the first use of the term "phlogiston", a word coined by Jonass Johann Joachim Becher in the 17th century to refer to what we now call oxygen. Phlogiston is the neutral form of "phlogistos", meaning "inflammable". The word comes from "phlogizein", meaning "put on fire, burning", and from "phlox" (in the genitive form "phlogos"), meaning "flame"; it was the hypothetical theory of fire and was a constituent of all combustible material.

What would now be described as oxidation was thought to be the release of "phlogiston", and the material left behind, such as ash, would be considered a "dephlogisticated" substance.

This understanding is not far from a thermodynamic perspective, in which something "on fire" has a different entropy than what remains after combustion—the so-called dephlogisticated substances. Oxygen or phlogiston is also currently considered an "epistemic object" and a number of preeminent scientists were involved in understanding it over the years, showing how much attention it still deserves [2–5].

This editorial builds upon the Special Issue "Oxygen Variations—2nd Edition" by integrating additional recent contributions addressing oxidative stress, redox regulation, and oxygen-driven adaptation across experimental, organ-specific, and clinical contexts that will propose new integrative insights from cellular models to clinical physiology [6,7].

All studies included can be interpreted through the dual lenses of hormesis, a beneficial adaptive zone lying between the "friend or foe" [8–15] nature of oxygen [16,17], and non-equilibrium thermodynamics, emphasizing oxygen variability as a structured biological stimulus rather than a static exposure [18].

1. Experimental and Cellular Models of Oxidative Stress

The tentative modeling of oxygen responses has been an objective for number of scientists. Sidorova et al. [19] provide a rigorous comparative framework for modeling oxidative stress in vivo using dietary, chemical, and physiological stressors in Wistar rats. From a hormetic standpoint, the study elegantly demonstrates that not all oxidative stressors are equivalent: diet-induced oxidative stress elicited the strongest redox response, characterized by concomitant increases in lipid peroxidation and antioxidant enzyme activity, while immobilization stress produced comparatively modest effects, opening up new perspectives on microgravity oxidative stress during spatial incursions.

Thermodynamically, these models represent distinct magnitudes and durations of entropy production, with dietary overload imposing a sustained metabolic disequilibrium, whereas acute stressors trigger transient adaptive responses.

This work provides a valuable platform for evaluating interventions that aim to shift oxidative stress from pathological to adaptive domains, as shown in other domains such as performance or physical training [20–22].

At the cellular level, Orzoł et al. [23] demonstrate that the modulation of oxidative stress can reverse premature senescence in equine adipose-derived stromal cells affected by metabolic syndrome.

Orientin treatment restored proliferation, migration, and clonogenicity while reducing senescence markers and oxidative load, paving a promising therapeutical path [24]. Within a hormetic framework, orientin appears to recalibrate redox signaling toward a low-stress adaptive zone.

Thermodynamically, the intervention reduces dissipative losses associated with chronic oxidative stress, allowing cellular energy fluxes to be reallocated toward regeneration rather than damage control.

2. Mitochondrial Dysfunction and Redox-driven Pathology

Pierro et al. [25] extend the discussion to clonal hematological disease, identifying oxidative stress and mitochondrial dysfunction as central drivers in myelodysplastic syndromes.

Persistent ROS (Reactive Oxygen Species) and RNS (Reactive Nitrogen Species) production destabilizes genomic integrity and promotes clonal evolution, representing a failure of hormetic containment. In thermodynamic terms, the bone marrow niche becomes trapped in a high-entropy state, where energy dissipation exceeds adaptive capacity. The review highlights redox-modulating therapies as potential tools to restore controlled signaling and re-establish a lower-entropy, functionally productive hematopoietic environment.

3. Brain, Vascular Tone, and Neuroenergetics

The brain constitutes a critical testbed for oxygen-driven hormesis. Salvagno et al. [26] analyze how ROS and RNS regulate cerebral vascular tone, emphasizing that species-specific redox signaling can induce vasodilation or vasoconstriction.

From a thermodynamic perspective, cerebral autoregulation emerges as a fine-tuned balance between oxygen delivery, mitochondrial efficiency, and entropy minimization in a high-demand organ.

From a therapeutical perspective, Münz et al. [27] provide experimental evidence that targeted moderate hyperoxemia improves neurological outcomes after combined subdural hematoma and hemorrhagic shock without exacerbating oxidative or nitrosative tissue damage.

This supports the concept that carefully dosed hyperoxia operates within a hormetic window, enhancing systemic organization rather than inducing oxidative collapse.

In the same direction, Damato et al. [28] further demonstrate that non-steady-state oxygen exposure produces distinct neurovascular and inflammatory responses compared to

https://doi.org/10.3390/ijms27041863

steady-state hyperoxia. Oscillating FiO_2 induced delayed cytokine responses and modulate cortical activation, underscoring the importance of temporal oxygen variability. Thermodynamically, these oscillations represent repeated controlled perturbations that reshape neurovascular coupling and inflammatory signaling.

4. Hyperoxia, (Relative) Hypoxia, and Systemic Adaptation

The concept of oxy-inflammation [29] is described by Vezzoli et al. [30] in underwater activities, where divers experience alternating hypoxic and hyperoxic conditions under hyperbaric stress. The diving response exemplifies a naturally occurring hormetic system in which oxygen fluctuations, pressure, and environmental stressors jointly modulate redox and inflammatory pathways [31–34].

Changing the classical hyperbaric levels clinically used, Cannellotto et al. [35] clarify that even mild-pressure hyperbaric oxygen therapy generates sufficient mitochondrial hyperoxia to activate hypoxia-related signaling pathways through relative post-exposure hypoxia.

This apparent paradox aligns with thermodynamic principles: transient oxygen excess increases electron flux, followed by adaptive signaling that enhances angiogenesis and tissue repair. As already proposed by Salvagno et al. [36], this relative hypoxia is a potent trigger for physiological adaptations.

Using higher oxygen levels, Nesovic Ostojic et al. [37] demonstrate that hyperbaric oxygen preconditioning reduces oxidative damage and DNA strand breaks in ischemia–reperfusion acute kidney injury while upregulating HIF-1α and suppressing NF-κB.

This dual action exemplifies hormesis [38,39], where controlled oxidative signaling primes antioxidant capacity and genomic stability, allowing the system to better withstand subsequent energetic insults [40–43].

5. Integrative Perspective and Conclusions

Taken together, the studies included in this Special Issue and its extensions converge on a unifying concept: oxygen variability, when precisely controlled, operates as a powerful regulator of biological organization.

Hormesis provides the dose–response framework, while thermodynamics explains how transient increases in entropy production can drive reorganization toward more efficient and resilient states.

Future research should focus on defining individualized oxygen dosing strategies and identifying biomarkers that discriminate adaptive from maladaptive redox responses. It should aim to characterize the multiscale biological effects of oxygen partial pressure variations. Controlled oscillations between hypoxia, normoxia, hyperoxia, and hyperbaric hyperoxia act as non-equilibrium perturbations driving hormetic adaptation [44–46].

At the molecular level, transient redox signaling modulates ROS-sensitive pathways (HIF-1α, NRF2, NF-κB) and mitochondrial function.

These signals propagate to organ-level responses affecting brain energetics, vascular tone, immune regulation, and tissue repair.

Clinically, optimized oxygen variability enhances resilience, functional recovery, and therapeutic outcomes, whereas excessive or prolonged exposure may lead to maladaptive oxidative stress. It seems that too-high or too-frequent doses may offer a sub-optimal response.

6. Conceptual Thermodynamic Framework of Oxygen-Driven Adaptation

From a thermodynamic perspective, biological systems operate far from equilibrium and rely on continuous energy fluxes to maintain organization.

Variations in oxygen availability introduce controlled perturbations that transiently increase entropy production (σ), forcing metabolic reorganization. When the perturbation

https://doi.org/10.3390/ijms27041863

magnitude remains within a hormetic window, adaptive responses emerge, leading to improved efficiency and resilience. Excessive or sustained perturbations exceed dissipative capacity [47,48] and result in non-compensated/prolonged/pathological oxidative stress (see Figure 1).

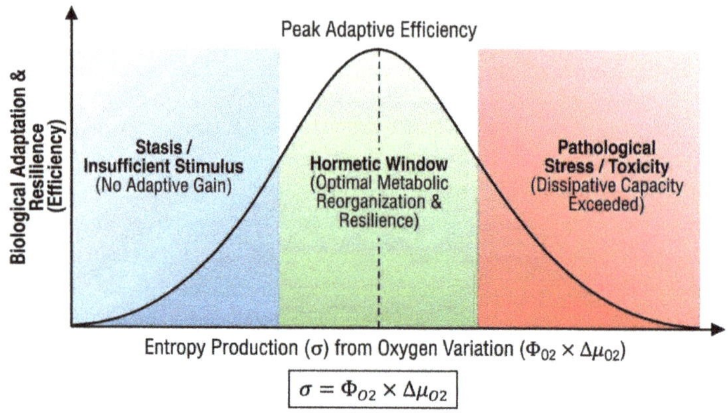

Figure 1. Conceptual relationship between entropy production (o), induced by variations in oxygen flux (Φ_{O2}) and the chemical potential gradient ($\Delta\mu_{O2}$), and the adaptive biological response, illustrating the concept of the hormetic window.

Conceptually, this relationship can be expressed in a simplified way:

$$\sigma = \Phi_{O2} \times \Delta\mu_{O2}$$

where σ represents entropy production, Φ_{O2} the oxygen flux, and $\Delta\mu_{O2}$ the chemical potential gradient of oxygen. Adaptive biological responses occur when σ remains within an optimal non-linear range, enabling reorganization toward lower effective entropy states following the perturbation.

The authors are confident that future research from several scientific fields will finetune "oxygen variations" [49,50] and reach specific, adaptative, hormetic, and personalized therapeutical approaches.

Author Contributions: Conceptualization, C.B. and S.M.-S.; methodology, C.B.; software, S.M.-S. and G.B.; validation, C.B., G.B. and S.M.-S.; formal analysis, C.B.; resources, C.B., G.B. and S.M.-S. data curation, C.B.; writing—original draft preparation, C.B.; writing—review and editing, C.B., S.M.-S. and G.B.; project administration, C.B. and G.B.; funding acquisition, G.B. All authors have read and agreed to the published version of the manuscript.

Conflicts of Interest: The authors declare no conflicts of interest.

References

1. Hancock, J.T. A Brief History of Oxygen: 250 Years on. *Oxygen* **2022**, *2*, 31–39. [CrossRef]
2. Gorriñobeaskoa, U. On the Historiography of Epistemic Objects: An Evolutionary Approach. *Ber. Wiss* **2025**, *48*, 180–198. [CrossRef]
3. Lanahan, J.K.; Alston, T.A. Oxygen Was Almost Named Nitrogen. *J. Anesth. Hist.* **2020**, *6*, 96–97. [CrossRef]
4. Severinghaus, J.W. The Most Important Discovery of Science. *Adv. Exp. Med. Biol.* **2016**, *876*, 1–16. [CrossRef]
5. Severinghaus, J.W. Eight sages over five centuries share oxygen's discovery. *Adv. Physiol. Educ.* **2016**, *40*, 370–376. [CrossRef] [PubMed]
6. Balestra, C.; Mrakic-Sposta, S.; Virgili, F. Oxygen Variations—Insights into Hypoxia, Hyperoxia and Hyperbaric Hyperoxia—Is the Dose the Clue? *Int. J. Mol. Sci.* **2023**, *24*, 13472. [CrossRef] [PubMed]

https://doi.org/10.3390/ijms27041863

7. Anbalagan, S. Oxygen is an essential gasotransmitter directly sensed via protein gasoreceptors. *Anim. Model. Exp. Med.* **2024**, *7*, 189–193. [CrossRef]
8. Jiang, Q.; Lin, X.; Zhai, M.; Gong, Y.; Li, Y.; Liu, S. The Role of ROS and Its Sources in Tumorigenesis: Friend or Foe? *Adv. Biol.* **2025**, *9*, e2400549. [CrossRef]
9. Glorieux, C.; Enríquez, C.; González, C.; Aguirre-Martínez, G.; Buc Calderon, P. The Multifaceted Roles of NRF2 in Cancer: Friend or Foe? *Antioxidants* **2024**, *13*, 70. [CrossRef] [PubMed]
10. Wang, R.; Liang, L.; Matsumoto, M.; Iwata, K.; Umemura, A.; He, F. Reactive Oxygen Species and NRF2 Signaling, Friends or Foes in Cancer? *Biomolecules* **2023**, *13*, 353. [CrossRef]
11. Cardoso, M.A.; Gonçalves, H.M.R.; Davis, F. Reactive oxygen species in biological media are they friend or foe? Major In vivo and In vitro sensing challenges. *Talanta* **2023**, *260*, 124648. [CrossRef]
12. Szarka, A.; Lőrincz, T.; Hajdinák, P. Friend or Foe: The Relativity of (Anti)oxidative Agents and Pathways. *Int. J. Mol. Sci.* **2022**, *23*, 5188. [CrossRef] [PubMed]
13. Shilovsky, G.A.; Ashapkin, V.V. Transcription Factor Nrf2 and Mitochondria—Friends or Foes in the Regulation of Aging Rate. *Biochemistry* **2022**, *87*, 1477–1486. [CrossRef]
14. Lesmana, R.; Parameswari, C.; Mandagi, G.F.; Wahyudi, J.F.; Permana, N.J.; Radhiyanti, P.T.; Gunadi, J.W. The Role of Exercise-Induced Reactive Oxygen Species (ROS) Hormesis in Aging: Friend or Foe. *Cell Physiol. Biochem.* **2022**, *56*, 692–706. [CrossRef]
15. Powers, S.K.; Deminice, R.; Ozdemir, M.; Yoshihara, T.; Bomkamp, M.P.; Hyatt, H. Exercise-induced oxidative stress: Friend or foe? *J. Sport. Health Sci.* **2020**, *9*, 415–425. [CrossRef]
16. Hafner, S.; Beloncle, F.; Koch, A.; Radermacher, P.; Asfar, P. Hyperoxia in intensive care, emergency, and peri-operative medicine: Dr. Jekyll or Mr. Hyde? A 2015 update. *Ann. Intensive Care* **2015**, *5*, 42. [CrossRef]
17. Asfar, P.; Calzia, E.; Huber-Lang, M.; Ignatius, A.; Radermacher, P. Hyperoxia during septic shock—Dr. Jekyll or Mr. Hyde? *Shock* **2012**, *37*, 122–123. [CrossRef]
18. Cano-Martínez, A.; Rubio-Ruiz, M.E.; Guarner-Lans, V. Homeostasis and evolution in relation to regeneration and repair. *J. Physiol.* **2024**, *602*, 2627–2648. [CrossRef]
19. Sidorova, Y.; Petrov, N.; Biryulina, N.; Sokolov, I.; Balakina, A.; Trusov, N.; Kochetkova, A. The Study of Approaches to Modeling Oxidative Stress in Male Wistar Rats: The Comparative Analysis of Diet-Induced, Chemically Induced, and Physiologically Induced Models. *Int. J. Mol. Sci.* **2025**, *26*, 6872. [CrossRef] [PubMed]
20. Suzuki, J. Exercise performance in well-trained male mice is promoted by intermittent hyperoxia via improving metabolic properties and capillary profiles. *Physiol. Rep.* **2025**, *13*, e70341. [CrossRef] [PubMed]
21. Suzuki, J. Effects of exercise training with intermittent hyperoxic intervention on endurance performance and muscle metabolic properties in male mice. *Physiol. Rep.* **2024**, *12*, e16117. [CrossRef]
22. Brugniaux, J.V.; Coombs, G.B.; Barak, O.F.; Dujic, Z.; Sekhon, M.S.; Ainslie, P.N. Highs and lows of hyperoxia: Physiological, performance, and clinical aspects. *Am. J. Physiol. Regul. Integr. Comp. Physiol.* **2018**, *315*, R1–R27. [CrossRef]
23. Orzoł, D.; Kępska, M.; Zyzak, M. Orientin Reverses Premature Senescence in Equine Adipose Stromal Cells Affected by Equine Metabolic Syndrome Through Oxidative Stress Modulation. *Int. J. Mol. Sci.* **2025**, *26*, 6867. [CrossRef]
24. Zheng, Y.; Chen, L.; Li, H.; Lin, J.; Ma, J. Orientin alleviates severe inflammation via regulating macrophage glycolysis and immune function in sepsis. *Free Radic. Biol. Med.* **2026**, *246*, 196–208. [CrossRef]
25. Pierro, F.; Fazio, M.; Murdaca, G.; Stagno, F.; Gangemi, S.; Allegra, A. Oxidative Stress and Mitochondrial Dysfunction in Myelodysplastic Syndrome: Roles in Development, Diagnosis, Prognosis, and Treatment. *Int. J. Mol. Sci.* **2025**, *26*, 6415. [CrossRef] [PubMed]
26. Salvagno, M.; Sterchele, E.D.; Zaccarelli, M.; Mrakic-Sposta, S.; Welsby, I.J.; Balestra, C.; Taccone, F.S. Oxidative Stress and Cerebral Vascular Tone: The Role of Reactive Oxygen and Nitrogen Species. *Int. J. Mol. Sci.* **2024**, *25*, 3007. [CrossRef] [PubMed]
27. Münz, F.; Datzmann, T.; Hoffmann, A.; Gröger, M.; Mathieu, R.; Mayer, S.; Zink, F.; Gässler, H.; Wolfschmitt, E.-M.; Hogg, M.; et al. The Effect of Targeted Hyperoxemia on Brain Immunohistochemistry after Long-Term, Resuscitated Porcine Acute Subdural Hematoma and Hemorrhagic Shock. *Int. J. Mol. Sci.* **2024**, *25*, 6574. [CrossRef] [PubMed]
28. Damato, E.G.; Piktel, J.S.; Margevicius, S.P.; Fillioe, S.J.; Norton, L.K.; Abdollahifar, A.; Strohl, K.P.; Burch, D.S.; Decker, M.J. Exposure to Non-Steady-State Oxygen Is Reflected in Changes to Arterial Blood Gas Values, Prefrontal Cortical Activity, and Systemic Cytokine Levels. *Int. J. Mol. Sci.* **2024**, *25*, 3279. [CrossRef] [PubMed]
29. Valacchi, G.; Virgili, F.; Cervellati, C.; Pecorelli, A. OxInflammation: From Subclinical Condition to Pathological Biomarker. *Front. Physiol.* **2018**, *9*, 858. [CrossRef]
30. Vezzoli, A.; Mrakic-Sposta, S.; Brizzolari, A.; Balestra, C.; Camporesi, E.M.; Bosco, G. Oxy-Inflammation in Humans during Underwater Activities. *Int. J. Mol. Sci.* **2024**, *25*, 3060. [CrossRef]
31. Rixen, M.; Weickmann, J.; Gebauer, R.A.; Weidenbach, M.; Markel, F.; Michaelis, A.; Dähnert, I.; Wüstenfeld, J.; Münch, D.; Poschart, M.; et al. First Real-Life Data on the Diving Response in Healthy Children. *Pediatr. Cardiol.* **2024**, *45*, 314–322. [CrossRef]

https://doi.org/10.3390/ijms27041863

32. Mulder, E.; Sieber, A.; Schagatay, E. Using underwater pulse oximetry in freediving to extreme depths to study risk of hypoxic blackout and diving response phases. *Front. Physiol.* **2021**, *12*, 651128. [CrossRef]
33. Lundell, R.V.; Tuominen, L.; Ojanen, T.; Parkkola, K.; Raisanen-Sokolowski, A. Diving Responses in Experienced Rebreather Divers: Short-Term Heart Rate Variability in Cold Water Diving. *Front. Physiol.* **2021**, *12*, 649319. [CrossRef]
34. Panneton, W.M. The mammalian diving response: An enigmatic reflex to preserve life? *Physiology* **2013**, *28*, 284–297. [CrossRef] [PubMed]
35. Cannellotto, M.; Yasells García, A.; Landa, M.S. Hyperoxia: Effective Mechanism of Hyperbaric Treatment at Mild-Pressure. *Int. J. Mol. Sci.* **2024**, *25*, 777. [CrossRef] [PubMed]
36. Salvagno, M.; Coppalini, G.; Taccone, F.S.; Strapazzon, G.; Mrakic-Sposta, S.; Rocco, M.; Khalife, M.; Balestra, C. The Normobaric Oxygen Paradox-Hyperoxic Hypoxic Paradox: A Novel Expedient Strategy in Hematopoiesis Clinical Issues. *Int. J. Mol. Sci.* **2022**, *24*, 82. [CrossRef] [PubMed]
37. Nesovic Ostojic, J.; Kovacevic, S.; Ivanov, M.; Brkic, P.; Zivotic, M.; Mihailovic-Stanojevic, N.; Karanovic, D.; Vajic, U.J.; Jeremic, R.; Jovovic, D.; et al. Hyperbaric Oxygen Reduces Oxidative Stress Impairment and DNA Damage and Simultaneously Increases HIF-1α in Ischemia–Reperfusion Acute Kidney Injury. *Int. J. Mol. Sci.* **2024**, *25*, 3870. [CrossRef]
38. Balestra, C.; Baldelli, S.; Virgili, F.; Salvagno, M.; Mrakic-Sposta, S.; Fratantonio, D. Pulsed Hyperoxia Acts on Plasmatic Advanced Glycation End Products and Advanced Oxidation Protein Products and Modulates Mitochondrial Biogenesis in Human Peripheral Blood Mononuclear Cells: A Pilot Study on the « Normobaric Oxygen Paradox ». *Int. J. Mol. Sci.* **2024**, *25*, 2394. [CrossRef]
39. Fratantonio, D.; Virgili, F.; Zucchi, A.; Lambrechts, K.; Latronico, T.; Lafere, P.; Germonpre, P.; Balestra, C. Increasing Oxygen Partial Pressures Induce a Distinct Transcriptional Response in Human PBMC: A Pilot Study on the "Normobaric Oxygen Paradox". *Int. J. Mol. Sci.* **2021**, *22*, 458. [CrossRef]
40. Marín-López, A.G.; Macias-Velez, R.J.; Jarero-Basulto, J.J.; Rivera-Cervantes, M.C. Evidence of a hormetic-like cytoprotective effect by erythropoietin in the SH-SY5Y cell model of oxygen-glucose deprivation. *Neuroscience* **2025**, *577*, 114–122. [CrossRef]
41. Chang, X.; Tamauchi, S.; Nakagawa, A.; Xinyuan, W.; Yoshida, K.; Yokoi, A.; Yoshikawa, N.; Kajiyama, H. Chemotherapeutic hormesis induced by the tumor microenvironment in refractory ovarian cancer. *Sci. Rep.* **2025**, *15*, 596. [CrossRef] [PubMed]
42. Bresilla, D.; Tawfik, I.; Hirtl, M.; Gabrijelčič, S.; Ostaku, J.; Mossegger, F.; Wurzer, L.; Lederer, S.; Kalinova, K.; Malle, E.; et al. Enhancing Late-Life Survival and Mobility via Mitohormesis by Reducing Mitochondrial Calcium Levels. *Aging Cell* **2025**, *24*, e70247. [CrossRef]
43. Burtscher, J.; Samaja, M. Healthy Aging at Moderate Altitudes: Hypoxia and Hormesis. *Gerontology* **2024**, *70*, 1152–1160. [CrossRef]
44. MacLaughlin, K.J.; Barton, G.P.; MacLaughlin, J.E.; Lamers, J.J.; Marcou, M.D.; O'Brien, M.J.; Braun, R.K.; Eldridge, M.W. 100% oxygen mobilizes stem cells and up-regulates MIF and APRIL in humans: A new point on the hormetic dose curve. *Front. Cell Dev. Biol.* **2025**, *12*, 1377203. [CrossRef]
45. MacLaughlin, K.J.; Barton, G.P.; Braun, R.K.; MacLaughlin, J.E.; Lamers, J.J.; Marcou, M.D.; Eldridge, M.W. Hyperbaric air mobilizes stem cells in humans; a new perspective on the hormetic dose curve. *Front. Neurol.* **2023**, *14*, 1192793. [CrossRef] [PubMed]
46. MacLaughlin, K.J.; Barton, G.P.; Braun, R.K.; Eldridge, M.W. Effect of intermittent hyperoxia on stem cell mobilization and cytokine expression. *Med. Gas. Res.* **2019**, *9*, 139–144. [CrossRef] [PubMed]
47. Prigogine, I.; George, C. The second law as a selection principle: The microscopic theory of dissipative processes in quantum systems. *Proc. Natl. Acad. Sci. USA* **1983**, *80*, 4590–4594. [CrossRef]
48. Prigogine, I.; Henin, F.; George, C. Dissipative processes, quantum States, and entropy. *Proc. Natl. Acad. Sci. USA* **1968**, *59*, 7–14. [CrossRef]
49. Leveque, C.; Mrakic Sposta, S.; Theunissen, S.; Germonpré, P.; Lambrechts, K.; Vezzoli, A.; Bosco, G.; Lévénez, M.; Lafère, P.; Guerrero, F.; et al. Oxidative Stress Response Kinetics after 60 Minutes at Different (1.4 ATA and 2.5 ATA) Hyperbaric Hyperoxia Exposures. *Int. J. Mol. Sci.* **2023**, *24*, 12361. [CrossRef]
50. Leveque, C.; Mrakic-Sposta, S.; Lafere, P.; Vezzoli, A.; Germonpre, P.; Beer, A.; Mievis, S.; Virgili, F.; Lambrechts, K.; Theunissen, S.; et al. Oxidative Stress Response's Kinetics after 60 Minutes at Different (30% or 100%) Normobaric Hyperoxia Exposures. *Int. J. Mol. Sci.* **2022**, *24*, 664. [CrossRef]

Disclaimer/Publisher's Note: The statements, opinions and data contained in all publications are solely those of the individual author(s) and contributor(s) and not of MDPI and/or the editor(s). MDPI and/or the editor(s) disclaim responsibility for any injury to people or property resulting from any ideas, methods, instructions or products referred to in the content.

https://doi.org/10.3390/ijms27041863

International Journal of
Molecular Sciences

MDPI

Article

The Study of Approaches to Modeling Oxidative Stress in Male Wistar Rats: The Comparative Analysis of Diet-Induced, Chemically Induced, and Physiologically Induced Models

Yuliya Sidorova *, Nikita Petrov, Nadezhda Biryulina, Ilya Sokolov, Anastasiya Balakina, Nikita Trusov and Alla Kochetkova

Federal Research Centre of Nutrition and Biotechnology, 109240 Moscow, Russia; petrov-nikita-y@mail.ru (N.P.); biryulina_nadezhda@mail.ru (N.B.); sokolov.iliya1993@gmail.com (I.S.); balakina.a.s@yandex.ru (A.B.); nikkitosu@yandex.ru (N.T.); kochetkova@ion.ru (A.K.)
* Correspondence: sidorova@ion.ru; Tel.: +7-495-698-53-71

Abstract

Oxidative stress can be caused by bad nutrition, psychoemotional stress, or other external influences in everyday life. The aim of this study is to develop and verify biological models using male Wistar rats that allow reproducing oxidative stress in vivo, in particular: food (diet with high cholesterol and fructose content), medical (injection of CCl_4), and physiological (immobilization stress). Diet with 1% cholesterol and fructose had the greatest impact on the antioxidant status of animals: a significant increase in serum malondialdehyde (by 1.8 times) and superoxide dismutase (by 2.4 times) as well as a significant decrease in the Cat gene expression by 35% were shown. The immobilization led only to a significant decrease in serum lipid peroxides by 29%. A single intraperitoneal administration of CCl_4 was accompanied by a significant increase in the blood lipid peroxides (by 1.3 times) and catalase (by 1.6 times), as well as a significant decrease in the *Cat* mRNA by 33% and *Gpx1* by 48%. The obtained data can be used to study the effectiveness of drugs, biologically active food supplements and functional nutrition in vivo.

Keywords: oxidative stress; biological model; antioxidant status; high-cholesterol diet; immobilization; CCl_4

1. Introduction

Oxidative stress occurs as a result of imbalanced production of reactive oxygen species (ROS). Excessive formation of ROS may lead to oxidative damage of molecules involved in aging and development of neurodegenerative and cardiovascular diseases. To increase a human organism's resistance to oxidative stress, it is necessary to provide it with antioxidants. It is necessary to select an appropriate biomodel that allows reproducing oxidative stress in laboratory rodents and obtaining reliable results.

Oxidative stress may be caused by bad nutrition, psycho-emotional stress or other external influences in everyday life. Excessive consumption of diets high in fat, especially saturated fatty acids, fried and smoked meats, baked goods, juices, and soda (sources of cholesterol and simple sugars) leads to the development of hyperlipidemia and obesity. The subsequent accumulation of adipose tissue in the body induces the development of oxidative stress, endothelial dysfunction, and excessive synthesis of adipokines, leading to other complications [1,2]. To simulate such conditions in vivo, diets with a high content of fat (45–60% fat by calories), easily digestible carbohydrates, and cholesterol are widely used.

The so-called "Cafeteria" diets, high in fat and sugar, simulate modern human obesogenic diets [3–6]. However, due to heterogeneity and a lack of standardization, this model is less effective. Obesity and associated diseases in animals develop slowly and generally replicate the corresponding human pathology when fat accumulates slowly, mainly due to excess energy intake and insufficient energy expenditure. The use of a high-cholesterol diet efficiently leads to conditions characterized by the accumulation of prooxidants and lipid peroxidation products [7].

Besides the diet-induced models, drug-based approaches using various chemical compounds have traditionally been used to model oxidative stress. Paracetamol (acetaminophen) [8], lipopolysaccharide [9], and carbon tetrachloride are most commonly used in in vivo studies. Paracetamol, which is a commonly used antipyretic and analgesic drug, is safe and effective at therapeutic doses. The main limitation of this model is the use of high doses to induce mitochondrial dysfunction, which leads to overproduction of ROS and further liver damage [10]. Lipopolysaccharide is a bacterial pathogen that imbalances oxidative stress status and immune system responses mainly through the overproduction of pro-inflammatory cytokines [11]. Carbon tetrachloride (CCl_4) is a well-known toxin associated with liver damage, causing oxidative stress and damage to cellular components [12–14]. It is a potent prooxidant agent that has been widely used in recent years to induce hepatotoxicity [15] and oxidative stress [16]. CCl_4 administration causes oxidative damage through the formation of free radicals and enhances lipid peroxidation [16]. Although carbon tetrachloride administration to animals is one of the most widely used in vivo models of oxidative stress/lipid peroxidation, it has several limitations. The induced oxidative stress is a consequence of poisoning and acute failure of vital organs, especially the liver [17]. The toxicity of CCl_4 depends on the dose and exposure time. At low doses, temporary effects prevail: disorders in lipid homeostasis, cytokine release, and apoptosis. At higher doses or longer exposure, fatty degeneration, fibrosis, cirrhosis, and even cancer may occur. At acute toxic doses irreversible liver injuries take place [18].

As an alternative for modeling oxidative stress, some studies use stress exposure [19,20]. Increased metabolic rate causes excessive formation of free radicals [21], in particular reactive oxygen species, accompanied by functional and structural damage to cells and tissues. For example, acute exercise on a treadmill causes a significant release of pro-inflammatory cytokines and free radicals from activated leukocytes and leads to muscle damage and tissue injury. Moreover, during prolonged exercise, oxygen consumption increases and produces reactive oxygen species (ROS). However, this method has limitations, like the necessity for preliminary training of animals and possible injuries during the test [22]. The forced swim test (FST) has been reported to increase rodent oxidative stress in the brain as well as tissue degeneration and oxidative stress in peripheral tissues, including the liver, which is regulated by the brain [23]. The necessity to warm and dry animals and potent injuries are also limitations of this method. To study physiological reactions caused by a state of chronic psychoemotional stress, a model of immobilization is used [24]. Stress caused by immobilization leads to behavioral changes such as anxiety, depression, anorexia, and decreased activity, similar to human reactions to crowding, frustration, and tension [25]. The model is easily reproduced and used to simulate acute or chronic stress [26].

The aim of the present study is to conduct a comprehensive comparative analysis of three distinct models of oxidative stress in male Wistar rats: dietary-induced stress, chemically induced stress via intraperitoneal injection of CCl_4, and physiologically induced stress through immobilization. This research seeks to evaluate and compare the extent and nature of oxidative stress elicited by each method, with particular focus on a panel of biochemical markers, including lipid peroxidation markers (LPO, MDA), antioxidant enzymes (SOD, catalase, glutathione peroxidaze), and antioxidant genes liver expression

(*Sod1*, *Gpx1*, *Cat*, *Nqo1*, and *Hmox1*). This investigation seeks to elucidate the differential effects and mechanisms underlying each model, thereby contributing to a more nuanced understanding of oxidative stress responses in preclinical research.

2. Results

2.1. Fatty Acid Composition

Table 1 presents the results of determining the fatty acid composition of sunflower and soybean oils used in diets.

Table 1. Fatty acid composition of soybean and sunflower oil, %.

Fatty Acid (FA)	FA Index	Soybean Oil	Sunflower Oil
Myristic	14:0	0.10	0.07
Pentadecanoic	15:0	0.02	0.01
Palmitic	16:0	10.29	6.14
Hexadecene	16:1	0.02	0.02
Palmitoleic	16:1 9-cis	0.08	0.04
Margarine	17:0	0.08	0.03
Heptadecenoic	17:1	0.04	0.03
Stearic	18:0	4.92	3.16
Oleic	18:1 9-cis	24.11	27.31
Vaccenic	18:1 11-cis	1.40	0.78
Octadecene	18:1 11-cis	0.06	0.00
cis, trans-linoleic	18:2 9-cis, 12-trans	0.05	0.24
trans, cis-linoleic	18:2 9-trans, 12-cis	0.00	0.19
Linoleic	18:2	47.22	60.58
Octadecatrienic	Total trans-isomers	0.13	0.00
α-linolenic	18:3 ω-3	10.17	0.08
Arachidic	20:0	0.49	0.24
gondoic (total isomers)	20:1	0.24	0.20
Behenic	22:0	0.43	0.72

Soybean oil is a source of linoleic, oleic, palmitic, α-linolenic, and stearic fatty acids. Sunflower oil is a source of linoleic, oleic, palmitic, and stearic fatty acids. Thus, the main difference in the fatty acid composition of soybean oil from sunflower oil is the content of α-linolenic ω-3 fatty acid.

2.2. In Vivo Study Results

The general condition of all animals in terms of appearance, fur quality, food and water consumption, and behavior during daily examination was satisfactory. Figure 1 shows the average cumulative feed and calorie consumption of animals throughout the experiment.

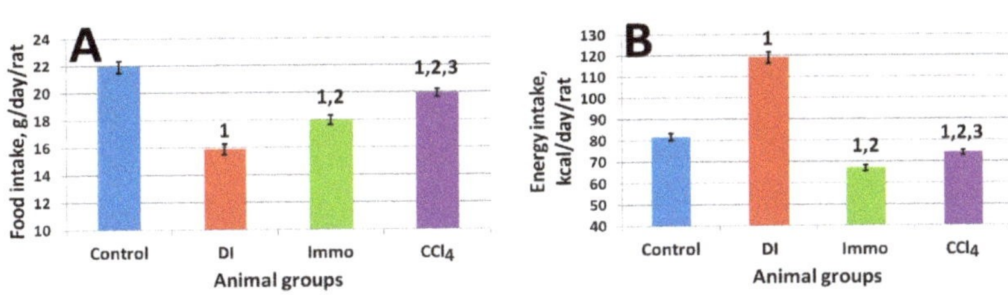

Figure 1. (**A**) Average food intake, g/day/rat (η^2 = 0.40); (**B**) average energy intake, kcal/day/rat (η^2 = 0.71). [1] differences are significant against control group; [2] differences are significant against DI group; [3] differences are significant against Immo group; $p < 0.01$.

Animals of the diet-induced (DI) group consumed significantly less food compared to animals of the control, Immo, and CCl_4 groups. However, in terms of caloric content, these animals, on the contrary, received significantly more energy than the others, since in addition to feed, they consumed an average of 50 ± 3 mL of a 30% fructose solution.

Animals of groups Immo and CCl_4 consumed significantly less food and energy compared to control animals, while animals of group Immo consumed less food compared to animals of group CCl_4. Thus, immobilization stress led to a significant decrease in animals' appetite compared to all other groups. Replacing the fat component in the diet, namely soybean oil, with sunflower oil also led to a significant decrease in appetite.

Figure 2 shows the body weight gain of animals throughout the experiment.

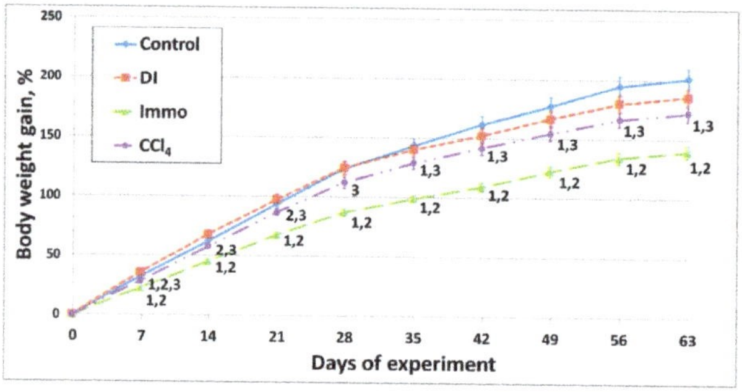

Figure 2. Body weight gain of experimental animals, %. [1] differences are significant against control group; [2] differences are significant against DI group; [3] differences are significant against Immo group; $p < 0.05$.

Starting from the 7th day, a significant lag in the body weight gain of Immo group animals was observed compared to the control, DI, and CCl_4 animals. The difference remained significant throughout the experiment. The body weight gain of CCl_4 animals, starting from day 35, was significantly lower compared to the control until the end of the experiment. The obtained result is consistent with the food intake data. The body weight gain of DI animals did not differ significantly from the control, despite higher calorie consumption.

Figure 3 shows the results of the elevated plus maze test.

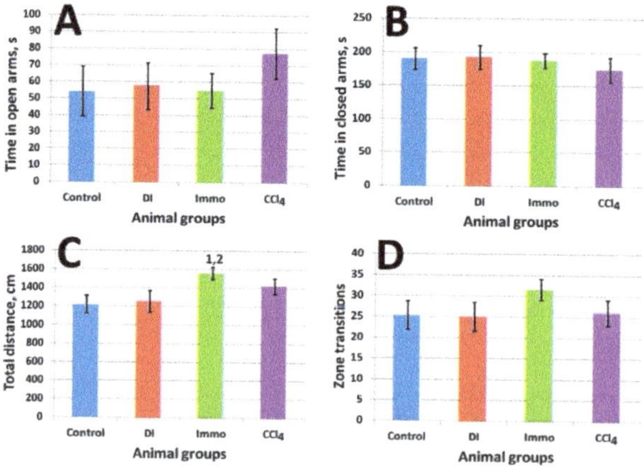

Figure 3. Elevated plus maze test results. [1] differences are significant against control group; [2] differences are significant against DI group; $p < 0.05$. (**A**) Time in open arms, s ($\eta^2 = 0.04$); (**B**) time in closed arms, s ($\eta^2 = 0.02$); (**C**) total distance ($\eta^2 = 0.170$); (**D**) zone transition number ($\eta^2 = 0.06$).

Animals of group Immo showed more activity, reflected by a significantly greater distance traveled, compared to the control ($p = 0.02$) and DI ($p = 0.03$) animals. The obtained result indicates the influence of immobilization on the component of exploratory and motor activity, characterized by the distance traveled, without changing the degree of anxiety.

Table 2 shows the body composition of experimental animals.

Table 2. Body composition of experimental animals.

Parameter	Group				Statistics	
	Control	DI	Immo	CCl_4	p	η^2
Fat mass, %	13.7 (11.8–15.9)	13.9 (9.7–15.2)	8.1 (6.7–11.7) [1,2]	12.3 (8.7–15.5)	0.05	0.17
Lean mass, %	79.8 ± 1.0	80.8 ± 1.1	85.1 ± 1.1 [1,2]	81.9 ± 1.5	0.02	0.20
Free water, %	0.25 (0.22–0.29)	0.20 (0.17–0.23) [1]	0.32 (0.29–0.35) [1,2]	0.21 (0.17–0.23) [1,3]	<0.01	0.39
Total water, %	67.8 ± 0.9	68.5 ± 0.9	72.3 ± 0.9 [1,2]	69.7 ± 1.2	0.02	0.21

[1] differences are significant compared to control group; [2] differences are significant compared to DI group; [3] differences are significant compared to Immo group; $p \leq 0.05$.

As can be seen from the presented data, the body fat mass of Immo animals was significantly lower compared to control animals and DI animals, while their lean mass, on the contrary, was significantly higher compared to these groups. Also, the total water content in the body of these animals was significantly higher compared to control and DI animals.

Table 3 shows the results of biochemistry blood test of experimental animals.

Table 3. Biochemistry blood test.

Parameter	Animal Groups				Statistics	
	Control	DI	Immo	CCl_4	p	η^2
Total protein, g/L	71.9 ± 1.4	77.4 ± 1.8 [1]	71.5 ± 1.1 [2]	72.7 ± 1.5 [2]	0.02	0.20
Albumin, g/L	30.5 ± 0.3	31.5 ± 0.5	30.6 ± 0.3	30.3 ± 0.4 [2]	0.04	0.12
Globulins, g/L	41.0 [38.0–44.0]	44.8 [43.4–49.2] [1]	40.1 [38.9–43.3] [2]	41.8 [39.9–43.8]	0.04	0.21
Cholesterol, mmol/L	1.65 [1.37–1.79]	2.52 [1.83–2.79] [1]	1.51 [1.38–1.76] [2]	1.11 [0.96–1.47] [1,2,3]	<0.01	0.49
Triglycerides, mmol/L	2.95 [2.29–3.86]	2.17 [1.38–2.85] [1]	1.36 [1.02–1.69] [1]	0.74 [0.53–1.07] [1]	<0.01	0.44
HDL, mmol/L	1.28 ± 0.09	1.33 ± 0.09	1.41 ± 0.05	1.10 ± 0.09 [2,3]	0.05	0.17
LDL, mmol/L	0.10 [0.09–0.11]	0.44 [0.33–0.70] [1]	0.15 [0.13–0.17] [1,2]	0.08 [0.07–0.12] [2,3]	<0.01	0.65
Total bilirubin, μmol/L	5.01 [4.79–5.46]	4.51 [4.36–5.38]	5.16 [5.00–5.43] [2]	5.30 [5.00–5.62] [2]	0.03	0.10
Creatinine, μmol/L	46.3 ± 0.8	46.3 ± 1.3	49.0 ± 0.8	46.3 ± 0.9	0.12	0.12
Alkaline phosphatase, U/L	159 [143–213]	191 [178–202]	154 [139–202]	144 [137–171] [2]	0.02	0.15
ALT, U/L	74.3 [60.9–84.4]	91.2 [72.5–148.1] [1]	89.5 [83.5–101.1] [1]	102.7 [79.0–109.7] [1]	0.02	0.17
AST, U/L	40.0 [34.2–172.8]	201.7 [52.2–230.7]	239.4 [81.7–258.7] [1]	62.5 [42.9–271.3]	0.03	0.04
Urea, mmol/L	6.33 ± 0.24	4.08 ± 0.29 [1]	5.59 ± 0.28 [2]	6.70 ± 0.36 [2,3]	<0.01	0.51
Uric acid, mmol/L	85.1 [81.3–92.8]	95.7 [81.6–107.1]	90.4 [87.1–103.5]	77.5 [73.3–93.9]	0.31	0.05
Phosphor, mmol/L	2.12 [2.04–2.74]	2.07 [1.91–2.32]	2.39 [2.22–2.53] [2]	2.39 [2.35–2.54] [2]	0.03	0.15

Table 3. *Cont.*

Parameter	Animal Groups				Statistics	
	Control	DI	Immo	CCl_4	p	η^2
Magnesium, mmol/L	0.90 [0.78–0.99]	0.73 [0.65–0.77] [1]	0.85 [0.82–1.02] [2]	0.79 [0.76–0.83]	<0.01	0.26
Calcium, mmol/L	2.45 [2.31–3.36]	2.42 [2.40–2.61]	2.38 [2.31–2.42]	2.45 [2.38–2.50]	0.51	0.04
Glucose, mmol/L	6.78 [5.91–7.19]	7.87 [7.63–8.25] [1]	6.10 [5.65–6.47] [2]	5.93 [5.84–6.27] [1,2]	<0.01	0.43
Glucose, mmol/L (whole blood)	5.85 [5.30–6.28]	7.30 [7.05–7.55] [1]	5.55 [5.18–6.33] [2]	5.95 [5.53–6.03] [2]	<0.01	0.53
Glycated hemoglobin, %	6.3 [5.4–6.8]	6.7 [5.7–7.5]	6.4 [5.9–7.8]	5.2 [5.0–5.4] [1,2,3]	0.03	0.05

[1] differences are significant against control group; [2] differences are significant against DI group; [3] differences are significant against Immo group; $p < 0.05$.

Animals of the DI group had a significant increase in total protein against the background of a significant increase in globulins compared to control animals. Consumption of exogenous cholesterol and fructose resulted in a significant increase in the blood cholesterol and LDL levels compared to control animals, while the triglyceride level was significantly lower. A significant increase in the serum ALT level and a decrease in serum urea were revealed compared to the control group. According to mineral metabolism, a reliable decrease in blood magnesium level of these animals was observed. The level of serum glucose and complete blood glucose in these animals was significantly higher compared to all groups, no changes in the glycated hemoglobin level were found.

In animals of Immo group with normal levels of total cholesterol, a significant decrease in triglyceride levels and an increase in LDL levels were found compared to animals of the control group. Also, animals of this group showed a significantly higher level of ALT compared to control animals.

A significantly lower concentration of serum cholesterol and triglycerides was found in animals of CCl_4 group compared to the control group. The ALT level was also significantly higher compared to animals of the control group. The animals of this experimental group had the lowest serum glucose: the differences are significant compared to the control group, while no difference was found in whole blood glucose. The level of glycated hemoglobin also differed significantly and was lower than in control animals.

Table 4 presents the biochemical parameters determined in the liver of animals.

Table 4. Liver biochemical parameters.

Parameter	Animal Groups				Statistics	
	Control	DI	Immo	CCl_4	p	η^2
Final body weight, g	479 [440–505]	449 [438–498]	369 [360–392] [1,2]	430 [404–448] [1,3]	<0.01	0.38
Liver weight, relative, %	2.72 [2.60–2.93]	4.33 [4.08–4.69] [1]	2.42 [2.27–2.53] [1,2]	2.68 [2.57–2.76] [2,3]	<0.01	0.87
Fat content, mg/g liver	89.4 [81.4–114.2]	189.6 [121.4–223.5] [1]	76.3 [63.3–83.3] [1,2]	93.9 [85.6–105.5] [2,3]	<0.01	0.49
Cholesterol, mg/g liver	5.79 [4.14–6.92]	14.2 [6.1–16.9] [1]	4.12 [3.38–5.19] [2]	17.3 [12.8–18.5] [1,3]	<0.01	0.62
Triglycerides, mg/g liver	44.0 [34.7–59.2]	64.2 [48.6–98.4] [1]	38.2 [32.0–42.2] [2]	33.3 [24.7–38.7] [1,2]	0.01	0.31

[1] differences are significant against control group; [2] differences are significant against DI group; [3] differences are significant against Immo group; $p < 0.01$.

Animals of the DI group had the highest relative liver weight and the highest liver fat content; the differences were significant with all groups. Cholesterol and triglyceride levels were significantly higher compared to those in the control group.

Animals of the Immo group at the end of the experiment had significantly lower body weight, relative liver weight, and liver fat content compared to the control group. Moreover, the levels of cholesterol and triglycerides did not differ significantly from those in the control group.

At the end of the experiment, the body weight of animals in the CCl_4 group was significantly lower compared to the control group. The level of cholesterol in the liver of these animals was significantly higher compared to the control group, and the level of triglycerides was significantly lower than the control group.

Biochemical parameters of blood serum determined by ELISA are shown in Table 5.

Table 5. Blood serum biochemical parameters determined by ELISA.

Parameters	Animal Groups				Statistics	
	Control	DI	Immo	CCl_4	p	η^2
Lipid peroxides, ng/mL	362.8 [318.9–438.5]	381.4 [345.3–544.4]	258.6 [246.2–291.1] [1]	482.8 [420.0–534.5] [1]	<0.01	0.31
MDA, ng/mL	190.4 [149.8–233.1]	352.4 [226.0–462.2] [1]	191.5 [146.2–295.8]	168.3 [120.6–218.9] [2]	0.05	0.13
Glutathione peroxidase, pg/mL	69.5 [55.5–82.1]	67.7 [58.2–72.5]	69.7 [55.6–87.2]	60.0 [49.9–81.2]	0.88	0.07
Catalase, ng/mL	1.42 [1.03–1.61]	1.58 [1.28–1.93]	1.03 [0.83–1.29] [2]	2.34 [1.81–2.44] [1,3]	<0.01	0.20
SOD, ng/mL	2.75 [2.31–3.07]	6.55 [3.91–9.78] [1]	4.65 [2.20–6.46]	2.46 [1.78–3,52] [2]	0.037	0.20

[1] differences are significant compared to control group, [2] differences are significant compared to DI group, [3] differences are significant compared to Immo group; $p \leq 0.05$.

A significant accumulation of MDA, a product of lipid peroxidation, was noted in DI animals. Also, SOD activation in the blood of these animals was shown; the accumulation of SOD levels in their blood was significantly different compared to control animals that received a standard diet. Daily forced immobilization resulted in a significant decrease in blood lipid peroxides of animals compared to the control group. As a result of a single intraperitoneal injection of CCl_4 a significant accumulation of lipid peroxide levels and activation of catalase were noted in experimental animals compared to control.

Figure 4 shows the results reflecting the excretion of catecholamines in urine: dopamine, noradrenaline, and adrenaline.

A significant increase in noradrenaline ($p = 0.03$) was found in the urine of DI animals compared to control animals, while there were no significant differences in other indicators. The obtained result may be a consequence of activation of the sympathicoadrenal system in response to the toxic effects of cholesterol and fructose. Animals of the CCl_4 group had a significant decrease ($p = 0.04$) in the adrenaline level compared to animals of the Immo group.

As shown by the PCR analysis (Table 6), a significant decrease in the expression of the *Cat* gene by 35% ($p = 0.013$) was found in animals of the DI group, relative to the control level, as well as a moderate decrease, at the level of trends, in the expression of the *Gpx1* gene by 20% ($p = 0.059$) and *Sod1* gene by 21% ($p = 0.092$) compared to the control group. At the same time, a high-calorie diet had no statistically significant effect on the expression of the transcription factor Nrf2 and Nf2-mediated antioxidant defense enzyme genes *Hmox1* and *Nqo1*. No statistically significant changes in the expression of the studied genes were detected in animals of the Immo group compared to the control. A single intraperitoneal injection of CCl_4 solution resulted in a significant decrease in the amount of *Cat* mRNA by 33% ($p = 0.02$) and *Gpx1* mRNA by 48% ($p = 0.003$) compared to the control. Moreover, a significant 5-fold increase in the expression of the *Nqo1* gene ($p = 0.004$) was found in the liver of these rats compared to the control group.

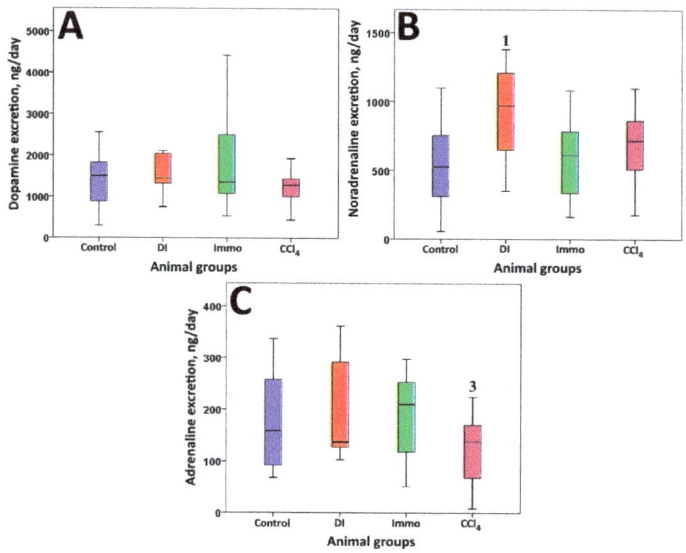

Figure 4. Catecholamine daily urine excretion. (**A**) Dopamine, ng/day; (**B**) noradrenaline, ng/day; (**C**) adrenaline, ng/day. [1] differences are significant compared to control group; [3] differences are significant compared to Immo group; $p < 0.05$. η^2 values are: (**A**) 0.12; (**B**) 0.18; (**C**) 0.11.

Table 6. Antioxidant gene and transcription factor expression in liver tissues.

Gene	Animal Group				Statistics	
	Control	DI	Immo	CCl_4	p	η^2
Cat	1.04 [0.90–1.12]	0.68 [0.66–0.80] [1]	0.96 [0.94–1.11] [2]	0.70 [0.61–0.79] [1,3]	<0.01	0.30
Sod1	0.98 [0.91–1.09]	0.77 [0.71–0.92]	1.13 [1.04–1.17] [2]	1.17 [1.01–1.51] [2]	0.02	0.53
Gpx1	1.04 [0.89–1.19]	0.83 [0.69–0.86]	0.76 [0.70–0.91]	0.54 [0.49–0.59] [1,3]	<0.01	0.44
Hmox1	0.94 [0.82–1.11]	1.05 [0.86–1.32]	0.64 [0.52–0.80]	0.80 [0.58–1.17]	0.34	0.18
Nqo1	1.36 [0.85–1.57]	1.61 [1.14–3.21]	1.64 [0.96–2.75]	7.13 [5.05–9.53] [1,2,3]	<0.01	0.44
Nrf2	1.06 [1.05–1.16]	0.96 [0.82–1.16]	1.07 [0.97–1.18]	0.87 [0.73–1.03]	0.43	0.18
Nfkb1	1.04 [0.95–1.95]	0.95 [0.84–1.03]	0.94 [0.90–1.01]	1.05 [1.00–1.12]	0.62	0.14

[1] differences are significant against control group; [2] differences are significant against DI group; [3] differences are significant against Immo group ($p < 0.05$).

3. Discussion

Rats treated with a diet high in cholesterol and fructose consumed significantly less food, despite receiving almost 1.5 times more energy due to fructose. However, the body weight gain, as well as the fat/lean mass ratio in these animals, did not differ significantly from the control. In our case, consumption of this diet did not lead to the development of obesity but only affected the metabolic processes.

Animals subjected to forced immobilization consumed significantly less food and energy (by 18%), which led to a significant reduction in body weight gain compared to all groups of animals. The fat mass in the body composition of these animals was also significantly lower. The immobilization model has a serious impact on the psycho-emotional state of animals. That is accompanied by loss of appetite, leading to an exhaustion of the body, a decrease in organ weight and a change in a number of biochemical parameters [27]. The ratio of both total and free water in the body of these animals was significantly higher compared to the control. The obtained result is consistent with the data presented in the study [28], where immobilization stress led to a decrease in daily diuresis of experimental rats, which led to water retention in the animals' bodies.

A decrease in both appetite and body weight gain was detected in animals of CCl_4 group. The obtained result is explained by differences in the diet: the animals of this group received a diet with the inclusion of sunflower oil, while control animals received soybean oil, a source of ω-3 PUFA, in particular α-linolenic acid (Table 1). The study [29] also showed that the introduction of ω-3 PUFAs into the diet of rats promotes the appetite and, accordingly, food consumption.

According to numerous studies, long-term consumption of a high-cholesterol diet causes lipid metabolism disorders and oxidative stress [30–32]. Feeding animals a diet containing 1% cholesterol for 9 weeks resulted in increased serum total cholesterol and LDL, indicating the development of hypercholesterolemia and dyslipidemia. This is also confirmed by extreme liver fat accumulation and increased liver cholesterol and triglyceride levels. Fructose consumption resulted in a significant increase in blood glucose level. A significant increase (by 60%) in the relative liver weight was also noted compared to the control group. The obtained results suggest that such a diet leads to disorders in internal organs and metabolic systems.

Rats subjected to chronic immobilization stress had decreased relative liver weight and liver fat content. The blood level of triglycerides was also significantly lower compared to control animals. As mentioned above, severe psycho-emotional stress leads to exhaustion of the body and a decrease in organ weight.

A single intraperitoneal injection of CCl_4 had a strong toxic effect on rats' metabolic processes. We observed a significant decrease in the blood levels of cholesterol, triglycerides, glucose, and glycated hemoglobin compared to the control. Similar results were obtained in the work [33]. Liver intoxication with CCl_4 leads to a decrease in glycogen stores, inhibiting gluconeogenesis and decreasing blood glucose level [34]. The content of glycated hemoglobin characterizes the average blood glucose level over the last 60 days, which corresponds to the average lifespan of erythrocytes in rats [35]. The reaction of glucose binding to hemoglobin is irreversible; therefore, glycated hemoglobin circulates in the blood until the death of the bound erythrocyte [36].

Excessive accumulation of reactive oxygen species (ROS) in the liver leads to injury of hepatocyte membranes. The process of lipid peroxidation (LPO) is activated there with the production of lipid peroxides and MDA [37,38].

The blood level of lipid hydroperoxides and MDA reflects the degree of cell damage due to lipid peroxidation processes [39]. A significantly higher level of blood MDA in the animals treated with a diet high in cholesterol and fructose indicates the activation of lipid peroxidation processes. Similar results were obtained in the works [40–43], where the consumption of high-cholesterol diets by laboratory rodents (rats, mice, hamsters, rabbits) led to an increase in the serum levels of MDA and lipid peroxides. We also revealed a significant increase in the blood levels of lipid peroxides in animals that received a single injection of CCl_4, compared to the control. CCl_4 is a potent hepatotoxin and is rapidly transformed by cytochrome P450 in the presence of oxygen into metabolites, that damage polyunsaturated fatty acids of membrane phospholipids, leading to the formation of peroxides and the initiation of lipid peroxidation [17,37,44].

Activation of lipid peroxidation provokes a response from the antioxidant defense system. A significant increase in the blood level of SOD was found in animals fed a high-cholesterol diet with fructose, compared to control animals. The obtained data show the activation of the antioxidant defense system since the synthesis of SOD increases in response to lipid peroxidation. The study [30] also noted an increase in the levels of antioxidant defense enzymes—SOD, glutathione reductase, and xanthine oxidase—in the blood of male Wistar rats fed a high-fat, high-fructose diet for 18 months. The activation of body's compensatory mechanisms is also confirmed by a significant increase in the blood total protein of animals, which is the marker of liver synthesizing activity [12]. Rats subjected to a single injection of CCl_4 showed significantly higher levels of catalase, which also indicates the activation of the antioxidant defense system in these animals. Catalase is one of the main enzymes that prevent cellular accumulation of hydrogen peroxide, which promotes the formation of the hydroxyl radical. The level of catalase increases in response to an increase in the level of hydrogen peroxide.

AST and ALT are deposited mainly in the heart and liver. An increase in their blood level may indicate a disruption in the functioning and integrity of hepatocytes [45]. The results showed a significant increase in the level of blood ALT in the animals of all experimental groups. Blood AST level was also significantly increased in animals subjected to forced immobilization. A significant increase in the level of blood transaminases and a more than 2.5-fold increase in the AST over ALT confirms the exhaustive effect of immobilization on the rats [46]. The obtained data are also consistent with the results of the work [12], where intraperitoneal administration of CCl_4 to mice and rats led to a significant increase in the levels of serum transaminases of the animals. We also noted a visible (but not significant, $p = 0.124$) increase in the blood AST level in animals receiving a diet high in cholesterol and fructose.

Catecholamines are the major neurotransmitters that mediate various central nervous system functions such as locomotor activity, cognition, emotion, memory, and endocrine regulation. These hormones have the ability to reduce oxidative stress by scavenging free radicals and binding metal ions. The presence of a catechol fragment in the structure determines the activity of catecholamines in removing free radicals [47]. A significant increase in the daily excretion of norepinephrine was found in animals fed a diet high in cholesterol and fructose compared to control animals. This is a consequence of increased activity of the sympathoadenal system in response to the toxic effects of exogenous cholesterol on the animal body [48]. Increased levels of catecholamines in the body may also be associated with increased production of reactive oxygen species [49].

On the other hand, the high reactivity of catecholamines to free radicals also means that these molecules will break down over time, losing their function and forming potentially toxic metabolites [47]. In animals that received a single injection of CCl_4, a tendency toward decreased adrenaline excretion was noted ($p = 0.222$ relative to the control group and $p = 0.106$ relative to the DI group), and the differences with animals subjected to immobilization stress were significant ($p < 0.05$).

As the level of ROS increases, protective antioxidant mechanisms activate to degrade them. Our study showed a decrease in the expression of key antioxidant enzyme genes *Cat*, *Gpx1* and *Sod1* in the liver of rats of the DI and CCl_4 groups. This indicates a weakening of the antioxidant defense system and the development of oxidative stress in these groups.

Thus, a single intraperitoneal injection of CCl_4 resulted in decreased activity of the GSH, SOD, and CAT [50]. In similar studies on male Wistar rats, a single administration of CCl_4 resulted in a significant decrease in the activity of SOD, CAT, and GSH and the expression of the *Sod1* gene. The authors attribute this decrease to the depletion of antioxidant enzymes as a result of oxidative stress caused by the administration of CCl_4 [51].

The Nrf2/Keap1/ARE signaling pathway plays a key role in protecting the cell from oxidative stress. The antioxidant and phase II detoxification enzymes regulated by this signaling pathway can eliminate ROS and suppress the biotransformation of xenobiotics. Activated transcription factor Nrf2 can induce expression of protective enzyme genes such as *Hmox1* and *Nqo1* to resist oxidative stress damage [52].

A single intraperitoneal administration of CCl_4 resulted in a moderate decrease in the expression of *Nrf2* and *Hmox1* genes and a 5-fold increase in the expression of *Nqo1*. A similar study in male Sprague-Dawley rats injected intraperitoneally with CCl_4 showed a decrease in *Nrf2*, *Hmox1*, and *Nqo1* mRNA levels in rat liver [53]. In the other study, oral administration of CCl_4 to male Sprague-Dawley rats for 6 weeks caused liver fibrosis, as well as a three-fold increase in the liver expression of NQO1 protein, while the amount of hemeoxygenase-1 protein did not change compared to the control [54]. The administration of CCl_4 was also accompanied by a significant increase in the expression of NQO1 protein in the rat liver. The authors suggest that increased NQO1 expression occurs in response to ROS generation caused by inflammation or xenobiotic transformation. NQO1 is associated with cellular redox balance, protecting the cell from free radicals inhibiting the one-electron reduction of quinines [55].

Limitations of the Study

The main limitation of this study is the difference in the fat component of the groups' diets. The standard AIN-93 diet contains soybean oil in the fat component. Soybean oil is a source of ω-3 PUFAs, whose consumption can prevent the development of oxidative stress. Accordingly, the diets of the experimental groups included sunflower oil, which does not contain ω-3/6 PUFAs. Moreover, the use of sunflower oil provides a closer approximation to the average human diet, which often includes sunflower oil as the most accessible product. Also, the combination of sunflower oil, margarine, cholesterol and fructose in our study is used to simulate an unhealthy diet with a high proportion of saturated fats and easily digestible carbohydrates.

The use of only one dose of CCl_4 in a single administration can also be considered as a limitation of the presented study. According to literature data, the toxic effect of CCl_4 depends on the dose and exposure time, from weaker reversible effects to severe irreversible injuries. We have chosen a single administration so that the toxic effect of CCl_4 would be reversible. Although studies using other doses, as well as chronic exposure to this substance, are of scientific interest and have been published repeatedly. Evaluation of the chronic effects of CCl_4 on the antioxidant system and internal organs of animals may become the subject of our further studies.

4. Materials and Methods

4.1. Experimental Animals

The experiment was conducted using 50 Wistar male rats (age 4 weeks) with an initial body weight of 100 ± 2 g. Animal studies were carried out in accordance with standard principles described in "Guide for the Care and Use of Laboratory Animals" [56] and approved by the Local Ethics Committee (Protocol No. 8 dated 6 September 2024). Animals were kept under controlled environmental conditions (temperature 20–24 °C, relative humidity 30–60%, 12 h lighting cycle).

The open field (OF) test was used to divide animals into groups [57].

The open field box was a black square arena (90 cm × 90 cm) surrounded by gray walls (40 cm) and divided into one central zone and two peripheral zones (Figure 5).

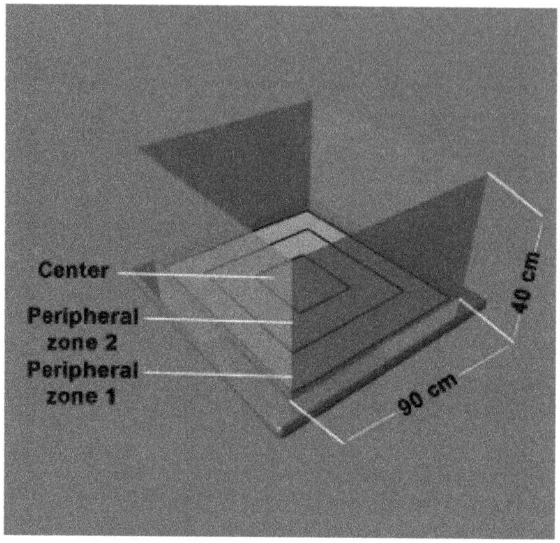

Figure 5. Open field box.

The animals were placed in the corner and allowed to explore the box for 3 min. To evaluate the behavior, the following parameters were used: horizontal (number of transitions between zones, total distance), the latency of the first move, the latency of the first entry into the central zone, time spent in different zones of the field. The test was conducted during the period of the animals' minimal activity (between 10 a.m. and 3 p.m.).

The movement of animals was recorded using the Smart 3.0.04 video-tracking system (Panlab, Barcelona, Spain).

4.2. Determination of Fatty Acid Composition of Oil Samples (Sunflower and Soybean)

About 10 mg of the lipophilic fraction of each sample was added to screw-capped tubes with a liner. Further, 2.0 mL of methanol (chemically pure, Aquametry, Moscow, Russia), 20 µL of hexane, and 20 µL of acetyl chloride (Acros organics, Geel, Belgium) were added to the samples. The test tubes were tightly closed with lids and, after brief vigorous shaking, were placed in a drying oven for 1 h at 80 °C to methylate the fatty acids. After cooling the samples to room temperature, 2.5 mL of hexane and 100 µL of deionized water were added to them, and they were vigorously mixed on a vortex shaker for about 10 s. After separation, 1.0 mL of the upper hexane layer containing methyl esters was transferred to vials for gas chromatographic analysis.

Gas Chromatography Conditions with Flame Ionization Detector

Sample injection volume 1 µL, flow split mode 50:1, carrier gas hydrogen, flow rate 1.65 mL/min. Injector temperature 200 °C, detector temperature 240 °C. Separation conditions: initial temperature 100 °C (isotherm for 3 min), then increase at a rate of 3 °C/min to 200 °C, isotherm for 3 min, then increase at a rate of 3 °C/min to 240 °C, isotherm for 6 min. Data collection and processing were carried out using Agilent ChemStation Rev.B.04.03 and Microsoft Excel 2007 software, respectively. The ratio of fatty acids was determined by the internal normalization method.

4.3. Experimental Design

Open Field testing of animals was conducted after seven days acclimatization prior to the start of the experiment. Animals were divided into 4 groups (n = 12) based on body weight and OF test results: control, diet-Induced (DI), Immo, and CCl_4. The groups were formed to achieve the same average weight and the same average OF activity of animals between the groups (Table 7).

Table 7. Animal groups.

Parameter	Animal Group			
	Control	**DI**	**Immo**	**CCl_4**
Body weight, g	157 ± 3	160 ± 3	160 ± 3	157 ± 3
	Open Field Test Results			
Time in center, s	1.4 ± 0.6	1.1 ± 0.5	1.9 ± 0.5	1.7 ± 0.8
Zone transitions	5.8 ± 1.0	5.5 ± 1.3	6.2 ± 0.9	5.7 ± 1.1
Total distance, cm	1581 ± 135	1729 ± 109	1768 ± 100	1741 ± 119

Animals of all groups received a standard semi-synthetic diet according to AIN93G with some modifications [58] and water ad libitum during the 63 days of the experiment.

The experimental design is presented in Figure 6.

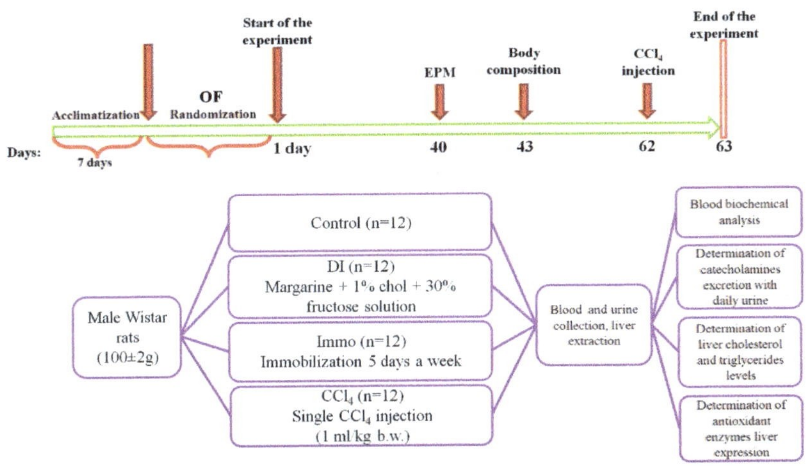

Figure 6. Design of the experiment.

Animals of the control group received a standard diet (lard and soybean oil as fat components, 375 ± 3 kcal). Animals of group DI received a standard semi-synthetic diet (lard and margarine as fat components) with the addition of 1% cholesterol (375 ± 3 kcal). The animals received a 30% fructose solution as their only source of drink. Animals of group Immo received a standard semi-synthetic diet (lard and sunflower oil as fat components, 375 ± 3 kcal). The fatty acid composition of oils used in diets is shown in Table 1. These animals were subjected to 30 min forced immobilization in plastic restrainers (Open Science, Moscow, Russia) for 5 days a week. Immobilization is a traditional model of stress in which, in addition to movement restriction, there is a pronounced emotional component associated with the inability to avoid a threatening situation. Rats of the experimental group CCl_4 received a standard semi-synthetic diet (lard and sunflower oil as fat components, 375 ± 3 kcal). On the 62nd day of the experiment, the animals were intraperitoneally injected with a 50% solution of CCl_4 in olive oil at a dose of 1 mL/kg body weight [59–62].

On the 43rd day of the experiment, we studied body composition using a quantitative magnetic resonance system (EchoMRI LLC, Houston, TX, USA) that allows measuring total body fat mass, lean body mass, free water content and total body water volume of rats in less than 1 min in a living animal without anesthesia or euthanasia.

We tested animals in the elevated plus maze on the 40th day of the experiment to assess their level of anxiety and exploratory behavior during periods of their minimum daily activity (from 10:00 to 15:00). The movement of rats in the maze, the time spent in the open and closed arms, the number of zone transitions, and the distance traveled were recorded with the Smart 3.0.04 video tracking system (Panlab Harvard Apparatus, Barcelona, Spain).

Twenty-four hours prior to the end of the experiment, animals were placed in metabolic cages to collect daily urine. On day 63 of the experiment, we measured the fasting glucose level in blood taken from the tail vein using an electrochemical glucometer (OneTouch Select, Malvern, PA, USA).

On the 63rd day, rats from all groups (deprived for 12 h) were decapitated under light anesthesia, and a pathological autopsy was performed. One milliliter of blood was collected in test tubes with K_2EDTA to determine glycated hemoglobin, the remaining blood collected after decapitation was incubated at 2–8 °C for 3 h, centrifuged for 30 min at 3000 rpm at 4 °C, and the resulting serum was stored at −20 °C. The liver was extracted by pathological dissection and weighed. A sample of liver (approximately 0.5 g) was collected to determine the expression of antioxidant enzymes; the remaining liver was additionally weighed, frozen, and lyophilized prior to fat extraction.

The content of glycated hemoglobin was determined spectrophotometrically using the commercial Glycohemotest Kit (ELTA, Moscow, Russia). The method is based on the principle of affinity separation of glycated and non-glycated fractions of hemoglobin of blood hemolysate on a sorbent with grafted 4-aminomethylphenylboronic acid.

Parameters of protein metabolism (total protein, albumin, globulins, urea, creatinine), lipid metabolism (total cholesterol, HDL cholesterol, LDL cholesterol, triglycerides), carbohydrate metabolism (glucose), purine metabolism (uric acid), mineral metabolism (calcium, phosphorus, magnesium), and liver function (total bilirubin, ALT, AST, alkaline phosphatase) were determined in blood serum using the automatic biochemical analyzer "Konelab 20i" (ThermoScientific, Waltham, MA, USA). Fat was extracted from the liver using the Folch method [63]. Samples of lyophilized liver were ground and transferred into test tubes. A mixture of chloroform and methanol (2:1) in a ratio of 1/10 was added to the samples. The samples were stirred for 1.5 h, then distilled water was added in a volume of 1/3 of the solvent volume, after which the mixture was centrifuged at 3500 rpm for 5 min. The fat dissolved in chloroform, which settled at the bottom of the test tube, was collected in pre-weighed flasks. After this, chloroform was added to the test tubes in a volume of 1/3 of the original volume of solvents, centrifuged at 3500 rpm for 5 min, and the fat dissolved in chloroform was again transferred into the flasks. The resulting combined fat extracts were evaporated on a rotary evaporator until the chloroform was completely removed. The flasks with fat were placed in a muffle furnace at 80 °C for 15 min. After cooling, the flasks were weighed and the mass of extracted fat was determined by the difference with the original flask mass. Before analysis, the fat sample was pre-dissolved in 95% ethanol at a concentration of 2.5 mg/mL. The content of triglycerides and cholesterol in fat extracted from the liver was determined photometrically using a Konelab 20i automatic biochemical analyzer (ThermoScientific, Waltham, MA, USA).

The catalase, glutathione peroxidase, and superoxide dismutase levels, as well as the degree of accumulation of lipid hydroperoxides and malondialdehyde (MDA), were determined in blood serum using the competitive ELISA analysis method according to the manufacturer's instructions (Elabscience, Cloud Clone, Fine Test, Houston, TX, USA).

Sample preparation of daily urine included catecholamine derivatization (epinephrine, norepinephrine, and dopamine) in order to separate them under reverse-phase chromatography conditions and achieve the required ranges of quantitative determination. Carbonate buffer and benzoyl chloride solution in acetonitrile were added to urine samples, mixed and incubated at room temperature. Obtained solutions were then analyzed using HPLC-MS/MS.

Catecholamine levels in daily urine were determined by HPLC-MS/MS using an Agilent 1200 Series chromatograph (Agilent Technologies, Santa Clara, CA, USA) and a Thermo LTQ Velos Pro mass spectrometer (Thermo Fisher Scientific, Waltham, MA, USA). Separation of catecholamine derivatives in the water–acetonitrile system was carried out on an Agilent ZORBAX Eclipse XDB-C18 chromatographic column in gradient elution mode.

4.4. Antioxidant System Gene Expression

The expression of the following genes was assessed in rat liver using real-time reverse transcription polymerase chain reaction (RT-PCR): anti-inflammatory nuclear transcription factor (*NfkB*), transcription factor Nrf2 (*Nrf2*), superoxide dismutase (*Sod1*), glutathione peroxidase (*Gpx1*), catalase (*Cat*), NAD(P)H-quinone oxidoreductase (*Nqo1*), and heme oxygenase-1 (*Hmox1*). Total RNA was isolated from liver tissue using the ExtractRNA reagent (Eurogen, Moscow, Russia), and complementary DNA was synthesized using the MMLV RT kit (Eurogen, Moscow, Russia) according to the manufacturers' protocol. For real-time PCR, primers and probes from DNA Synthesis LLC (Moscow, Russia) were used; the primer sequences are shown in Table 8.

Table 8. The primer sequences.

Primer	Sequence
NfkB	F CGTGGAGTACGACAACATCTC R GAGGTGTCGTCCCATCGTA FAM CTGCTCCTGGAGGGTGACGC-BHQ1
Nrf2	F CACATCCAGACAGACACCAGT R GAATGTCTCTGCCAAAAGC FAM CTCCCAGGTTGCCCACATTCCC-BHQ1
Hmox1	F CCAGCCTGAACTAGCCCA R CCTTGGTGGCCTCCTTC FAM CCACAGCTCGACAGCATGTCC-BHQ1
Sod1	F GACAATACACAAGGCTGTACCA R CAGGTCTCCAACATGCCTC FAM CTCACTCTAAGAAACATGGCGGTC-BHQ1
Cat	F GTCTGGGACTTCTGGAGTCTT R CATAGCCATTCATGTGCCG FAM CCATCAGGTTACTTTCTTGTTCAG-BHQ1
Gpx1	F TCAGTTCGGACATCAGGAGA R CATTCACCTCGCACTTCTCAA FAM CCCTCAAGTATGTCCGACCCG-BHQ1
Nqo1	F GGGACATGAACGTCATTCTC R CACCAGTTGAGGTTCTAAGACC FAM CAATTCAGAGTGGCATTCTGCGC-BHQ1

The PCR reaction mixture with a total volume of 25 μL contained 2.5 μL of cDNA (diluted 1:10) obtained in the reverse transcription reaction from 2 μg of total RNA, 2.5 μL of 10X Taq Turbo buffer for HS Taq DNA polymerase (with 2.5 mM $MgCl_2$) (Eurogen, Moscow, Russia), 1 μL of (F + R) primers (10 μM), 0.5 μL of FAM probe (10 μM), 1.0 μL of dNTPs mixture (10 mM) (Eurogen, Moscow, Russia), 0.25 μL of HS Taq DNA polymerase (5 U/mL) (Eurogen, Moscow, Russia), and 17.25 μL of nuclease-free water (Thermo Scientific, Waltham, MA, USA). Amplification was performed on a CFX 96 device (Bio-Rad, Hercules, CA, USA). Gene expression was assessed by the threshold cycle value and normalized relative to the reference genes *Actb* and *Gapdh* using the $2^{-\Delta\Delta Ct}$ method.

4.5. Statistical Analysis

We used the sample homogenous by sex, age, and line to reliably identify a significant biological response through statistical analysis.

Statistical processing of the obtained results was carried out using the SPSS Statistics 20 (IBM) software package. The sample was tested for normality using the Kolmogorov–Smirnov test at $p = 0.05$. In the case of normal distribution, parametric research methods were used: ANOVA according to plan 4^1 (single-factor, four-level, balanced experiment). In case of rejection of the null hypothesis, the method of multiple comparison of means was used—Tukey's criterion (q-test). The mean (M) and standard error of the mean (SEM) were calculated; data are presented as the M ± SEM. If the sample did not correspond to a normal distribution, nonparametric goodness-of-fit tests were used: Kruskal–Wallis test. In case of rejection of the null hypothesis, the multiple comparison method was used–Duncan's test (MRT). The median (Me) and lower (Q1) and upper (Q3) quartiles were determined. Data are presented as Me (Q1–Q3). Differences were considered statistically significant at $p < 0.05$.

We calculated η^2. The classification and interpretation of η^2 (the strength of the effect) are presented in Table 9.

Table 9. Classification of the effect strength for η^2.

Effect Strength	Value of η^2	Interpretation
Weak	0.01–0.06	The factor explains only a small part of the variation in the dependent variable. The effect may be statistically significant with a large sample size.
Average	0.06–0.14	The factor explains a moderate part of the variation in the dependent variable. The effect can be practically significant.
Strong	≥0.14	The factor explains a significant part of the variance in the dependent variable. The effect is likely to have practical meaning.

5. Conclusions

The combined consumption of sunflower oil, margarine, cholesterol, and fructose by animals resulted in the development of non-alcoholic fatty liver disease, characterized by an increase in the relative organ weight and extreme accumulation of fat, cholesterol, and triglycerides in the liver. In addition, a significant increase in the alanine aminotransferase serum concentration was revealed, accompanied by significant changes in the antioxidant status of rats: accumulation of serum MDA and activation of SOD. A significant increase in serum total cholesterol and LDL point at the development of hyperlipidemia in these animals.

Immobilization stress had a strong effect on the animals' appetite, which led to a significant loss of their body weight; lean mass predominated in the body composition of these animals, with a significant decrease in the fat quota. The relative liver weight of these animals was significantly reduced against the background of weight loss; the fat content in the liver was also significantly lower. Immobilization had no effect on the liver levels of cholesterol and triglycerides. The blood biochemistry test showed a decrease in cholesterol level along with an increase in LDL and ALT. The effect of immobilization on the antioxidant system is shown only by a decrease in blood lipid peroxides.

Partial replacement of the diet lipid component with sunflower oil led to a significant decrease in animals' appetite and a decrease in body weight, without changing the body composition, expressed in relative units. A single intraperitoneal injection of CCl_4 against the background of sunflower oil consumption led to a significant increase in lipid peroxidation in the blood, characterized by the lipid peroxide accumulation and catalase activation. The significant increase in blood ALT and liver cholesterol shows the rapid development of toxic liver injury. In addition, a disturbance in carbohydrate metabolism was detected, expressed by a decrease in blood glucose and glycated hemoglobin.

The immobilization model has a serious impact on the psycho-emotional state of animals, which is accompanied by a loss of appetite, further leading to body exhaustion, a decrease in organ weight and changes in a number of biochemical parameters. However, in case of oxidative stress, it provides the least effect, resulting only in decreased levels of lipid peroxides. This model can be effectively used to evaluate the effects of adaptogens with anti-anxiety properties.

We have found that treating animals with a misbalanced diet containing sunflower oil, margarine, cholesterol, and fructose has the greatest impact on the rats' bodies. The obtained data may be of interest in modeling hyperlipidemia; the model can be effectively used to reproduce non-alcoholic fatty liver disease in vivo and to assess the state of oxidative stress in the body of animals.

A single intraperitoneal administration of CCl_4 against the background of a decrease in the omega-3 fatty acid quota in the animal's body is accompanied by a change in a number of biochemical parameters characterizing oxidative stress, and can be effectively used to study the effects of antioxidants in an in vivo experiment.

Author Contributions: Conceptualization, Y.S. and A.K.; methodology, Y.S., N.P. and N.B.; formal analysis, Y.S., N.P. and N.B.; investigation, Y.S., N.P., N.B., I.S., N.T. and A.B.; writing—original draft preparation, Y.S., N.P. and A.B.; writing—review and editing, Y.S. and A.K. All authors have read and agreed to the published version of the manuscript.

Funding: This research was funded by Russian Science Foundation, grant number 24-16-00171. https://rscf.ru/project/24-16-00171/ (accessed on 28 May 2025).

Institutional Review Board Statement: The animal study protocol was approved by the Local Ethics Committee of the Federal Research Center of Nutrition and Biotechnology (Protocol No. 8 dated 6 September 2024).

Informed Consent Statement: Not applicable.

Data Availability Statement: The data presented in this study are available on request from the corresponding author.

Conflicts of Interest: The authors declare no conflicts of interest.

Abbreviations

The following abbreviations are used in this manuscript:

ALT	Alanine aminotransferase
ALP	Alkaline phosphatase
AST	Aspartate aminotransferase
HDL	High-density lipoprotein
LDL	Low-density lipoprotein
MDA	Malon dialdehyde
OF	Open Field
PCR	Polymerase chain reaction
ROS	Reactive oxygen species
SOD	Superoxide dismutase

References

1. Wilson, O.W.A.; Garra, S.; Bopp, M.; Bopp, C.M. Incorporating the American College of Cardiology/American Heart Association Hypertension Diagnostic Criteria into Metabolic Syndrome Criteria Will Significantly Increase the Prevalence of Metabolic Syndrome among College Students. *J. Hum. Hypertens.* **2021**, *35*, 517–523. [CrossRef] [PubMed]
2. Zhang, H.; Sairam, M.R. Sex Hormone Imbalances and Adipose Tissue Dysfunction Impacting on Metabolic Syndrome; a Paradigm for the Discovery of Novel Adipokines. *Horm. Mol. Biol. Clin. Investig.* **2014**, *17*, 89–97. [CrossRef] [PubMed]
3. Tan, B.L.; Norhaizan, M.E. Effect of High-Fat Diets on Oxidative Stress, Cellular Inflammatory Response and Cognitive Function. *Nutrients* **2019**, *11*, 2579. [CrossRef] [PubMed]
4. Doulberis, M.; Papaefthymiou, A.; Polyzos, S.A.; Katsinelos, P.; Grigoriadis, N.; Srivastava, D.S.; Kountouras, J. Rodent Models of Obesity. *Minerva Endocrinol.* **2020**, *45*, 243–263. [CrossRef] [PubMed]
5. Shang, Z.; Gao, Y.; Xue, Y.; Zhang, C.; Qiu, J.; Qian, Y.; Fang, M.; Zhang, X.; Sun, X.; Kong, X.; et al. Shenge Formula Attenuates High-Fat Diet-Induced Obesity and Fatty Liver via Inhibiting ACOX1. *Phytomedicine* **2024**, *123*, 155183. [CrossRef] [PubMed]
6. Zhang, Z.; Yuan, Y.; Hu, L.; Tang, J.; Meng, Z.; Dai, L.; Gao, Y.; Ma, S.; Wang, X.; Yuan, Y.; et al. ANGPTL8 Accelerates Liver Fibrosis Mediated by HFD-Induced Inflammatory Activity via LILRB2/ERK Signaling Pathways. *J. Adv. Res.* **2023**, *47*, 41–56. [CrossRef] [PubMed]
7. Malakul, W.; Seenak, P.; Jumroon, N.; Arikit, S.; Kumphune, S.; Nernpermpisooth, N. Novel Coconut Vinegar Attenuates Hepatic and Vascular Oxidative Stress in Rats Fed a High-Cholesterol Diet. *Front. Nutr.* **2022**, *9*, 835278. [CrossRef] [PubMed]
8. Kandemir, F.; Kucukler, S.; Eldutar, E.; Caglayan, C.; Gülçin, İ. Chrysin Protects Rat Kidney from Paracetamol-Induced Oxidative Stress, Inflammation, Apoptosis, and Autophagy: A Multi-Biomarker Approach. *Sci. Pharm.* **2017**, *85*, 4. [CrossRef] [PubMed]
9. Kadiiska, M.B.; Peddada, S.; Herbert, R.A.; Basu, S.; Hensley, K.; Jones, D.P.; Hatch, G.E.; Mason, R.P. Biomarkers of Oxidative Stress Study VI. Endogenous Plasma Antioxidants Fail as Useful Biomarkers of Endotoxin-Induced Oxidative Stress. *Free Radic. Biol. Med.* **2015**, *81*, 100–106. [CrossRef] [PubMed]
10. Li, Q.; Zhang, W.; Cheng, N.; Zhu, Y.; Li, H.; Zhang, S.; Guo, W.; Ge, G. Pectolinarigenin Ameliorates Acetaminophen-Induced Acute Liver Injury via Attenuating Oxidative Stress and Inflammatory Response in Nrf_2 and PPARa Dependent Manners. *Phytomedicine* **2023**, *113*, 154726. [CrossRef] [PubMed]
11. Mortazavi, A.; Mohammad Pour Kargar, H.; Beheshti, F.; Anaeigoudari, A.; Vaezi, G.; Hosseini, M. The Effects of Carvacrol on Oxidative Stress, Inflammation, and Liver Function Indicators in a Systemic Inflammation Model Induced by Lipopolysaccharide in Rats. *Int. J. Vitam. Nutr. Res.* **2023**, *93*, 111–121. [CrossRef] [PubMed]
12. Ullah, H.; Khan, A.; Baig, M.W.; Ullah, N.; Ahmed, N.; Tipu, M.K.; Ali, H.; Khan, S. Poncirin Attenuates CCL_4-Induced Liver Injury through Inhibition of Oxidative Stress and Inflammatory Cytokines in Mice. *BMC Complement. Med. Ther.* **2020**, *20*, 115. [CrossRef] [PubMed]
13. Jiang, M.; Huang, C.; Wu, Q.; Su, Y.; Wang, X.; Xuan, Z.; Wang, Y.; Xu, F.; Ge, C. Sini San Ameliorates CCl_4-Induced Liver Fibrosis in Mice by Inhibiting AKT-Mediated Hepatocyte Apoptosis. *J. Ethnopharmacol.* **2023**, *303*, 115965. [CrossRef] [PubMed]
14. Wang, M.; Zhang, S.-S.; An, M.; Xia, Y.; Fan, M.-S.; Sun, Z.; Zhang, L.-J.; Zhao, Y.; Sheng, J.; Wang, X.-J. Neferine Ameliorates Nonalcoholic Steatohepatitis through Regulating AMPK Pathway. *Phytomedicine* **2023**, *114*, 154798. [CrossRef] [PubMed]
15. Fareed, M.M.; Khalid, H.; Khalid, S.; Shityakov, S. Deciphering Molecular Mechanisms of Carbon Tetrachloride- Induced Hepatotoxicity: A Brief Systematic Review. *Curr. Mol. Med.* **2024**, *24*, 1124–1134. [CrossRef] [PubMed]
16. Unsal, V.; Cicek, M.; Sabancilar, İ. Toxicity of Carbon Tetrachloride, Free Radicals and Role of Antioxidants. *Rev. Environ. Health* **2021**, *36*, 279–295. [CrossRef] [PubMed]

17. Tsikas, D. Assessment of Lipid Peroxidation by Measuring Malondialdehyde (MDA) and Relatives in Biological Samples: Analytical and Biological Challenges. *Anal. Biochem.* **2017**, *524*, 13–30. [CrossRef] [PubMed]
18. Weber, L.W.D.; Boll, M.; Stampfl, A. Hepatotoxicity and Mechanism of Action of Haloalkanes: Carbon Tetrachloride as a Toxicological Model. *Crit. Rev. Toxicol.* **2003**, *33*, 105–136. [CrossRef] [PubMed]
19. Karna, K.; Soni, K.; You, J.; Choi, N.; Kim, H.; Kim, C.; Lee, S.; Shin, Y.; Park, J. MOTILIPERM Ameliorates Immobilization Stress-Induced Testicular Dysfunction via Inhibition of Oxidative Stress and Modulation of the Nrf_2/HO-1 Pathway in SD Rats. *Int. J. Mol. Sci.* **2020**, *21*, 4750. [CrossRef] [PubMed]
20. Kolesnikova, L.I.; Kolesnikov, S.I.; Korytov, L.I.; Suslikova, M.I.; Darenskaya, M.A.; Grebenkina, L.A.; Kolesnikova, L.R. Oxidative Stress as a Mechanisms of Reduced Glucose Absorption under Conditions of Immobilization Stress. *Bull. Exp. Biol. Med.* **2017**, *164*, 132–135. [CrossRef] [PubMed]
21. Samarghandian, S.; Azimi-Nezhad, M.; Farkhondeh, T.; Samini, F. Anti-Oxidative Effects of Curcumin on Immobilization-Induced Oxidative Stress in Rat Brain, Liver and Kidney. *Biomed. Pharmacother.* **2017**, *87*, 223–229. [CrossRef] [PubMed]
22. Suzuki, K.; Tominaga, T.; Ruhee, R.T.; Ma, S. Characterization and Modulation of Systemic Inflammatory Response to Exhaustive Exercise in Relation to Oxidative Stress. *Antioxidants* **2020**, *9*, 401. [CrossRef] [PubMed]
23. Naoe, S.; Fujimoto, Y.; Murakami, K.; Yukimine, R.; Tanaka, A.; Yamaoka, K.; Kataoka, T. Effects of Low-Dose/High-Dose-Rate X-Irradiation on Oxidative Stress in Organs Following Forced Swim Test and Its Combined Effects on Alcohol-Induced Liver Damage in Mice. *J. Radiat. Res.* **2023**, *64*, 635–643. [CrossRef] [PubMed]
24. Al-Sowayan, N.S. Possible Modulation of Nervous Tension-Induced Oxidative Stress by Vitamin E. *Saudi J. Biol. Sci.* **2020**, *27*, 2563–2566. [CrossRef] [PubMed]
25. Wang, X.; Fang, C.; Wu, J.; Wang, S.; Zhao, R.; Ma, J. Xiaoyaosan Decoction Regulates Food Intake and Body Weight via the Leptin-Leptin Receptor-Proopiomelanocortin Pathway in Rats with Chronic Immobilization Stress. *J. Tradit. Chin. Med. Chung I Tsa Chih Ying Wen Pan* **2019**, *39*, 34–44. [PubMed]
26. Molina, P.; Andero, R.; Armario, A. Restraint or Immobilization: A Comparison of Methodologies for Restricting Free Movement in Rodents and Their Potential Impact on Physiology and Behavior. *Neurosci. Biobehav. Rev.* **2023**, *151*, 105224. [CrossRef] [PubMed]
27. Zhu, H.-Z.; Liang, Y.-D.; Ma, Q.-Y.; Hao, W.-Z.; Li, X.-J.; Wu, M.-S.; Deng, L.-J.; Li, Y.-M.; Chen, J.-X. Xiaoyaosan Improves Depressive-like Behavior in Rats with Chronic Immobilization Stress through Modulation of the Gut Microbiota. *Biomed. Pharmacother.* **2019**, *112*, 108621. [CrossRef] [PubMed]
28. Michajlovskij, N.; Lichardus, B.; Kvetnanský, R.; Ponec, J. Effect of Acute and Repeated Immobilization Stress on Food and Water Intake, Urine Output and Vasopressin Changes in Rats. *Endocrinol. Exp.* **1988**, *22*, 143–157. [PubMed]
29. Kizilaslan, N.; Zekiye Erdem, N.; Katar, M.; Gevrek, F. The Effects of Probiotics and Omega-3 Fatty Acids in Liver Steatosis Induced in Rats by High-Fructose Corn Syrup. *Int. J. Clin. Pract.* **2022**, *2022*, 7172492. [CrossRef] [PubMed]
30. Zhao, Y.; Wang, Q.-Y.; Zeng, L.-T.; Wang, J.-J.; Liu, Z.; Fan, G.-Q.; Li, J.; Cai, J.-P. Long-Term High-Fat High-Fructose Diet Induces Type 2 Diabetes in Rats through Oxidative Stress. *Nutrients* **2022**, *14*, 2181. [CrossRef] [PubMed]
31. Chávez-Gutiérrez, E.; Fuentes-Venado, C.E.; Rodríguez-Páez, L.; Guerra-Araiza, C.; Larqué, C.; Martínez-Herrera, E.; Ocharan-Hernández, M.E.; Lomelí, J.; Loza-Mejía, M.A.; Salazar, J.R.; et al. High Fructose and High Fat Diet Impair Different Types of Memory through Oxidative Stress in a Sex- and Hormone-Dependent Manner. *Metabolites* **2022**, *12*, 341. [CrossRef] [PubMed]
32. Miles, T.K.; Odle, A.K.; Byrum, S.D.; Lagasse, A.; Haney, A.; Ortega, V.G.; Bolen, C.R.; Banik, J.; Reddick, M.M.; Herdman, A.; et al. Anterior Pituitary Transcriptomics Following a High-Fat Diet: Impact of Oxidative Stress on Cell Metabolism. *Endocrinology* **2023**, *165*, bqad191. [CrossRef] [PubMed]
33. Yang, N.; Ko, M.; Ahn, M.; Shin, T. Hepatoprotective Effects of Norgalanthamine on Carbon Tetrachloride Induced-Hepatotoxicity in Mice. *Drug Chem. Toxicol.* **2023**, *46*, 144–154. [CrossRef] [PubMed]
34. Krähenbühl, S.; Reichen, J. Decreased Hepatic Glucose Production in Rats with Carbon Tetrachloride-Induced Cirrhosis. *J. Hepatol.* **1993**, *19*, 64–70. [CrossRef] [PubMed]
35. Ramaiah, L.; Bounous, D.I.; Elmore, S.A. Hematopoietic System. In *Haschek and Rousseaux's Handbook of Toxicologic Pathology*; Elsevier: Amsterdam, The Netherlands, 2013; pp. 1863–1933. [CrossRef]
36. Santos, R.D.; Shapiro, M.D.; Ballantyne, C.M. Glycated Hemoglobin to Detect Subclinical Atherosclerosis in People Without Diabetes. *J. Am. Coll. Cardiol.* **2021**, *77*, 2792–2795. [CrossRef] [PubMed]
37. Islam, M.A.; Al Mamun, M.A.; Faruk, M.; Ul Islam, M.T.; Rahman, M.M.; Alam, M.; Rahman, A.F.M.T.; Reza, H.; Alam, M.A. Astaxanthin Ameliorates Hepatic Damage and Oxidative Stress in Carbon Tetrachloride-Administered Rats. *Pharmacogn. Res.* **2017**, *9*, 84. [CrossRef] [PubMed]
38. Ilderbayev, O.; Okassova, A.; Rakhyzhanova, S.; Ilderbayeva, G.; Zhazykbayeva, L. The Levels of Oxidative Stress in a Combination of Stress Factors. *J. Med. Life* **2022**, *15*, 927–931. [CrossRef] [PubMed]

39. Ayala, A.; Muñoz, M.F.; Argüelles, S. Lipid Peroxidation: Production, Metabolism, and Signaling Mechanisms of Malondialdehyde and 4-Hydroxy-2-Nonenal. *Oxidative Med. Cell. Longev.* **2014**, *2014*, 360438. [CrossRef] [PubMed]
40. Pengnet, S.; Prommaouan, S.; Sumarithum, P.; Malakul, W. Naringin Reverses High-Cholesterol Diet-Induced Vascular Dysfunction and Oxidative Stress in Rats via Regulating LOX-1 and NADPH Oxidase Subunit Expression. *Biomed Res. Int.* **2019**, *2019*, 3708497. [CrossRef] [PubMed]
41. Wang, J.; Jiang, Y.; Jin, L.; Qian, C.; Zuo, W.; Lin, J.; Xie, L.; Jin, B.; Zhao, Y.; Huang, L.; et al. Alantolactone Attenuates High-Fat Diet-Induced Inflammation and Oxidative Stress in Non-Alcoholic Fatty Liver Disease. *Nutr. Diabetes* **2024**, *14*, 41. [CrossRef] [PubMed]
42. Wu, W.-T.; Hsu, T.-H.; Chen, W.-L.; Yang, C.-K.; Lo, H.-C. Polysaccharides of Grifola Frondosa Ameliorate Oxidative Stress and Hypercholesterolaemia in Hamsters Fed a High-Fat, High-Cholesterol Diet. *J. Pharm. Pharmacol.* **2022**, *74*, 1296–1306. [CrossRef] [PubMed]
43. Salehi, I.; Mohammadi, M.; Mirzaei, F.; Soufi, F.G. Amlodipine Attenuates Oxidative Stress in the Heart and Blood of High-Cholesterol Diet Rabbits. *Cardiovasc. J. Afr.* **2012**, *23*, 18–22. [CrossRef] [PubMed]
44. Dai, Y.; Cederbaum, A.I. Inactivation and Degradation of Human Cytochrome P4502E1 by CCl_4 in a Transfected HepG2 Cell Line. *J. Pharmacol. Exp. Ther.* **1995**, *275*, 1614–1622. [CrossRef] [PubMed]
45. Cohen, S.M.; Bevan, C.; Gollapudi, B.; Klaunig, J.E. Evaluation of the Carcinogenicity of Carbon Tetrachloride. *J. Toxicol. Environ. Health Part B* **2023**, *26*, 342–370. [CrossRef] [PubMed]
46. Amini, R.; Asle-Rousta, M.; Aghazadeh, S. Hepatoprotective Effect of Limonene against Chronic Immobilization Induced Liver Damage in Rats. *Naunyn Schmiedebergs. Arch. Pharmacol.* **2020**, *393*, 2053–2059. [CrossRef] [PubMed]
47. Álvarez-Diduk, R.; Galano, A. Adrenaline and Noradrenaline: Protectors against Oxidative Stress or Molecular Targets? *J. Phys. Chem. B* **2015**, *119*, 3479–3491. [CrossRef] [PubMed]
48. Labban, R.S.M.; Alfawaz, H.; Almnaizel, A.T.; Hassan, W.M.; Bhat, R.S.; Moubayed, N.M.; Bjørklund, G.; El-Ansary, A. High-Fat Diet-Induced Obesity and Impairment of Brain Neurotransmitter Pool. *Transl. Neurosci.* **2020**, *11*, 147–160. [CrossRef] [PubMed]
49. Chainy, G.B.N.; Sahoo, D.K. Hormones and Oxidative Stress: An Overview. *Free Radic. Res.* **2020**, *54*, 1–26. [CrossRef] [PubMed]
50. Yan, Y.; Jun, C.; Lu, Y.; Jiangmei, S. Combination of Metformin and Luteolin Synergistically Protects Carbon Tetrachloride-induced Hepatotoxicity: Mechanism Involves Antioxidant, Anti-inflammatory, Antiapoptotic, and Nrf_2/HO-1 Signaling Pathway. *BioFactors* **2019**, *45*, 598–606. [CrossRef] [PubMed]
51. Ojeaburu, S.; Oriakhi, K. Hepatoprotective, Antioxidant and, Anti-Inflammatory Potentials of Gallic Acid in Carbon Tetrachloride-Induced Hepatic Damage in Wistar Rats. *Toxicol. Rep.* **2021**, *8*, 177–185. [CrossRef] [PubMed]
52. Li, L.; Dong, H.; Song, E.; Xu, X.; Liu, L.; Song, Y. Nrf_2/ARE Pathway Activation, HO-1 and NQO1 Induction by Polychlorinated Biphenyl Quinone Is Associated with Reactive Oxygen Species and PI3K/AKT Signaling. *Chem. Biol. Interact.* **2014**, *209*, 56–67. [CrossRef] [PubMed]
53. Han, C.; Sun, T.; Xv, G.; Wang, S.; Gu, J.; Liu, C. Berberine Ameliorates CCl_4-induced Liver Injury in Rats through Regulation of the Nrf_2-Keap1-ARE and P53 Signaling Pathways. *Mol. Med. Rep.* **2019**, *20*, 3095–3102. [CrossRef] [PubMed]
54. Fan, J.; Chen, Q.; Wei, L.; Zhou, X.; Wang, R.; Zhang, H. Asiatic Acid Ameliorates CC L4-Induced Liver Fibrosis in Rats: Involvement of Nrf_2/ARE, NF-KB/IκBα, and JAK1/STAT3 Signaling Pathways. *Drug Des. Devel. Ther.* **2018**, *12*, 3595–3605. [CrossRef] [PubMed]
55. Bona, S.; Rodrigues, G.; Moreira, A.J.; Di Naso, F.C.; Dias, A.S.; Da Silveira, T.R.; Marroni, C.A.; Marroni, N.P. Antifibrogenic Effect of Melatonin in Rats with Experimental Liver Cirrhosis Induced by Carbon Tetrachloride. *JGH Open* **2018**, *2*, 117–123. [CrossRef] [PubMed]
56. National Research Council. *Guide for the Care and Use of Laboratory Animals*; National Academies Press: Washington, DC, USA, 2011. [CrossRef]
57. Kraeuter, A.-K.; Guest, P.C.; Sarnyai, Z. The Open Field Test for Measuring Locomotor Activity and Anxiety-Like Behavior. *Methods Mol. Biol.* **2019**, *1916*, 99–103. [CrossRef] [PubMed]
58. Reeves, P.G. Components of the AIN-93 Diets as Improvements in the AIN-76A Diet. *J. Nutr.* **1997**, *127* (Suppl. S5), 838S–841S. [CrossRef] [PubMed]
59. Rahmani, A.H.; Almatroudi, A.; Allemailem, K.S.; Alharbi, H.O.A.; Babiker, A.Y.; Althwab, S.A.; Alsuhaymi, N.; Alsugoor, M.H.; Khan, A.A.; Al-Megrin, W.A.I. Oleuropein, a Phenolic Component of *Olea europaea* L. Ameliorates CCl_4-Induced Liver Injury in Rats through the Regulation of Oxidative Stress and Inflammation. *Eur. Rev. Med. Pharmacol. Sci.* **2024**, *28*, 1259–1271. [CrossRef] [PubMed]
60. Sun, Y.; Demagny, H.; Faure, A.; Pontanari, F.; Jalil, A.; Bresciani, N.; Yildiz, E.; Korbelius, M.; Perino, A.; Schoonjans, K. Asparagine Protects Pericentral Hepatocytes during Acute Liver Injury. *J. Clin. Investig.* **2023**, *133*, e163508. [CrossRef] [PubMed]
61. Li, Y.; Guo, Z.; Cui, H.; Wang, T.; Xu, Y.; Zhao, J. Urantide Prevents CCl_4-induced Acute Liver Injury in Rats by Regulating the MAPK Signalling Pathway. *Mol. Med. Rep.* **2021**, *24*, 688. [CrossRef] [PubMed]

62. Frank, D.; Savir, S.; Gruenbaum, B.F.; Melamed, I.; Grinshpun, J.; Kuts, R.; Knyazer, B.; Zlotnik, A.; Vinokur, M.; Boyko, M. Inducing Acute Liver Injury in Rats via Carbon Tetrachloride (CCl_4) Exposure Through an Orogastric Tube. *J. Vis. Exp.* **2020**, *158*, e60695. [CrossRef] [PubMed]
63. Holman, B.W.B.; Bailes, K.L.; Meyer, R.G.; Hopkins, D.L. Effect of Modified Soxhlet (Soxtec) and Folch Extraction Method Selection on the Total Lipid Determination of Aged Beef. *J. Food Sci. Technol.* **2019**, *56*, 3957–3961. [CrossRef] [PubMed]

Disclaimer/Publisher's Note: The statements, opinions and data contained in all publications are solely those of the individual author(s) and contributor(s) and not of MDPI and/or the editor(s). MDPI and/or the editor(s) disclaim responsibility for any injury to people or property resulting from any ideas, methods, instructions or products referred to in the content.

International Journal of
Molecular Sciences

MDPI

Article

Orientin Reverses Premature Senescence in Equine Adipose Stromal Cells Affected by Equine Metabolic Syndrome Through Oxidative Stress Modulation

Dominika Orzoł, Martyna Kępska and Magdalena Zyzak *

Department of Experimental Biology, Institute of Biology, Wrocław University of Environmental and Life Sciences, C. K. Norwida 25, 50-375 Wrocław, Poland; 121656@student.upwr.edu.pl (D.O.); martyna.kepska@upwr.edu.pl (M.K.)

* Correspondence: magdalena.zyzak@upwr.edu.pl

Abstract

Equine metabolic syndrome (EMS) is a prevalent endocrine disorder associated with insulin dysregulation, oxidative stress, and impaired regenerative capacity of adipose-derived stem cells (ASCs). The aim of this study was to evaluate the effects of orientin—a plant-derived flavonoid with known antioxidant properties—on equine ASCs (EqASCs) derived from both clinically healthy and diagnosed EMS-affected mares. EqASCs were treated with orientin to evaluate its biological effects. The analysis included key cellular functions such as proliferative capacity, viability, apoptosis, oxidative stress, senescence, clonogenicity, and migration. Orientin significantly enhanced the proliferative activity of EqASCs, as evidenced by increased Ki67 expression and favorable alterations in cell cycle distribution. In addition, the treatment improved overall cell viability, reduced apoptotic activity, and restored both the clonogenic potential and migratory capacity of the cells, with particularly pronounced effects observed in EqASCs isolated from EMS-affected horses. Importantly, orientin also led to a marked reduction in cellular senescence and oxidative stress, further suggesting its potential as a protective and regenerative agent in metabolically impaired ASCs. These findings indicate that orientin can exert comprehensive cytoprotective effects on EqASCs, with pronounced benefits in cells derived from EMS-affected animals. By improving multiple functional parameters, orientin emerges as a promising candidate for therapeutic strategies aimed at restoring the regenerative potential of ASCs compromised by metabolic dysregulation in horses.

Keywords: orientin; ASCs; equine metabolic syndrome; senescence; ROS; oxidative stress

1. Introduction

Equine metabolic syndrome (EMS) represents a significant and growing concern within veterinary medicine, affecting an increasing proportion of the global equine population [1]. This endocrine disorder, analogous in many respects to human metabolic syndrome, is defined by a constellation of clinical and metabolic abnormalities, including regional adiposity, increased risk of endocrinopathic laminitis, and insulin dysregulation manifesting as hyperinsulinemia or an exaggerated insulin response [2,3]. First systematically described by Johnson, EMS shares clinical features with peripheral Cushing's syndrome, particularly in terms of insulin resistance and abnormal fat deposition [4,5]. The pathogenesis of EMS is complex and multifactorial, arising from the interplay of genetic predisposition, inappropriate dietary practices, and lack of physical activity [5–8].

Emerging evidence has also highlighted the involvement of accelerated cellular aging, or premature senescence, particularly in adipose-derived stromal cells (ASCs), which impairs tissue regeneration and may exacerbate disease progression [5,9].

An emerging and critical dimension of EMS pathophysiology is the progression of premature cellular senescence, a process characterized by irreversible cell cycle arrest accompanied by functional deterioration and altered secretory profiles [10]. Recent evidence suggests that EMS is not merely a metabolic condition but also a disease of accelerated cellular aging, particularly affecting ASCs, which are essential for tissue repair and homeostasis [1,5].

In horses affected by EMS, ASCs exhibit markers of early senescence, including increased expression of senescence-associated β-galactosidase (SA-β-Gal), elevated levels of p53 and p21, and a pro-inflammatory senescence-associated secretory phenotype (SASP) [9]. This cellular phenotype not only limits the regenerative capacity of these progenitor cells but also contributes to a pro-inflammatory microenvironment that exacerbates systemic insulin resistance and local tissue dysfunction. The accumulation of senescent cells within adipose and other metabolic tissues may thus play a pivotal role in the perpetuation and progression of EMS, linking metabolic stress to impaired cellular resilience. Mechanistically, oxidative stress, mitochondrial dysfunction, and chronic low-grade inflammation—common features of EMS—are recognized drivers of premature senescence [1]. The overproduction of reactive oxygen species (ROS) in metabolically stressed adipocytes and stromal cells induces DNA damage responses that activate senescence signaling cascades. Moreover, insulin dysregulation itself may promote senescence by modulating key pathways such as mTOR and FOXO, which regulate cellular metabolism, growth, and longevity [1,11]. Targeting senescence pathways may offer novel therapeutic avenues in the management of EMS. Interventions aimed at reducing oxidative stress, enhancing mitochondrial function, or selectively eliminating senescent cells (senolytics) are under investigation in both human and veterinary contexts and hold promise for restoring metabolic balance and cellular vitality in affected horses [5,9].

Given the central role of premature cellular senescence in the pathogenesis EMS, the identification of bioactive compounds capable of mitigating this process has garnered increasing scientific interest. Among such compounds, orientin, a flavonoid glycoside belonging to the flavone subclass and commonly found in plants such as *Ocimum sanctum* (holy basil) and *Passiflora edulis*, has demonstrated significant antioxidant, anti-inflammatory, and cytoprotective properties that position it as a promising candidate for combating cellular aging in metabolic disorders [5,12].

Recent preclinical studies have shown that orientin attenuates oxidative stress-induced senescence in various cell types by scavenging reactive oxygen species (ROS) and enhancing endogenous antioxidant defenses, such as superoxide dismutase (SOD) and glutathione peroxidase (GPx) [13]. This is particularly relevant in the context of EMS, where elevated oxidative stress within adipose tissue and ASCs contributes to DNA damage and mitochondrial dysfunction—two principal triggers of senescence [9,14–16]. At the molecular level, orientin exerts regulatory effects on key signaling pathways associated with longevity and metabolic homeostasis, including the PI3K/Akt, AMPK, and FOXO signaling axes. By modulating of these cascades, orientin supports mitochondrial homeostasis, inhibits of pro-senescent gene expression (such as *p16INK4a* and *p21*), and enhances autophagic flux, thereby promoting cellular resilience and extending the functional lifespan of progenitor cells [5,17]. Furthermore, orientin has been shown to suppress the senescence-associated secretory phenotype (SASP), leading to reduced secretion of inflammatory cytokines like IL-6 and TNF-α, which are known to exacerbate systemic inflammation and insulin resistance in EMS [9,18,19]. Additionally, orientin's favorable pharmacological profile—including low toxicity, good bioavailability, and the ability to cross cellular membranes—further supports its therapeutic potential [9,20]. Although most existing data are derived from in vitro and rodent studies, its mechanism of action aligns with the major pathological processes identified in EMS, warranting translational investigation in equine models.

This study aims to explore the potential of orientin as a therapeutic agent for EMS, focusing on its protective effects against oxidative stress and premature senescence in EqASCs. Given its pleiotropic actions, we hypothesized that orientin may attenuate the progression of EMS-related cellular impairments and contribute to restoring homeostasis in metabolically compromised stromal cells. Further research is needed to validate these effects in vivo and assess their clinical relevance in equine practice.

2. Results

2.1. Evaluation of the Cytotoxicity and Biocompatibility of Orientin and GI_{50} Determination

To assess the cytotoxicity and biocompatibility of orientin on ASCs after 24 h of treatment with increasing orientin concentrations, the MTT assay was performed. The dose-response curve demonstrated a sigmoidal relationship between orientin concentration (μM) and cell viability (%), with a progressive increase in cell viability observed up to approximately 60 μM, after which the curve plateaus, indicating a saturation effect (Figure 1).

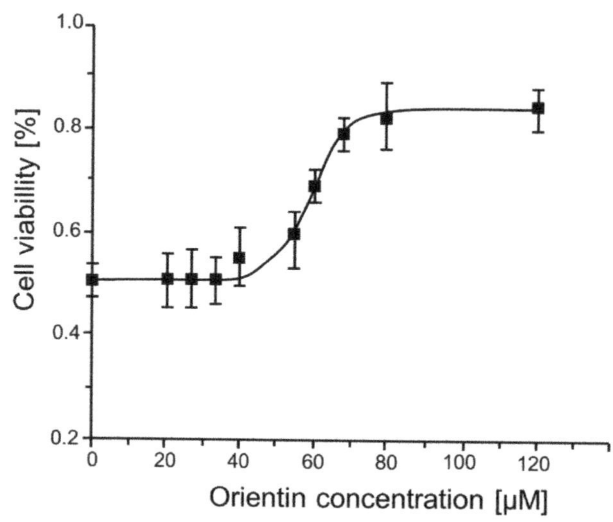

Figure 1. Effect of orientin on equine ASCs viability. Dose-response curve showing cell viability (%) in relation to increasing concentrations of orientin (15 to 130 μM). Data represent mean ± SD from three independent experiments.

Nonlinear regression analysis was conducted to determine the GI_{50} value (the concentration at which cell viability reaches 50% of the maximal response), which was calculated to be approximately 60 μM. This concentration was subsequently selected for further experiments. The fit of the model is statistically significant ($p < 0.0001$), and the high R^2 value (close to 0.99) confirms a strong correlation between orientin concentration and cell viability (Supplementary Material).

2.2. *Orientin Restores Proliferative Capacity and Promotes Cell Cycle Re-Entry in EMS-Derived EqASCs*

Nuclear Ki67 immunostaining revealed significantly reduced proliferative activity in EqASCs derived from EMS-affected horses compared to healthy controls. Ki67 staining showed that EMS cells treated with orientin had a stronger signal compared to the EMS control group (Figure 2A) Quantitative analysis confirmed that orientin significantly increased the proliferation rate compared to EMS cells (Figure 2B; $p < 0.001$). Interestingly, orientin application to control, healthy cells showed similar potentiation of cell proliferation (Figure 2A,B; $p < 0.001$). To assess whether orientin influences cell cycle dynamics, microcapillary flow cytometry-based analysis was performed to establish the differential distribution of EqASCs across G0/G1, S, and G2/M cell cycle phases (Figure 2C). In the G0/G1 stage, a significantly lower proportion of EMS-derived EqASCs was observed compared to healthy controls ($p < 0.001$). In contrast, orientin did not significantly alter the G0/G1 distribution in both healthy and EMS ASCs cells (Figure 2C). In the S phase, orientin markedly increased the proportion of EMS-EqASCs undergoing DNA replication compared to native cells ($p < 0.01$), but no significant changes were observed in G2/M phase entry upon orientin treatment compared to healthy cells with orientin treatment and EMS and orientin-treated cells (Figure 2C).

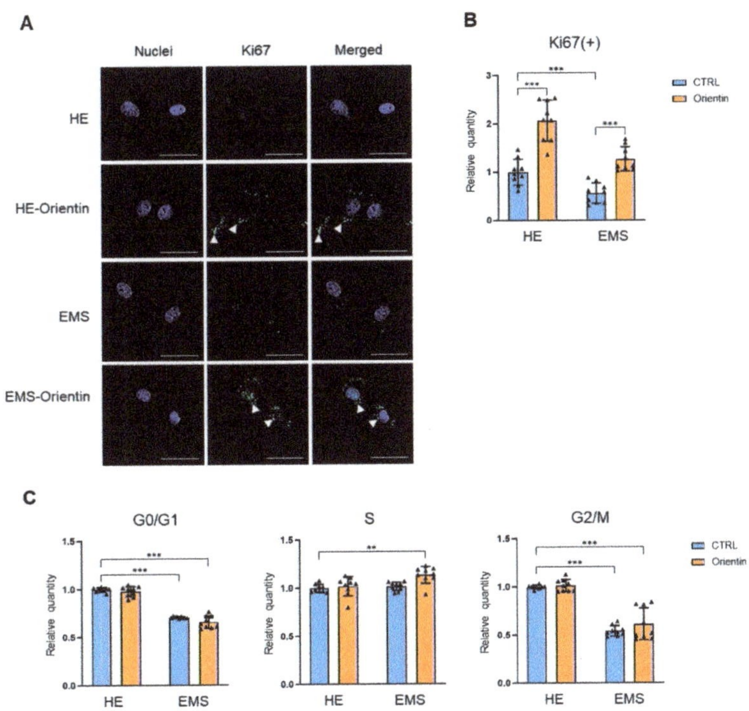

Figure 2. Orientin promotes proliferation and cell cycle progression in EqASCs from EMS-affected horses. (**A**) Representative confocal photomicrographs showing immunofluorescence staining of Ki67 protein (green) and DAPI nuclear counterstaining (blue) in ASCs derived from healthy (HE) and EMS horses, with or without orientin treatment. White arrowheads indicate additional intense Ki67 expression after orientin treatment. Scale bar: 30 µm. (**B**) Quantification of Ki67-positive cells shows a significant increase in proliferative activity following orientin treatment. (**C**) Histograms depicting the distribution of experimental cells across cell cycle stages. Data are presented as mean ± SD, with individual data points shown as triangles; ** $p < 0.01$., *** $p < 0.001$.

2.3. Orientin Attenuates Cellular Senescence and Enhances Clonogenic and Migratory Potential in EMS-Derived EqASCs

Senescence-associated β-galactosidase (SA-β-gal) staining was performed to assess the extent of cellular aging in healthy and EMS EqASCs cells and following orientin treatment (Figure 3A). As illustrated in Figure 3A, EMS-EqASCs displayed a pronounced increase in the number of SA-β-gal-positive cells. In contrast, both control and EMS-affected EqASCs treated with orientin exhibited a marked reduction in senescence-associated staining (Figure 3A). Quantitative analysis (Figure 3B) confirmed a significant decrease in the percentage of SA-β-gal-positive cells upon orientin treatment in the healthy ($p < 0.001$) and EMS group ($p < 0.001$), rejuvenating the senescence profile toward levels comparable with healthy controls, even though the level remained significantly higher ($p < 0.05$).

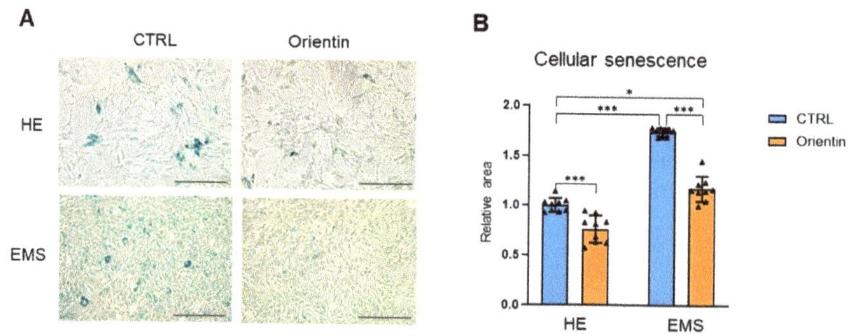

Figure 3. Orientin reduces cellular senescence of EMS-derived EqASCs. (**A**) Representative images of senescence-associated β-galactosidase (SA-β-gal) staining in EqASCs from healthy (HE) and EMS horses, with or without orientin treatment. Blue-stained cells indicate a senescent phenotype. Scale bar: 100 μm. (**B**) Quantification of SA-β-gal-positive cells. Data are presented as mean ± SD, with individual data points shown as triangles; * $p < 0.05$, *** $p < 0.001$.

To further investigate the functional impact of orientin on the regenerative potential of aged EqASCs, a colony-forming unit (CFU) assay was conducted. The representative images (Figure 4A) highlight that EMS-derived EqASCs exhibited reduced clonogenic capacity. Treatment with orientin significantly increased the number and size of colonies in both native and EMS-EqASCs cells, as evidenced by pararosaniline staining. Quantification (Figure 4B) revealed a statistically significant increase in clonogenicity following orientin treatment in healthy ($p < 0.001$) and EMS ($p < 0.001$) compared to the untreated cells.

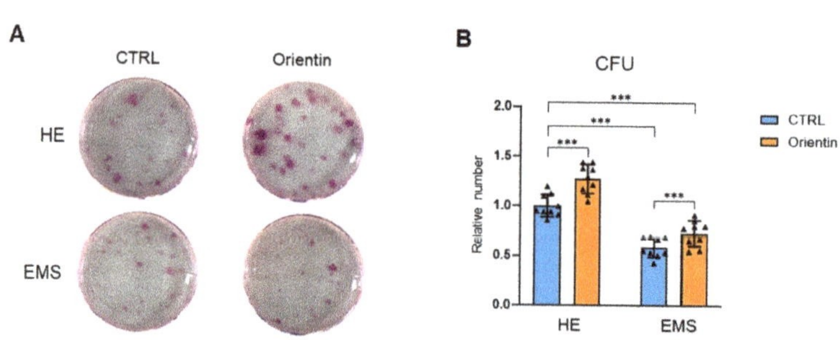

Figure 4. Orientin enhances the clonogenic potential of EMS-derived EqASCs. (**A**) Representative pararosaniline-stained plates from colony-forming unit fibroblast (CFU) assays and (**B**) quantification of colony number in healthy (HE) and EMS-derived EqASCs before (CTRL) and after orientin treatment. Data are presented as mean ± SD, with individual data points shown as triangles; *** $p < 0.001$.

Cell migration is a key feature of stromal cell regenerative performance and tissue repair. A wound healing (scratch) assay was therefore performed to examine the migratory capacity of EqASCs in response to orientin (Figure 5A). Untreated EMS-EqASCs cells displayed limited migration into the scratch area after over 24 h post-wound induction compared to the native cells ($p < 0.01$). Conversely, orientin-treated cells showed pronounced closure of the wound area, especially after 6 h (Figure 5A,B) in both healthy ($p < 0.001$) and EMS ($p < 0.001$) cells, leading to a higher efficiency of this process in EMS cells compared to native cells ($p < 0.001$). After 24 h (Figure 5A,C), a significant increase in wound closure was similarly observed in both orientin-treated healthy ($p < 0.001$) and EMS groups ($p < 0.001$). However, orientin-treated EMS cells were still characterized by reduced migration rates when compared to healthy ASCs ($p < 0.01$).

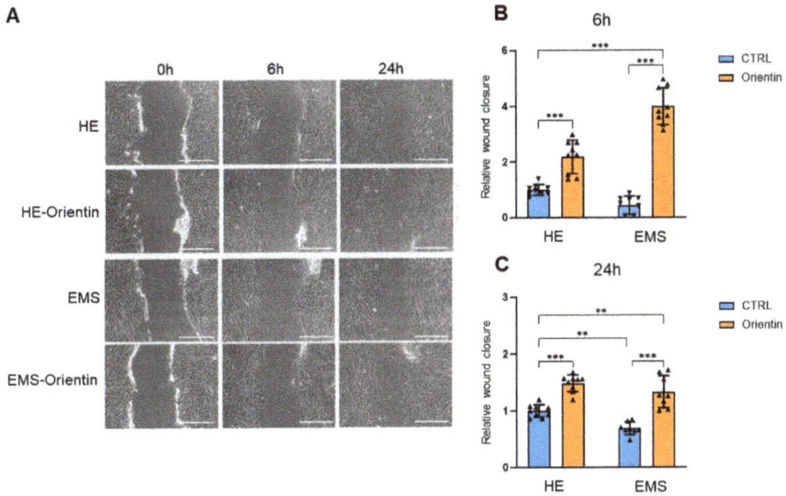

Figure 5. Orientin enhances the migratory potential of EMS-derived EqASCs. (**A**) Representative images of wound healing assay at 0, 6, and 24 h after scratch. Scale bar: 400 µm. (**B**) Quantification of wound closure after 6 and (**C**) 24 h. Data are presented as mean ± SD, with individual data points shown as triangles; ** $p < 0.01$, *** $p < 0.001$.

2.4. Orientin Reduces Apoptosis and Modulates the Expression of Key Apoptotic and Cell Cycle Regulatory Genes in EMS-EqASCs

To assess the pro-survival effects of orientin in EqASCs cells obtained from healthy and EMS horses, cell viability was quantified using the Muse® Annexin V & Dead Cell assay. As shown in Figure 6A–C, EMS-derived EqASCs exhibited a significantly increased proportion of dead (Figure 6A; $p < 0.001$) and total dead (Figure 6C; $p < 0.001$) cells compared to healthy controls and a lower proportion of live cells (Figure 6B; $p < 0.001$). Treatment with orientin led to a marked reduction in the number of dead (Figure 6A) cells in both the healthy ($p < 0.001$) and EMS group ($p < 0.001$). In correlation with this result, an increase in viable cells was noted after orientin treatment (Figure 6B), both in native ($p < 0.001$) and EMS ($p < 0.001$) cells relative to untreated cells.

To further validate the protective effect of orientin against cell death, a detailed quantitative analysis of cell distribution across various apoptosis stages was performed. (Figure 6D–J). The analysis distinguished between early apoptotic, late apoptotic, and live cell populations. Figure 6D shows a significant decrease in early apoptotic cells in EqASCs derived from EMS horses compared to healthy controls ($p < 0.001$). Importantly, treatment with orientin did not reduce the proportion of early apoptotic cells in both healthy and EMS-derived cells. EMS-EqASCs also displayed a markedly elevated number of total apoptotic cells compared to healthy cells ($p < 0.001$). Upon orientin treatment, this population was significantly decreased in both healthy ($p < 0.01$) and EMS-EqASCs ($p < 0.01$) cells, further supporting the compound's anti-apoptotic efficacy under metabolic stress conditions. Next, a significant increase in the late apoptotic/dead ratio (Figure 6F) of cells in the EMS group compared to healthy controls ($p < 0.001$) was observed. Noteworthy, orientin treatment significantly restored cell viability in healthy ($p < 0.001$) and EMS-EqASCs ($p < 0.001$) cells and also moderately increased viability in EMS orientin-treated cells compared to healthy cells ($p < 0.01$).

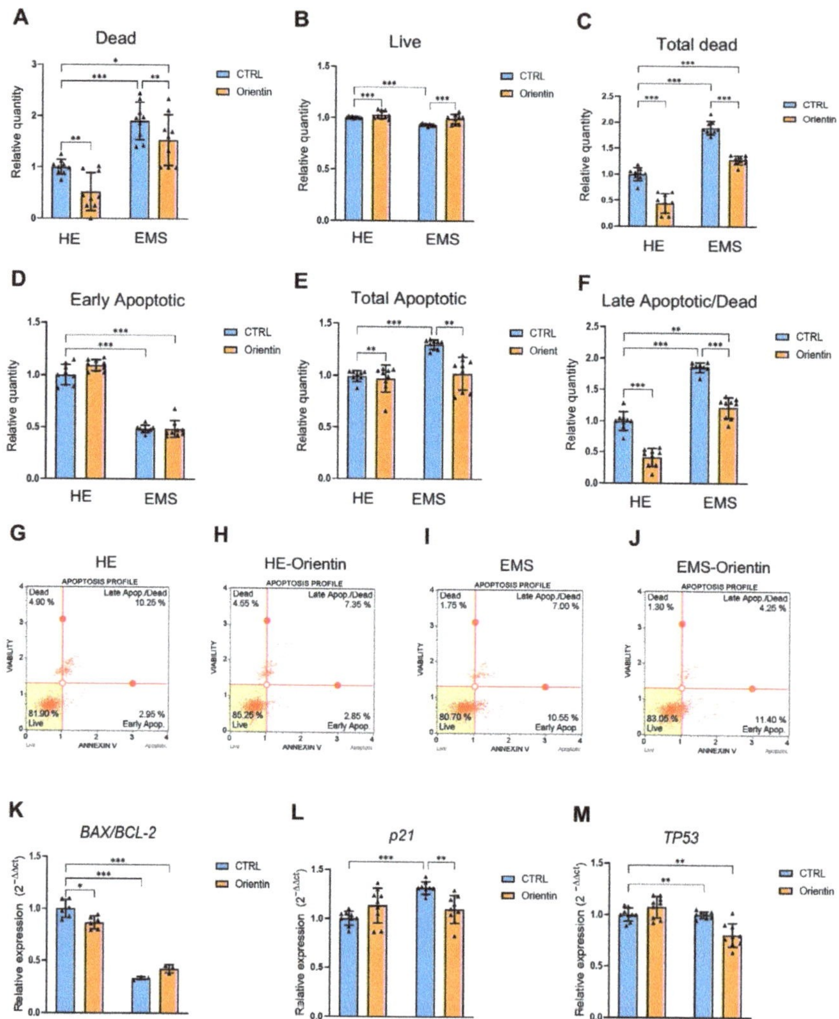

Figure 6. Orientin attenuates apoptosis and modulates the expression of key apoptotic and senescence-related genes in EMS-derived EqASCs. Quantification of (**A–C**) live and dead cells and (**D–F**) apoptotic healthy (HE) and EMS-derived EqASCs cells. (**G–J**) Representative plots from MUSE® Cell Analyzer. (**K–M**) Gene expression analysis of *BAX/BCL-2* ratio, *p21*, and *TP53*. Data are expressed as mean ± SD, with individual data points shown as triangles; * $p < 0.05$, ** $p < 0.01$, *** $p < 0.001$.

Then, changes in the expression levels of key genes involved in apoptosis regulation were analyzed. The expression ratio of *BAX* to *BCL-2* (Figure 6K), a key indicator of the pro-apoptotic to anti-apoptotic signaling balance, was significantly reduced in healthy EqASCs cells following orientin treatment ($p < 0.05$). In contrast, EMS-derived EqASCs exhibited an overall lower basal *BAX/BCL-2* ratio compared to healthy controls ($p < 0.001$. Importantly, orientin treatment did not significantly alter the *BAX/BCL-2* expression in EMS-EqASCs. Gene expression analysis revealed that *p21* mRNA levels (Figure 6L) were significantly elevated in EqASCs derived from EMS horses compared to healthy controls ($p < 0.001$). Treatment with orientin resulted in a significant reduction in *p21* expression only in EMS-derived EqASCs ($p < 0.01$). *TP53*, a central regulator of the DNA damage response and cellular senescence, showed significantly elevated expression in EMS-derived EqASCs compared to healthy controls (Figure 6M $p < 0.001$). In healthy ASCs, orientin treatment did not significantly alter *TP53* expression. Conversely, orientin treatment significantly reduced *TP53* expression in EMS-derived EqASCs ($p < 0.01$) compared to the healthy cells.

2.5. Orientin Reduces Oxidative Stress in EMS-Derived EqASCs

Oxidative stress in EqASCs was assessed using MUSE-based analysis of ROS-positive and ROS-negative cell populations, CM-H2DCFDA fluorescence imaging, flow cytometry, and gene expression analysis of key antioxidant enzymes.

Microfluidic flow cytometry (Figure 7A–C) showed a significantly lowered number of ROS-negative cells (Figure 7A; $p < 0.001$) and a substantially higher number of ROS-positive cells (Figure 7B; $p < 0.001$) in EqASCs isolated from horses with EMS compared to healthy controls. Orientin treatment significantly increased the ROS-negative population in EMS-derived EqASCs ($p < 0.01$), and decreased the intracellular accumulation of ROS in treated cells ($p < 0.001$).

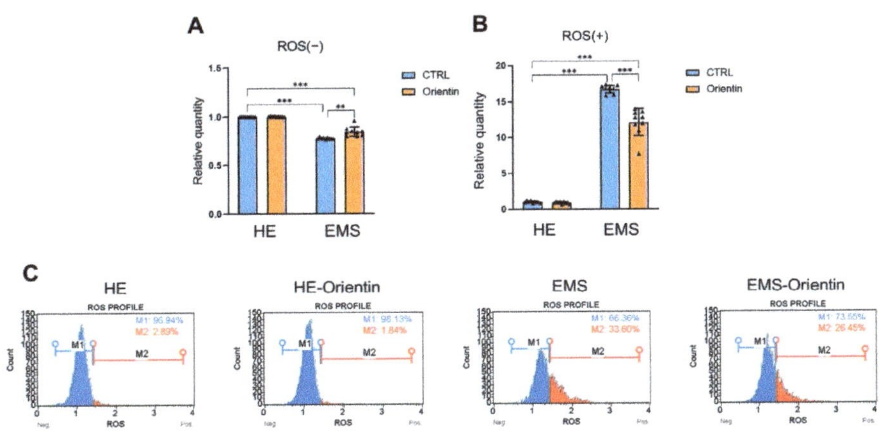

Figure 7. Orientin reduces oxidative stress in EMS-derived EqASCs. (**A–C**) Analysis of ROS-positive and ROS-negative cell populations using the MUSE® Cell Analyzer in healthy (HE) and EMS-derived EqASCs. Data are expressed as mean ± SD, with individual data points shown as triangles; ** $p < 0.01$, *** $p < 0.001$.

The elevated oxidative status in EMS-ASCs was further confirmed by fluorescence microscopy using the CM-H2DCFDA probe (Figure 8A,B). EMS cells showed an intense fluorescence signal indicating ROS accumulation, which was significantly reduced after orientin treatment (Figure 8A). Quantitative analysis (Figure 8B) confirmed a significant increase in the relative fluorescence intensity in the group of EMS-derived EqASCs cells compared to native cells ($p < 0.001$). Importantly, treatment of both groups reduced fluorescence levels in both healthy ($p < 0.001$) and EMS ($p < 0.001$) cells. However, EMS EqASCs treated with orientin presented a consistently higher ROS signal relative to control EqASCs ($p < 0.01$). Flow cytometry analysis using CM-H2DCFDA (Figure 8C,D) corroborated these findings, showing a significantly higher mean fluorescence intensity in EMS cells ($p < 0.001$), which was effectively attenuated by orientin treatment ($p < 0.05$). Orientin treatment reduced this level in both EMS ($p < 0.001$) and native ($p < 0.001$) cells.

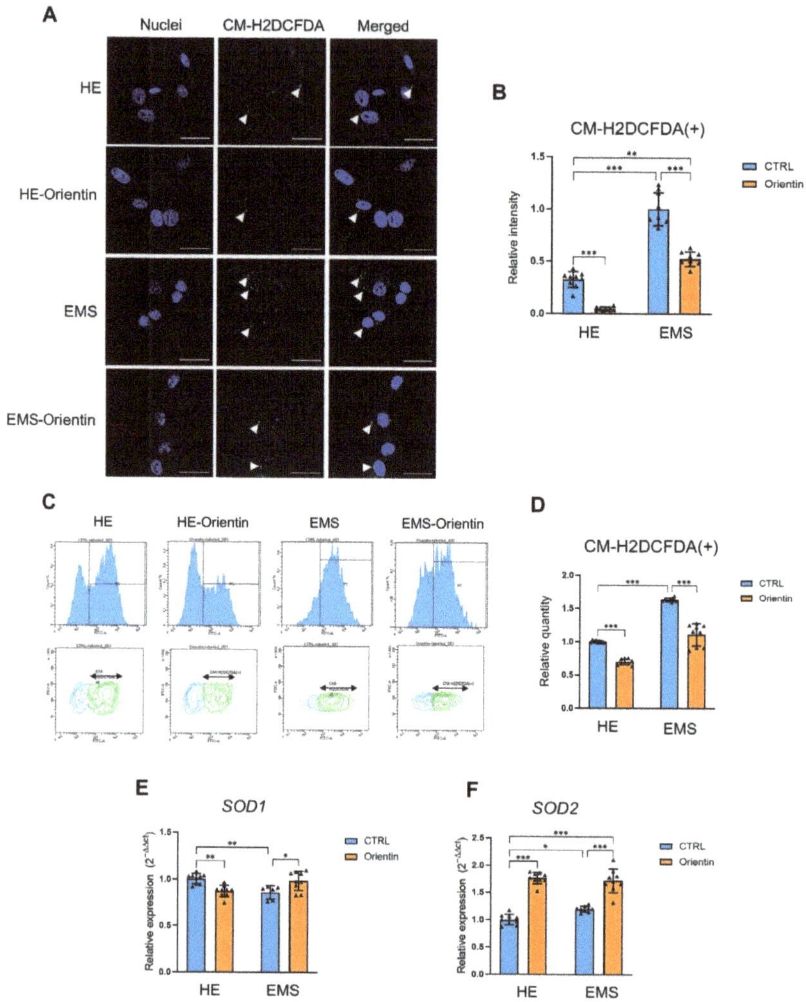

Figure 8. Orientin reduces oxidative stress in EMS-derived EqASCs. (**A**) Representative fluorescence images of ROS accumulation in healthy (HE) and EMS-derived cells, before and after orientin treatment, detected by CM-H2DCFDA staining; green—ROS, blue—DAPI. White arrowheads indicate additional intense CM-H2DCFDA expression before and after orientin treatment. Scale bar: 30 µm. (**B**) Quantification of ROS fluorescence intensity from (**A**). (**C**,**D**) Flow cytometric analysis of ROS levels using CM-H2DCFDA probe. (**E**,**F**) Relative mRNA expression levels of *SOD1* and *SOD2* determined by qPCR. Data are expressed as mean ± SD, with individual data points shown as triangles; * $p < 0.05$, ** $p < 0.01$, *** $p < 0.001$.

To investigate the underlying molecular mechanisms by which orientin influences cellular redox status, the expression of key antioxidant genes *SOD1* and *SOD2* was analyzed

(Figure 8E,F). EMS-derived EqASCs showed decreased expression of *SOD1* (Figure 8E; $p < 0.01$) mRNA level compared to healthy cells. Orientin treatment significantly decreased *SOD1* expression in healthy cells (Figure 8E; $p < 0.01$), whereas, on the contrary, it increased the expression of this gene in EMS cells ($p < 0.5$). The expression level of the *SOD2* mRNA was increased in EMS cells (Figure 8F; $p < 0.05$). Orientin treatment additionally increased this level in both healthy (Figure 8F; $p < 0.001$) and EMS-derived cells ($p < 0.001$).

3. Discussion

This study provided compelling evidence that orientin, a flavonoid glycoside, exerts multifaceted cytoprotective effects on EqASCs, particularly those derived from horses suffering from equine metabolic syndrome (EMS). The compound appears to significantly influence several key cellular mechanisms, including modulation of apoptosis, enhancement of cell cycle progress, attenuation of oxidative stress, and restoration of regenerative capacity. These properties highlighted orientin's potential as a supportive agent in regenerative therapies, especially in cases where stromal cell function was compromised due to metabolic dysfunctions.

The results of the present study demonstrated that orientin significantly enhanced Ki67 expression and increased the number of cells in the S phase of the cell cycle in EqASCs obtained from horses affected by EMS. Ki67 is a well-established marker of cellular proliferation, expressed during the active phases of the cell cycle (G1, S, G2, and M), but absent in quiescent (G0) cells, making it a reliable indicator of proliferative activity [21,22]. The observed increase in S-phase cells suggests that orientin facilitated the transition from the G1 to S phase, potentially through modulation of cyclin-dependent kinases (CDKs) and their associated cyclins. Previous studies showed that orientin can induce G0/G1 cell cycle arrest in human colorectal carcinoma HT29 cells by upregulating the CDK inhibitor $p21^{WAF1/CIP1}$ and downregulating cyclins D1 and E, as well as CDK2 and CDK4 [23]. Although our study focused on EqASCs rather than cancer cells, it is plausible that orientin exerts similar regulatory effects on the cell cycle machinery in EqASCs. Interestingly, despite the pronounced increase in S phase cells, no significant change was observed in the G2/M cell population following orientin treatment. This apparent discrepancy may be explained by the relatively short incubation period of 24 h. The population doubling time of EqASCs in vitro typically ranges from 48 to 72 h, and in cells derived from metabolically compromised animals, such as those with EMS, this time might have been even longer due to senescent-like features and decreased metabolic activity [24,25]. Consequently, the cells may not have had sufficient time to progress into mitosis during the experimental window, although the observed increase in S phase cells strongly indicated preparation for cell cycle entry and active DNA replication.

The observed enhancement of clonogenic potential in both healthy and EMS-derived ASCs following orientin treatment underscored its role in promoting self-renewal and stemness. Clonogenic assays, which evaluated a cell's capacity for unlimited division, were pivotal in assessing stem cell functionality. The increase in both the number and size of colonies suggests that orientin might have activated signaling pathways supporting stem cell maintenance and proliferation. Several key signaling pathways are known to regulate stem cell self-renewal and clonogenicity. For instance, the Wnt/β-catenin pathway is integral in maintaining the undifferentiated state and promoting proliferation in various stem cell types [26]. Inhibition of Wnt signaling was shown to reduce colony formation in human embryonic stem cells [27], highlighting its role in self-renewal processes. Similarly, the PI3K/Akt pathway is crucial for stem cell survival and proliferation, with studies demonstrating that its activation supports the self-renewal of embryonic stem cells [28,29]. Moreover, the JNK signaling pathway was implicated in regulating the traits of various stem cells, including their self-renewal and differentiation capacities [30]. Activation of these pathways might have underlain the observed effects of orientin on ASC clonogenicity. Phytochemicals, such as orientin, were recognized for their potential to modulate these signaling pathways [20,31]. For example, certain flavonoids can enhance stem cell proliferation and counteract senescence by influencing pathways like Wnt/β-catenin and PI3K/Akt [32]. Therefore, the effects of orientin on EqASCs clonogenicity might have been attributed to its capacity to modulate these critical signaling cascades, thereby promoting stem cell self-renewal and proliferation. These findings provided a basis for further investigation into orientin's therapeutic potential in regenerative medicine.

The observed enhancement in migratory capacity of orientin-treated ASCs, as evidenced by accelerated wound closure in scratch assays, indicated improved cell motility and potential for tissue repair. Cell migration is a critical component of tissue re-generation, involving intricate coordination of cytoskeletal dynamics and interactions with the extracellular matrix. Orientin, a flavonoid compound, was shown to modulate signaling pathways associated with cell migration [33]. In MCF-7 breast cancer cells, orientin inhibited migration and invasion by suppressing the PKCα/ERK/AP-1/STAT3 signaling axis, leading to decreased expression of matrix metalloproteinase-9 (MMP-9) and interleukin-8 (IL-8) [34]. These findings suggest that orientin can influence key pathways governing cell motility. Furthermore, orientin has demonstrated the ability to inhibit the MAPK signaling pathway, which plays a pivotal role in regulating cell migration. In studies involving fibroblast-like synovial cells from rheumatoid arthritis patients, orientin treatment resulted in reduced phosphorylation of ERK, JNK, and p38 MAPKs, correlating with decreased migratory and invasive behaviors [33]. In addition to its effects on signaling pathways, orientin was reported to promote wound healing processes [35]. In 3T3 fibroblast cells, orientin enhanced cell proliferation and migration, contributing to improved wound closure in vitro [36]. Similarly, isoorientin, a structurally related compound, facilitated excisional skin wound healing in mice by modulating inflammatory responses and promoting tissue remodeling [35,36]. Collectively, these findings support the notion that orientin can also affect the EqASCs' migratory capacity through modulation of key signaling pathways and promotion of wound healing mechanisms, but further investigations are warranted to elucidate the precise molecular mechanisms underlying orientin's effects on EqASCs migration and to explore its potential therapeutic applications in regenerative medicine.

Mesenchymal stromal cells (MSCs), including ASCs, are increasingly utilized in both human and veterinary regenerative medicine owing to their multipotency, paracrine activity, and immunomodulatory capacity [37,38]. However, in metabolically dysregulated environments such as EMS, the therapeutic efficacy of ASCs may be impaired due to increased levels of oxidative stress, mitochondrial dysfunction, and apoptosis [39]. Therefore, strategies aimed at preserving ASCs viability and functionality in such pathophysiological states are of paramount importance. One of the most striking findings of this study was orientin's capacity to modulate apoptosis in both healthy and EMS-affected EqASCs. The observed reduction in the BAX/BCL-2 expression ratio indicates a shift in the cellular equilibrium towards survival, suggesting that orientin may inhibit the intrinsic apoptotic pathway [23]. This shift is particularly beneficial in EMS-ASCs, where elevated pro-apoptotic signaling contributed to the depletion of the stromal cell pool and a subsequent decline in regenerative performance. Previous studies have confirmed that orientin exerts anti-apoptotic effects via mitochondrial pathways, notably through suppression of cytochrome c release and inhibition of caspase-3 activation. In models of oxidative and metabolic stress, orientin has been shown to increase *BCL-2* expression while down-regulating *BAX*, thereby stabilizing mitochondrial membranes and reducing the loss of mitochondrial potential [40]. Furthermore, orientin can modulate the PI3K/Akt pathway, which plays a key role in regulating cell survival and response to oxidative stress [41]. In the context of endothelial cells, orientin may affect the activation of the PI3K/Akt/eNOS pathway, leading to increased nitric oxide (NO) production and improved endothelial function. Although direct studies on the effects of orientin on endothelial cells are limited, there is evidence for its beneficial effects in the context of oxidative stress and apoptosis in other cell types [42].

Oxidative stress is a key pathophysiological factor in EMS, contributing to cellular dysfunction, accelerated senescence, and impaired regenerative capacity of stromal cells. In our study, we observed that orientin, a natural flavonoid, significantly reduced the levels of reactive oxygen species (ROS) in EqASCs from EMS-affected horses (EMS-EqASCs), indicating its potent antioxidant properties. The mechanism of action of orientin involves the activation of the Nrf2/HO-1 signaling pathway, which plays a crucial role in regulating the cellular antioxidant response [40]. In models of oxidative injury, orientin promoted the translocation of the transcription factor Nrf2 into the nucleus, leading to increased expression of antioxidant enzymes such as heme oxygenase-1 (HO-1), NAD(P)H quinone dehydrogenase 1 (NQO1), and glutamate–cysteine ligase catalytic subunit (GCLC). This cascade ultimately reduces oxidative stress and protects cells from damage [43]. Furthermore, orientin was shown to enhance the activity of superoxide dismutase (SOD) enzymes, including both cytoplasmic SOD1 and mitochondrial SOD2. The upregulation of SOD2 is particularly important, as this enzyme plays a critical role in neutralizing superoxide anions within mitochondria, thereby safeguarding cells against oxidative injury [44]. In addition, orientin exhibited protective effects in various models of oxidative damage, including liver injury induced by d-galactosamine and lipopolysaccharide (d-GalN/LPS). In these models, orientin activated the Nrf2/Keap1 axis, resulting in decreased serum levels of liver enzymes ALT and AST and improved liver histopathology [45].

Reduction in senescence-associated β-galactosidase (SA-β-gal) staining in orientin-treated ASCs suggests a reversal of senescent phenotypes. Cellular senescence, characterized by irreversible cell cycle arrest, is a hallmark of aging and metabolic disorders, often leading to diminished regenerative capacity [1]. The ability of orientin to attenuate senescence markers in our studies indicates its potential in rejuvenating aged or metabolically compromised cells. In the context of senescence, orientin has been reported to possess antioxidant properties that mitigate cellular aging processes. Previous studies have demonstrated that orientin can reduce oxidative stress by scavenging free radicals and enhancing the activity of antioxidant enzymes. For instance, in D-galactose-induced aging models, orientin administration improved antioxidant enzyme levels and reduced markers of oxidative damage, thereby delaying aging-related changes [13,46]. Furthermore, orientin was shown to improve mitochondrial function, which is closely linked to cellular senescence [20]. Mitochondrial dysfunction is a key contributor to the onset of senescence, as it leads to increased production of reactive oxygen species (ROS) and subsequent cellular damage. By enhancing mitochondrial homeostasis, orientin might have alleviated senescence and promote cellular longevity. Recent research indicated that orientin can improve mitochondrial function and inhibit chondrocyte senescence via the PI3K/AKT/NF-κB signaling pathway [20]. In summary, the anti-senescent effects of orientin in ASCs may be mediated through its antioxidant properties and its ability to enhance mitochondrial function. These findings suggest that orientin holds promise as a therapeutic agent for rejuvenating aged or metabolically compromised stem cells, thereby improving their regenerative potential.

While this study provides evidence for the cytoprotective and anti-apoptotic effects of orientin in ASCs under metabolic stress, it is important to note that the findings are based solely on in vitro cellular models. The absence of in vivo validation represents a limitation that must be addressed in future research. Cellular systems, although useful for mechanistic insight, do not fully replicate the complex physiological and metabolic environment present in living organisms, particularly in the context of metabolic syndrome and its systemic effects. Therefore, to better understand the therapeutic potential and biological behavior of orientin, future studies should incorporate animal models of EMS or comparable mammalian models that simulate the metabolic, inflammatory, and oxidative stress conditions observed in the disease. Such studies would allow for assessment of orientin's bioavailability, pharmacokinetics, tissue-specific effects, and long-term safety profile. Moreover, investigating orientin's influence on systemic oxidative stress, insulin sensitivity, inflammatory markers, and adipose tissue remodeling in vivo would provide critical translational insight and support the development of orientin-based therapies for metabolic disorders.

4. Materials and Methods

4.1. Equine ASC Cell Culture and Orientin Treatment

Healthy and EMS-affected Equine ASCs were obtained from the cell collection of the Department of Experimental Biology, University of Environmental and Life Sciences, Wrocław, Poland. ASCs cultures were maintained in 75 cm^2 flasks and cultured in Dulbecco's modified Eagle's medium (DMEM) containing 1000 mg/L glucose (Life Technologies, Paisley, UK), supplemented with 5% of fetal bovine serum (FBS; Sigma-Aldrich, St. Louis, MO, USA), and 1% of a penicillin and streptomycin solution (PS; Sigma-Aldrich, St. Louis, MO, USA), and incubated at 37 °C in a humidified 5% CO_2, 95% air atmosphere. Cultured cells were harvested every three days (80–90% of confluence) and detached from the flasks with a trypsin–EDTA solution (Sigma-Aldrich, St. Louis, MO, USA). The media were changed every second day.

The orientin was purchased from Cayman Chemicals (Ann Arbor, MI, USA) in the form of a crystalline solid and for this study it was dissolved in a sodium hydroxide solution (NaOH). After the determination of cytotoxic activity of orientin, described below, the cells were treated with orientin with the final concentration of 60 μM under standard conditions for 24 h before testing.

For each experimental method, data were obtained from three independent biological replicates (cells isolated from three healthy and three EMS horses), each analyzed in at least three technical replicates. For most methods, technical replicates were performed in separate wells, except for assays using microscopy techniques, where technical replicates referred to different fields of view on the same sample.

4.2. Determination of Cytotoxic Activity of Orientin

The determination of cytotoxic activity of orientin was examined by the MTT assay [47]. The MTT assay was performed in a 96-well flat-bottomed plate; 200 μL of culture medium containing 0.2×10^5 cells was distributed among the wells and incubated for 24 h. The culture medium was then removed, washed with DPBS solution (Sigma-Aldrich, St. Louis, MO, USA), and 200 μL each of fresh medium with the appropriate concentration of orientin was added. The effect of orientin on EqASCs was studied at successive concentrations of 15, 45, 50, 60, 70, 80, 100, 120, and 130 μM. A solution of NaOH (sodium hydroxide) was added to one of the wells as a control. Cells were incubated for 24 h under standard conditions.

After incubation, the medium with orientin was removed and 200 μL of culture medium with MTT reagent (Sigma-Aldrich, St. Louis, MO, USA) at a concentration of 5 mg/mL was added to each well. The cell culture was carried out for 2 h under the same standard conditions. The solution was removed from the wells, after which 100 μL of DMSO solution (AppliChem, Darmstadt, Germany) was added to each well and incubated for 20 min. Absorbance measurements of solutions with dissolved formazan were performed spectrophotometrically at 570 nm using a Synergy H1 plate reader (BioTek® Instruments, Inc., Winooski, VT, USA).

4.3. Evaluation of Oxidative Stress

(a) Quantification of ROS accumulation using Muse® Oxidative Stress assay

The reactive oxygen species accumulation (ROS) was measured using the Muse® Oxidative Stress Assay Kit (Luminex, Austin, TX, USA) according to the manufacturer's protocol. After trypsinization, 200 μL of Muse Oxidative Stress Working Solution was added to the cell pellet and incubated 30 min at 37 °C. Then, the ROS-negative and ROS-positive cells were counted using a Muse™ Cell Analyzer (EMD Millipore, Temecula, CA, USA).

(b) Fluorescence microscopy-based detection of intracellular ROS with CM-H_2DCFDA

Furthermore, the reactive oxygen species were stained in cells using the CM-H2DCFDA fluorescent dye (General Oxidative Stress Indicator) (Invitrogen Life Technologies, Eugene, OR, USA). The cells were stained according to manufacturers' instructions. Four hundred microliters of medium containing 0.6×10^5 EqASCs were seeded on coverslips in a 24-well plate. After treating the cells with orientin for 24 h, they were washed with DPBS and then CM-H2DCFDA staining solution (10 μM, prepared in culture medium without FBS and without PS) was added. The cells were then incubated for 30 min in an incubator, and after washing again with DPBS, they were fixed in 4% PFA (Sigma-Aldrich, St. Louis, MO, USA) for 15 min at room temperature (RT). Afterward, they were washed with DPBS three times and the slides were closed using the Fluoroshield™ with DAPI (Sigma-Aldrich, St. Louis, MO, USA). Microscopic preparations were observed using a Leica DMi8 (Leica Microsystems, Wetzlar, Germany) confocal microscope with a magnification of ×630. The photomicrographs were finally analyzed in Fiji using ImageJ Software (version 1.52n, Wayne Rasband, National Institutes of Health, Bethesda, MD, USA) with the 'Color Pixel Counter' plugin. The average number of green pixels per cell was measured using a fixed threshold value that was applied consistently across all images.

(c) Flow cytometric analysis of CM-H_2DCFDA-stained cells

For analysis on a flow cytometer, cells were seeded on a 6-well plate. After trypsinization and centrifugation at 300× *g*, 5 min, the pellets were washed with DPBS and then centrifuged again at 300× *g*, 5 min. The pellets were resuspended in DPBS, and then the suspension was transferred to another tube as a control sample (unstained), and then centrifuged as before. A 100 μL volume of DPBS was added to the control sample after the supernatant was drawn off, and 100 μL of the prepared reagent was added to the test sample; both samples were then incubated for 30 min in an incubator. After incubation, the cells were washed three times with DPBS and finally resuspended in 350 μL of DPBS. CM-H2DCFDA-positive cells were counted on a BD LSRFortessa™ Cell Analyzer (Becton, Dickinson and Company, BD Biosciences, San Jose, Belgium) using an FITC detector.

4.4. Senescence Analysis

Cellular senescence was analyzed using the β-galactosidase hydrolysis kit (Senescence Cells Histochemical Staining Kit, Sigma Aldrich, St. Louis, MO, USA) according to the manufacturer's instructions. The cells were seeded in a 12-well plate, and were first treated with fixation buffer and incubated for 6 min at RT. Next, the cells were treated with staining mixture and incubated overnight at 37 °C. The photos were taken the next day using the Leica DMi1 inverted microscope (Leica Microsystems, Wetzlar, Germany). Color analysis was performed in Fiji using ImageJ Software (version 1.52n, Wayne Rasband, National

Institutes of Health, USA) using the 'Color Pixel Counter' plugin to measure the total area of green pixels in each image.

4.5. Evaluation of Viability and Apoptosis

Cell viability and apoptosis were analyzed using the Muse® Annexin V & Dead Cell Kit (Luminex, Austin, TX, USA), following the manufacturer's instructions. Briefly, approximately 0.3×10^6 cells were suspended in 100 μL of Annexin V & Dead Cell Reagent. Cells were incubated for 20 min in the dark at RT and then analyzed using the Muse™ Cell Analyzer (EMD Millipore, Temecula, CA, USA). The analysis provided the percentage of live, early apoptotic, late apoptotic, and dead cells.

4.6. Evaluation of Cell Proliferation

(a) Immunocytochemical detection of Ki67 expression

The viability of EqASCs was assessed by examining the expression level of the Ki67 cell proliferation marker [48]. Initially, 400 μL of medium containing 0.6×10^5 cells was seeded on coverslips in a 24-well plate. After treating the cells with orientin for 24 h, they were fixed in 4% PFA solution for 20 min at RT. The wells were then washed twice with cold DPBS solution and the cell membranes were next permeabilized using 0.1% Triton X-100 (Sigma-Aldrich, St. Louis, MO, USA) for 5 min at RT, after which they were again washed twice with cold DPBS solution. Removing excess DPBS, the slides were treated with a blocking solution (1% BSA, Sigma-Aldrich, St. Louis, MO, USA, 10% Normal Goat Serum, Abcam, Cambridge, UK, 0.3M Glycine, Sigma-Aldrich, St. Louis, MO, USA, 0.1% Tween® 20, Sigma-Aldrich, St. Louis, MO, USA in DPBS) for 1 h at RT. After blocking, the cells were washed twice with cold DPBS, and after removing the DPBS, Ki67 primary antibody solution (#ab15580, Abcam, Cambridge, UK) was added to the coverslips at a concentration of 0.5 μg/mL (1:250 in DPBS) and incubated overnight at 4 °C. After incubation, the coverslips were washed twice with cold DPBS and a solution of secondary antibody (anti-Rabbit) conjugated with Alexa Fluor 488 fluorochrome (#111-545-003, Jackson ImmunoResearch, Ely, UK) at a dilution of 1:800 in DPBS was added. The coverslips were again incubated for 1 h in the dark at RT. After incubation, the coverslips were rinsed twice with cold DPBS and sealed in 4′,6-Diamidino-2′- phenylindole dihydrochloride (DAPI) mounting medium (Fluoroshield™ with DAPI, Sigma-Aldrich, St. Louis, MO, USA). Preparations were observed and imaged using a confocal laser scanning microscope (Leica DMi8, Leica Microsystems, Wetzlar, Germany) and micrographs processed with the Fiji ImageJ software (Version 1.52n, Wayne Rasband, National Institutes of Health, USA). The mean green pixel area per cell was determined using the same threshold value for all images.

(b) Cell cycle distribution analysis by flow cytometry

The percentage of cells in the G0/G1, S, and G2/M phases of cell cycle was analyzed using the Muse® Cell Cycle Kit (Luminex, Austin, TX, USA). In accordance with the manufacturer's protocol, approximately 0.3×10^6 cells were suspended in 200 μL of ice cold 70% ethanol and incubated for 3 h at −20 °C. After incubation, the cells were centrifuged at $300\times g$ for 5 min and washed once with DPBS. Next, 200 μL of Muse® Cell Cycle Reagent was added to each tube and incubated for 30 min at RT in the dark and then analyzed using the Muse™ Cell Analyzer (EMD Millipore, Temecula, CA, USA).

(c) Clonogenic potential assessed by colony-forming unit (CFU) assay

The colony unit forming (CFU) assay was used to evaluate the clonogenic property of the studied ASCs [49]. Approximately 250 cells were seeded into a 6-well plate and after 24 h they were treated with orientin, as previously described. After 11 days the cells were washed with DPBS and stained with 0.02% pararosaniline solution (Sigma-

Aldrich, St. Louis, MO, USA), allowing the colonies to be counted manually based on visual assessment.

(d) Cell migration and interaction asessed by scratch assay

A scratch assay was used to evaluate cell migration and intercellular interactions [48]. Cells were seeded into a 12-well plate and treated with orientin, as previously described. Once a uniform, confluent monolayer was formed, a sterile pipette tip was used to create a scratch across the center of each well, simulating a wound. The distance between the wound edges was measured using the Leica DMi1 inverted microscope (Leica Microsystems, Wetzlar, Germany) at 6- and 24-h post-scratch.

4.7. Reverse Transcription Quantitative Real-Time PCR Analysis

Total RNA was isolated using the phenol–chloroform method following cell homogenization in EXTRAzol solution (Blirt, Gdańsk, Poland). The RNA concentration was measured using a nanospectrophotometer (Synergy H1, BioTek® Instruments, Inc., Winooski, VT, USA) at 260 nm. Genomic DNA (gDNA) was digested using the Precision™ DNase Kit (Primerdesign Ltd., Chandler's Ford, UK). The cDNA was synthesized using the RevertAid RT Reverse Transcription Kit (Thermo Fisher Scientific, Vilnius, Lithuania) in a T100™ Thermal Cycler (Bio-Rad Laboratories, Singapore). qRT-PCR reactions were prepared using the SensiFAST™ SYBR® & Fluorescein Kit (Meridian, Cincinnati, OH, USA) and analyzed in a CFX Connect™ Real-Time PCR Detection System (Bio-Rad Laboratories, Singapore). All procedures were carried out in accordance with the respective manufacturers' instructions. Primers used in the qRT-PCR were designed using the Primer-BLAST tool provided by the National Center for Biotechnology Information (NCBI), U.S. National Library of Medicine. The relative expression of genes (Table 1) was normalized to GAPDH (glyceraldehydes-3-phosphate, housekeeping gene) expression and calculated using the $2^{-\Delta\Delta Cq}$ method.

Table 1. Primers used for gene expression analysis.

Gene	Primer	Sequence 5′-3′	Amplicon Length (bp)	Accession No.
GAPDH	F: R:	GATGCCCCAATGTTTGTGA AAGCAGGGATGATGTTCTGG	250	NM_001163856.1
p21	F: R:	GAAGAGAAACCCCCAGCTCC TGACTGCATCAAACCCCACA	241	XM_023633878.1
SOD1	F: R:	CATTCCATCATTGGCCGCAC GAGCGATCCCAATCACACCA	130	NM_001081826.3
SOD2	F: R:	GGACAAACCTGAGCCCCAAT TTGGACACCAGCCGATACAG	125	NM_001082517.2
TP53	F: R:	TTTCGACATAGCGTGGTGGT CTCAAAGCTGTTCCGTCCCA	180	NM_001202405.1
BAX	F: R:	CGAGTGGCAGCTGAGATGTT AAGGAAGTCCAGTGTCCAGC	153	XM_023650076.1
BCL2	F: R:	TTCTTTGAGTTCGGTGGGGT GGGCCGTACAGTTCCACAA	164	XM_001490436.4

4.8. Statistical Analyses

The results were presented as mean ± SD. The statistics were performed using GraphPad Prism version 10.5.0 for Windows (GraphPad Software, Boston, MA, USA). The Shapiro–Wilk test was used to confirm the normality of distribution, and the homogeneity of variances was verified using Bartlett's test. Two-way analysis of variance (ANOVA) was applied, focusing on the main effects only, with 'health status' (HE vs. EMS) and 'treatment' (CTRL vs. Orientin) as the two independent factors. Tukey's post hoc test was used for multiple comparisons. All results were expressed as relative values, where the mean value obtained for the untreated healthy control group was set as 1, and the values of the other groups were expressed relative to this reference. The differences were considered as statistically significant at $p < 0.05$.

5. Conclusions

The present study suggests that orientin can exert multifaceted cytoprotective and regenerative effects on EqASCs, particularly those derived from horses affected by EMS. Orientin treatment enhanced proliferative activity and favorable modulation of the cell cycle, improved cell viability, reduced apoptosis, and restored both clonogenic and migratory capacity. Importantly, orientin significantly reduced markers of oxidative stress and cellular senescence, two key factors contributing to impaired regenerative function in EMS-associated stromal cells. These findings indicate that orientin's therapeutic potential lies in mitigating cellular dysfunction associated with metabolic disorders in equine models. However, further studies are needed to fully elucidate the molecular mechanisms underlying orientin's action, particularly in relation to oxidative stress response pathways and the regulation of senescence. Future research should explore the involvement of key signaling axes such as AMPK, PI3K/Akt, and FOXO, as well as assess orientin's long-term effects and therapeutic efficacy in vivo. A deeper understanding of these mechanisms may facilitate development of targeted strategies to restore cellular homeostasis and regenerative potential in metabolically impaired tissues.

Supplementary Materials: The following supporting information can be downloaded at: https://www.mdpi.com/article/10.3390/ijms26146867/s1.

Author Contributions: Conceptualization, M.Z.; methodology, D.O. and M.Z.; software, M.Z. and M.K.; validation, D.O., M.K. and M.Z.; formal analysis, D.O. and M.K.; investigation, M.Z.; resources, M.Z.; data curation, D.O., M.K. and M.Z.; writing—original draft preparation, D.O., M.K. and M.Z.; writing—review and editing, M.Z. and M.K.; visualization, D.O. and M.K.; supervision, M.Z.; project administration, M.Z.; funding acquisition, D.O. and M.Z. All authors have read and agreed to the published version of the manuscript.

Funding: The research is co-financed under the individual student research project "Młode umysły—Young Minds Project" from the subsidy increased for the period 2020–2026 in the amount of 2% of the subsidy referred to Art. 387 (3) of the Law of 20 July 2018 on Higher Education and Science, obtained in 2019. The APC/BPC is co-financed by Wrocław University of Environmental and Life Sciences.

Institutional Review Board Statement: Adipose tissue collection used for the isolation of EqASCs was approved by the Local Ethics Commission, agreement no. 058/2021/P1, on 23 September 2021.

Informed Consent Statement: Not applicable.

Data Availability Statement: The data presented in this study are available on request from the corresponding author.

Acknowledgments: We would like to thank Lynda Bourebaba from the Department of Experimental Biology, Institute of Biology, Wrocław University of Environmental and Life Sciences, for valuable comments concerning the manuscript.

Conflicts of Interest: The authors declare no conflicts of interest.

Abbreviations

The following abbreviations are used in this manuscript:

EMS	Equine Metabolic Syndrome
ASCs	Adipose-Derived Mesenchymal Stromal Cells
SA-β-Gal	Senescence-Associated β-Galactosidase
SASP	Senescence-Associated Secretory Phenotype
ROS	Reactive Oxygen Species
mTOR	Mammalian Target of Rapamycin
FOXO	Forkhead Box O (transcription factors)
TNF-α	Tumor Necrosis Factor Alpha
IL-6	Interleukin 6
MMPs	Matrix Metalloproteinases
SOD	Superoxide Dismutase
GPx	Glutathione Peroxidase
PI3K	Phosphoinositide 3-Kinase
Akt	Protein Kinase B
AMPK	AMP-Activated Protein Kinase
p16^INK4a	Cyclin-Dependent Kinase Inhibitor 2A (also known as p16INK4a)
p21	Cyclin-Dependent Kinase Inhibitor 1A (CDKN1A)
TP53	Tumor Protein P53
CM-H2DCFDA	5-(and-6)-Chloromethyl-2′,7′-Dichlorodihydrofluorescein Diacetate, Acetyl Ester
DAPI	4′,6-Diamidino-2-Phenylindole

References

1. Marycz, K.; Kornicka, K.; Basinska, K.; Czyrek, A. Equine metabolic syndrome affects viability, senescence, and stress factors of equine adipose-derived mesenchymal stromal stem cells: New insight into EqASCs isolated from EMS horses in the context of their aging. *Oxidative Med. Cell Longev.* **2016**, *2016*, 4710326. [CrossRef] [PubMed]
2. Durham, A.E.; Frank, N.; McGowan, C.M.; Menzies-Gow, N.J.; Roelfsema, E.; Vervuert, I.; Feige, K.; Fey, K. ECEIM consensus statement on equine metabolic syndrome. *J. Vet. Intern. Med.* **2019**, *33*, 335–349. [CrossRef] [PubMed]
3. Dyson, J. Practical management of equine metabolic syndrome. *Livestock* **2014**, *19*, 186–193. [CrossRef]
4. Johnson, P.J. The equine metabolic syndrome: Peripheral Cushing's syndrome. *Vet. Clin. Equine Pract.* **2002**, *18*, 271–293. [CrossRef] [PubMed]
5. Stefaniuk-Szmukier, M.; Piórkowska, K.; Ropka-Molik, K. Equine metabolic syndrome: A complex disease influenced by multifactorial genetic factors. *Genes* **2023**, *14*, 1544. [CrossRef] [PubMed]
6. Frank, N.; Geor, R.J.; Bailey, S.; Durham, A.; Johnson, P. Equine metabolic syndrome. *J. Vet. Intern. Med.* **2010**, *24*, 467–475. [CrossRef] [PubMed]
7. Geor, R.J. Metabolic predispositions to laminitis in horses and ponies: Obesity, insulin resistance and metabolic syndromes. *J. Equine Vet. Sci.* **2008**, *28*, 753–759. [CrossRef]
8. McCue, M.E.; Geor, R.J.; Schultz, N. Equine metabolic syndrome: A complex disease influenced by genetics and the environment. *J. Equine Vet. Sci.* **2015**, *35*, 367–375. [CrossRef]
9. Fahmy, M.I.; Sadek, M.A.; Abdou, K.; El-Dessouki, A.M.; El-Shiekh, R.A.; Khalaf, S.S. Orientin: A comprehensive review of a promising bioactive flavonoid. *Inflammopharmacology* **2025**, *33*, 1713–1728. [CrossRef] [PubMed]
10. Campisi, J.; d'Adda di Fagagna, F. Cellular senescence: When bad things happen to good cells. *Nat. Rev. Mol. Cell Biol.* **2007**, *8*, 729–740. [CrossRef] [PubMed]
11. Loos, C.M.; McLeod, K.R.; Vanzant, E.S.; Stratton, S.A.; Bohannan, A.D.; Coleman, R.J.; van Doorn, D.A.; Urschel, K.L. Differential effect of two dietary protein sources on time course response of muscle anabolic signaling pathways in normal and insulin dysregulated horses. *Front. Vet. Sci.* **2022**, *9*, 896220. [CrossRef] [PubMed]
12. Kumar, S.; Pandey, A.K. Chemistry and biological activities of flavonoids: An overview. *Sci. World J.* **2013**, *2013*, 162750. [CrossRef] [PubMed]
13. An, F.; Yang, G.; Tian, J.; Wang, S. Antioxidant effects of the orientin and vitexin in Trollius chinensis Bunge in D-galactose-aged mice. *Neural Regen. Res.* **2012**, *7*, 2565–2575. [PubMed]
14. Tchkonia, T.; Morbeck, D.E.; Von Zglinicki, T.; Van Deursen, J.; Lustgarten, J.; Scrable, H.; Khosla, S.; Jensen, M.D.; Kirkland, J.L. Fat tissue, aging, and cellular senescence. *Aging Cell* **2010**, *9*, 667–684. [CrossRef] [PubMed]

15. Kornicka, K.; Śmieszek, A.; Szłapka-Kosarzewska, J.; Irwin Houston, J.M.; Roecken, M.; Marycz, K. Characterization of apoptosis, autophagy and oxidative stress in pancreatic islets cells and intestinal epithelial cells isolated from equine metabolic syndrome (EMS) horses. *Int. J. Mol. Sci.* **2018**, *19*, 3068. [CrossRef] [PubMed]
16. Liu, J.; Ding, Y.; Liu, Z.; Liang, X. Senescence in mesenchymal stem cells: Functional alterations, molecular mechanisms, and rejuvenation strategies. *Front. Cell Dev. Biol.* **2020**, *8*, 258. [CrossRef] [PubMed]
17. Salminen, A.; Kaarniranta, K. Control of p53 and NF-κB signaling by WIP1 and MIF: Role in cellular senescence and organismal aging. *Cell Signal.* **2011**, *23*, 747–752. [CrossRef] [PubMed]
18. Coppe, J.-P.; Patil, C.K.; Rodier, F.; Krtolica, A.; Beausejour, C.M.; Parrinello, S.; Hodgson, J.G.; Chin, K.; Desprez, P.-Y.; Campisi, J. A human-like senescence-associated secretory phenotype is conserved in mouse cells dependent on physiological oxygen. *PLoS ONE* **2010**, *5*, e9188. [CrossRef] [PubMed]
19. Zak, A.; Siwinska, N.; Elzinga, S.; Barker, V.; Stefaniak, T.; Schanbacher, B.; Place, N.; Niedzwiedz, A.; Adams, A. Effects of equine metabolic syndrome on inflammation and acute-phase markers in horses. *Domest. Anim. Endocrinol.* **2020**, *72*, 106448. [CrossRef] [PubMed]
20. Chen, H.; Liu, S.; Xing, J.; Wen, Y.; Chen, L. Orientin alleviates chondrocyte senescence and osteoarthritis by inhibiting PI3K/AKT pathway. *Bone Jt. Res.* **2025**, *14*, 245–258. [CrossRef] [PubMed]
21. Gerdes, J.; Lemke, H.; Baisch, H.; Wacker, H.-H.; Schwab, U.; Stein, H. Cell cycle analysis of a cell proliferation-associated human nuclear antigen defined by the monoclonal antibody Ki-67. *J. Immunol.* **1984**, *133*, 1710–1715. [CrossRef] [PubMed]
22. Sun, X.; Kaufman, P.D. Ki-67: More than a proliferation marker. *Chromosoma* **2018**, *127*, 175–186. [CrossRef] [PubMed]
23. Thangaraj, K.; Balasubramanian, B.; Park, S.; Natesan, K.; Liu, W.; Manju, V. Orientin induces G0/G1 cell cycle arrest and mitochondria mediated intrinsic apoptosis in human colorectal carcinoma HT29 cells. *Biomolecules* **2019**, *9*, 418. [CrossRef] [PubMed]
24. Zuk, P.A.; Zhu, M.; Ashjian, P.; De Ugarte, D.A.; Huang, J.I.; Mizuno, H.; Alfonso, Z.C.; Fraser, J.K.; Benhaim, P.; Hedrick, M.H. Human adipose tissue is a source of multipotent stem cells. *Mol. Biol. Cell* **2002**, *13*, 4279–4295. [CrossRef] [PubMed]
25. Vidal, M.A.; Kilroy, G.E.; Lopez, M.J.; Johnson, J.R.; Moore, R.M.; Gimble, J.M. Characterization of equine adipose tissue-derived stromal cells: Adipogenic and osteogenic capacity and comparison with bone marrow-derived mesenchymal stromal cells. *Vet. Surg.* **2007**, *36*, 613–622. [CrossRef] [PubMed]
26. Nusse, R.; Fuerer, C.; Ching, W.; Harnish, K.; Logan, C.; Zeng, A.; Ten Berge, D.; Kalani, Y. Wnt signaling and stem cell control. In *Cold Spring Harbor Symposia On Quantitative Biology*; Cold Spring Harbor Laboratory Press: New York, NY, USA, 2008; pp. 59–66.
27. Merrill, B.J. Wnt pathway regulation of embryonic stem cell self-renewal. *Cold Spring Harb. Perspect. Biol.* **2012**, *4*, a007971. [CrossRef] [PubMed]
28. Xu, Z.; Robitaille, A.M.; Berndt, J.D.; Davidson, K.C.; Fischer, K.A.; Mathieu, J.; Potter, J.C.; Ruohola-Baker, H.; Moon, R.T. Wnt/β-catenin signaling promotes self-renewal and inhibits the primed state transition in naïve human embryonic stem cells. *Proc. Natl. Acad. Sci. USA* **2016**, *113*, E6382–E6390. [CrossRef] [PubMed]
29. Fu, Y.; Li, H.; Hao, X. The self-renewal signaling pathways utilized by gastric cancer stem cells. *Tumor Biol.* **2017**, *39*, 1010428317697577. [CrossRef] [PubMed]
30. Semba, T.; Sammons, R.; Wang, X.; Xie, X.; Dalby, K.N.; Ueno, N.T. JNK signaling in stem cell self-renewal and differentiation. *Int. J. Mol. Sci.* **2020**, *21*, 2613. [CrossRef] [PubMed]
31. Vasudevan Sajini, D.; Thaggikuppe Krishnamurthy, P.; Chakkittukandiyil, A.; Mudavath, R.N. Orientin Modulates Nrf2-ARE, PI3K/Akt, JNK-ERK1/2, and TLR4/NF-kB Pathways to Produce Neuroprotective Benefits in Parkinson's Disease. *Neurochem. Res.* **2024**, *49*, 1577–1587. [CrossRef] [PubMed]
32. Yuan, T.-J.; Xu, X.-H.; Zhou, N.; Yan, G.; Gu, T.-W.; Peng, L.-H. Phytochemicals as new therapeutic candidates simultaneously stimulate proliferation and counteract senescence of stem cells. *Biomed. Pharmacother.* **2022**, *151*, 113170. [CrossRef] [PubMed]
33. Ji, W.; Xu, W. Orientin inhibits the progression of fibroblast-like synovial cells in rheumatoid arthritis by regulating MAPK-signaling pathway. *Allergol. Immunopathol.* **2022**, *50*, 154–162.
34. Kim, S.-J.; Pham, T.-H.; Bak, Y.; Ryu, H.-W.; Oh, S.-R.; Yoon, D.-Y. Orientin inhibits invasion by suppressing MMP-9 and IL-8 expression via the PKCα/ERK/AP-1/STAT3-mediated signaling pathways in TPA-treated MCF-7 breast cancer cells. *Phytomedicine* **2018**, *50*, 35–42. [CrossRef] [PubMed]
35. Hora, A.B.; Biano, L.S.; Nascimento, A.C.S.; Camargo, Z.T.; Heiden, G.I.; Albulquerque-Júnior, R.L.; Grespan, R.; Aragão, J.M.; Camargo, E.A. Isoorientin Improves Excisional Skin Wound Healing in Mice. *Pharmaceuticals* **2024**, *17*, 1368. [CrossRef] [PubMed]
36. Che Zain, M.S.; Lee, S.Y.; Sarian, M.N.; Fakurazi, S.; Shaari, K. In Vitro wound healing potential of flavonoid c-glycosides from oil palm (*Elaeis guineensis* Jacq.) leaves on 3t3 fibroblast cells. *Antioxidants* **2020**, *9*, 326. [CrossRef] [PubMed]
37. Squillaro, T.; Peluso, G.; Galderisi, U. Clinical trials with mesenchymal stem cells: An update. *Cell Transplant.* **2016**, *25*, 829–848. [CrossRef] [PubMed]
38. Gugjoo, M.B.; Sharma, G.T. Equine mesenchymal stem cells: Properties, sources, characterization, and potential therapeutic applications. *J. Equine Vet. Sci.* **2019**, *72*, 16–27. [CrossRef] [PubMed]

39. Marycz, K.; Weiss, C.; Śmieszek, A.; Kornicka, K. Evaluation of oxidative stress and mitophagy during adipogenic differentiation of adipose-derived stem cells isolated from equine metabolic syndrome (EMS) horses. *Stem Cells Int.* **2018**, *2018*, 5340756. [CrossRef] [PubMed]
40. Xiao, Q.; Piao, R.; Wang, H.; Li, C.; Song, L. Orientin-mediated Nrf_2/HO-$_1$ signal alleviates H_2O_2-induced oxidative damage via induction of JNK and PI3K/AKT activation. *Int. J. Biol. Macromol.* **2018**, *118*, 747–755. [CrossRef] [PubMed]
41. Li, F.; Zong, J.; Zhang, H.; Zhang, P.; Xu, L.; Liang, K.; Yang, L.; Yong, H.; Qian, W. Orientin reduces myocardial infarction size via eNOS/NO signaling and thus mitigates adverse cardiac remodeling. *Front. Pharmacol.* **2017**, *8*, 926. [CrossRef] [PubMed]
42. Liang, Y.; Li, J.; Lin, Q.; Huang, P.; Zhang, L.; Wu, W.; Ma, Y. Research progress on signaling pathway-associated oxidative stress in endothelial cells. *Oxidative Med. Cell Longev.* **2017**, *2017*, 7156941. [CrossRef] [PubMed]
43. Xiao, Q.; Cui, Y.; Zhao, Y.; Liu, L.; Wang, H.; Yang, L. Orientin relieves lipopolysaccharide-induced acute lung injury in mice: The involvement of its anti-inflammatory and anti-oxidant properties. *Int. Immunopharmacol.* **2021**, *90*, 107189. [CrossRef] [PubMed]
44. Fukui, M.; Zhu, B.T. Mitochondrial superoxide dismutase SOD2, but not cytosolic SOD1, plays a critical role in protection against glutamate-induced oxidative stress and cell death in HT22 neuronal cells. *Free Radic. Biol. Med.* **2010**, *48*, 821–830. [CrossRef] [PubMed]
45. Li, F.; Liao, X.; Jiang, L.; Zhao, J.; Wu, S.; Ming, J. Orientin attenuated d-GalN/LPS-induced liver injury through the inhibition of oxidative stress via nrf2/keap1 pathway. *J. Agric. Food Chem.* **2022**, *70*, 7953–7967. [CrossRef] [PubMed]
46. Qu, Y.; Shi, L.; Liu, Y.; Huang, L.; Luo, H.-R.; Wu, G.-S. Orientin prolongs the longevity of caenorhabditis elegans and postpones the development of neurodegenerative diseases via nutrition sensing and cellular protective pathways. *Oxidative Med. Cell Longev.* **2022**, *2022*, 8878923. [CrossRef] [PubMed]
47. Fan, H.; Wang, L.; Zhao, K.; Li, N.; Shi, Z.; Ge, Z.; Jin, Z. Fabrication, mechanical properties, and biocompatibility of graphene-reinforced chitosan composites. *Biomacromolecules* **2010**, *11*, 2345–2351. [CrossRef] [PubMed]
48. Bourebaba, L.; Zyzak, M.; Sikora, M.; Serwotka-Suszczak, A.; Mularczyk, M.; Al Naem, M.; Marycz, K. Sex hormone-binding globulin (SHBG) maintains proper equine adipose-derived stromal cells (ASCs)' Metabolic functions and negatively regulates their basal adipogenic potential. *Stem Cell Rev. Rep.* **2023**, *19*, 2251–2273. [CrossRef] [PubMed]
49. Frazier, T.P.; Gimble, J.M.; Devay, J.W.; Tucker, H.A.; Chiu, E.S.; Rowan, B.G. Body mass index affects proliferation and osteogenic differentiation of human subcutaneous adipose tissue-derived stem cells. *BMC Cell Biol.* **2013**, *14*, 34. [CrossRef] [PubMed]

Disclaimer/Publisher's Note: The statements, opinions and data contained in all publications are solely those of the individual author(s) and contributor(s) and not of MDPI and/or the editor(s). MDPI and/or the editor(s) disclaim responsibility for any injury to people or property resulting from any ideas, methods, instructions or products referred to in the content.

International Journal of
Molecular Sciences

MDPI

Review

Oxidative Stress and Mitochondrial Dysfunction in Myelodysplastic Syndrome: Roles in Development, Diagnosis, Prognosis, and Treatment

Federico Pierro [1], Manlio Fazio [1], Giuseppe Murdaca [2,3,*], Fabio Stagno [1], Sebastiano Gangemi [4] and Alessandro Allegra [1]

1 Division of Hematology, Department of Human Pathology in Adulthood and Childhood "Gaetano Barresi", University of Messina, Via Consolare Valeria, 98125 Messina, Italy; federico.pierro@studenti.unime.it (F.P.); manliofazio@hotmail.it (M.F.); fabio.stagno@unime.it (F.S.); aallegra@unime.it (A.A.)
2 Department of Internal Medicine, University of Genova, 16126 Genova, Italy
3 Allergology and Clinical Immunology, San Bartolomeo Hospital, 19038 Sarzana, Italy
4 Allergy and Clinical Immunology Unit, Department of Clinical and Experimental Medicine, University of Messina, Via Consolare Valeria, 98125 Messina, Italy; gangemis@unime.it
* Correspondence: giuseppe.murdaca@unige.it

Abstract

Myelodysplastic syndromes are a group of clonal hematopoietic stem cell disorders characterized by ineffective hematopoiesis, peripheral cytopenia, and dysplasia in one or more myeloid lineages, with a variable risk of progression to acute myeloid leukemia. In addition to well-characterized genetic and epigenetic abnormalities, oxidative stress has emerged as a critical contributor to the pathophysiology of myelodysplastic syndrome. Reactive oxygen species and reactive nitrogen species can induce cumulative DNA damage, mitochondrial dysfunction, and altered redox homeostasis, promoting genomic instability and clonal evolution. Elevated oxidative stress in patients with myelodysplastic syndromes has been linked to increased apoptosis of hematopoietic stem and progenitor cells, disruption of the bone marrow microenvironment, and progression toward leukemic transformation. Moreover, ROS-related pathways, such as TP53 mutations and epigenetic dysregulation, interact with the key molecular drivers of myelodysplastic syndrome. Given these findings, oxidative stress is now recognized not only as a hallmark of disease biology but also as a potential therapeutic target. Antioxidant-based strategies and agents that modulate redox signaling are being investigated for their ability to restore hematopoietic function and enhance treatment efficacy. This review provides an overview of the current biology of myelodysplastic syndrome, highlights the connections between oxidative stress and disease mechanisms, and explores emerging redox-targeted therapeutic approaches.

Keywords: myelodysplastic syndromes; oxidative stress; reactive oxygen species; iron overload; hematopoietic stem cells; DNA damage; epigenetic regulation; mitochondrial dysfunction; redox-targeted therapy

1. Introduction

General Considerations for Myelodysplastic Syndromes

Myelodysplastic syndromes (MDS) are hematological disorders characterized by peripheral cytopenias and hypercellular marrow, mainly affecting the elderly, and possibly progressing to acute myeloid leukemia (AML) through clonal evolution [1,2].

Over time, the classification of MDS has evolved. To enhance diagnostic accuracy, the 2016 WHO Classification incorporated molecular data into MDS diagnosis and management [3], notably identifying MDS with ring sideroblasts (MDS-RS) by SF3B1 mutations and ≥5% ring sideroblasts. Isolated del(5q) is a distinct subtype with good prognosis and response to lenalidomide, whereas TP53 mutations have poor outcomes [3]. Building on this, the 2022 WHO Classification redefined MDS into two main categories: genetically defined (MDS-5q, MDS-SF3B1, and MDS-biTP53) and morphologically defined (MDS with Low Blasts, MDS with Hypocellularity, and MDS with Increased Blasts) [4]. Key updates include reclassifying NPM1-mutated cases as AML and former MDS-U cases as Clonal Cytopenia of Undetermined Significance (CCUS) [5], underscoring the growing importance of genetic profiling in disease categorization.

However, differentiating MDS from related conditions remains challenging owing to overlapping features, making genetic analysis essential for prognosis and treatment decisions [6]. A variety of genetic alterations, including cytogenetic abnormalities, somatic mutations, and gene expression changes, drive MDS pathogenesis [7]. Frequent abnormalities have included del(5q), del(7q), trisomy 8, and complex karyotypes [7]. In addition, promoter hypermethylation and mutations in genes that regulate DNA methylation and histone modifications are commonly observed [7]. Particularly relevant are mutations in RNA splicing genes (*SF3B1, SRSF2, U2AF1,* and *ZRSR2*) and epigenetic regulators (TET2, ASXL1, and DNMT3A); spliceosome mutations are present in approximately 50% of cases [8,9]. Mutations affecting signal transduction pathways (e.g., NRAS and JAK2) and transcriptional regulators (e.g., RUNX1 and TP53) are also frequently encountered [8,9].

Gene expression profiling has contributed to the identification of dysregulated genes, and altered signaling pathways and prognostic molecular signatures [8]. Moreover, mutations in genes such as *DNMT3A, ASXL1,* and *TET2* may predict better responses to hypomethylating agents, supporting the integration of genomic, transcriptional, and clinical data to guide patient management [8].

Furthermore, in a therapeutical context, mutations in SF3B1 and IDH1/2 provide opportunities for targeted interventions. Consequently, molecular profiling using NGS has become one of the cornerstones of diagnosis and therapeutic planning for MDS [10].

In the context of pathogenesis, beyond genetic alterations, immune dysregulation plays a key role in MDS pathogenesis; it is often described as the "Yin–Yang theory" of immune activation and suppression, and is characterized by immune hyperactivity and increased apoptosis in low-risk MDS (LR-MDS), while high-risk MDS (HR-MDS) exhibits immune suppression [11].

Both innate and adaptive immune responses are hyperactive in the bone marrow of MDS patients, and autoimmune diseases are frequently observed, indicating a strong immunological component [12].

Supporting this, a 2012 study described autoimmune manifestations (AIMs) in some MDS patients that contributed to ineffective hematopoiesis via immune-mediated attacks on hematopoietic clones [13].

Therapeutic approaches often involve the use of steroids or immunosuppressants. Notably, azacytidine has shown potential in reducing steroid dependence in select cases [14].

2. Risk Stratification and Treatment Options

Prognostic Tools and Standard Treatment Approaches

Building on these diagnostic and pathogenic considerations, treatment decisions for MDS are strongly influenced by risk stratification tools.

The Revised International Prognostic Scoring System (IPSS-R), introduced in 2012, improves prognostic accuracy by adding new risk groups, refining blast and cytopenia evaluation, and classifying patients into five risk levels; it has improved prognostic precision by refining blast and cytopenia evaluation and dividing patients into five risk categories [15]. Additional prognostic indicators such as age, performance status, and ferritin and LDH levels have been associated with survival; although correlated with survival, they are not necessarily correlated with AML transformation [15]. More recently, Molecular IPSS (IPSS-M) has incorporated mutational data from mutations in over 30 genes (e.g., *TP53*, *ASXL1*, *RUNX1*, and *TET2*) to better predict survival, AML progression and disease evolution [16].

These tools reflect the growing role of next-generation sequencing (NGS) in MDS diagnosis, classification, prognosis, and treatment selection [17]. Treatment strategies are risk-adapted, and guided by IPSS-R or IPSS-M scores [18].

In low-risk MDS (LR-MDS), marked by dysplasia, low blast counts, and favorable genetics, therapy is largely supportive [19]. This includes transfusions, growth factors, and approved agents such as lenalidomide, HMAs (azacitidine, decitabine), and luspatercept. However, HSCT (hematopoietic stem cell transplantation) remains underutilized, despite curative potential [19,20].

Erythropoiesis-stimulating agents (ESAs), including EPO and darbepoetin alfa, are first-line treatments for anemia in patients with EPO < 500 U/L and low transfusion needs, improving hemoglobin and reducing transfusion burden [21].

Luspatercept increases transfusion independence in MDS-RS and is effective in ESAs-refractory cases [22].

Lenalidomide is particularly effective in del(5q) MDS, with 67% achieving transfusion independence and ~50% cytogenetic response [23]. Epoetin-α p shows erythroid responses in 32–46% of patients, far exceeding the percentages for placebo [24].

In contrast, in high-risk MDS (HR-MDS), the goal is to delay AML progression and improve survival. Standard care includes azacitidine and decitabine [25]. Notably, azacitidine improves survival in patients with chromosome 7 abnormalities [25].

The oral formulation of CC-486 (oral azacitidine) has also attracted attention. While it enhances transfusion independence and bilineage response in LR-MDS, it has also been associated with reports of increased early infection-related mortality [26]. In elderly AML patients, CC-486 extends survival by 10 months and reduces relapse [27].

Given the limitations of parenteral HMAs, oral formulations improve convenience and patient adherence [28,29].

Meanwhile, the bone marrow microenvironment (BME) in MDS supports malignant clones over healthy hematopoiesis. Azanucleotides may affect both malignant and stromal components; lenalidomide benefits patients with specific deletions, while luspatercept enhances erythropoiesis without clonal expansion [30].

Finally, the immunosuppressive BME also facilitates malignant persistence. Myeloid-derived suppressor cells (MDSCs), often expanded in MDS, correlate with progression and induce dysplasia in models, making them promising therapeutic targets [31,32].

3. New Treatment Approaches

Overview of Innovative Therapies Under Clinical Development

New agents such as roxadustat, imetelstat, oral HMAs, TP53 modulators, and magrolimab are being developed to overcome current treatment limitations and address molecular targets in MDS [21].

For example, splicing modulators aim to correct the common splicing defects in MDS. Inhibition of CHRM4 in early erythroid progenitors has emerged as a novel strategy with encouraging preclinical results. Splicing modulators and CHRM4 inhibitors in early erythroid progenitors also show promise [33].

Roxadustat, an oral Hypoxia-Inducible Factor–Prolyl Hydroxylase (HIF-PH) inhibitor, represents a mechanistically distinct approach to treating anemia, compared with ESAs. Clinical trials have demonstrated that it achieved 37.5% transfusion independence at both 28 and 52 weeks, with over 50% of patients experiencing a ≥50% reduction in transfusion requirements, particularly at a dose of 2.5 mg/kg [34].

Additionally, roxadustat has shown efficacy in improving anemia and lowering transfusion dependency in MDS patients with concurrent chronic kidney disease [35].

Roxadustat, an oral HIF-PH inhibitor, differs mechanistically from ESAs. It achieved 37.5% transfusion independence at both 28 and 52 weeks, with over half of patients reducing transfusion needs ≥50%, especially at 2.5 mg/kg [34]. It has also shown benefits in MDS patients with chronic kidney disease [35].

Imetelstat, a telomerase inhibitor, interferes with telomere maintenance by targeting the RNA component hTR, effectively impairing malignant hematopoietic stem cells (HSCs), hematopoietic progenitor cells (HPCs), and leukemic stem cells (LSCs), while sparing normal cells [36]. Currently approved for LR-MDS patients with transfusion-dependent anemia, imetelstat (7.1 mg/kg every 4 weeks) demonstrated improved red blood cell transfusion independence at 8 and 24 weeks, compared to placebo [36].

Targeting immune checkpoints is an emerging strategy. CD47, a key innate immune checkpoint, has become a compelling therapeutic target for MDS and AML, while magrolimab, an anti-CD47 monoclonal antibody, has shown synergistic effects when combined with azacitidine, particularly in high-risk patients with TP53 mutations [37].

Finally, sabatolimab, an anti-TIM-3 antibody, has also demonstrated durable responses when administered alongside HMAs in HR-MDS and AML patients. One study reported a complete remission (CR) rate of 33% and an overall response rate (ORR) of 75%, indicating robust clinical efficacy; additionally, it shows efficacy in ESA-refractory cases [36,38,39].

This review presents an overview of the contemporary biology of myelodysplastic syndrome, emphasizes the relationships between oxidative stress and disease processes, and examines novel redox-targeted therapy strategies.

4. Oxidative Stress: Mechanisms and Disease Connections

4.1. Oxidative Stress Plays a Role in Both Physiological and Pathological Contexts

Reactive oxygen species (ROS) and reactive nitrogen species (RNS) are byproducts of normal cellular metabolism and serve dual roles as damaging agents and essential signaling molecules. While excess ROS/RNS levels induce oxidative and nitrosative stress, damaging DNA, proteins, and lipids, physiological levels are crucial for redox homeostasis, immune responses, and intracellular signaling, as discussed by Valko et al. [40].

Oxidative stress has been implicated in a wide range of diseases, including cancer, cardiovascular and neurodegenerative disorders, diabetes, and aging [40]. ROS-induced damage contributes to chronic disease progression via lipid peroxidation, protein oxidation, and DNA strand breaks, as shown in studies by Cabello-Verrugio et al. and Kudryavtseva et al. [41,42]. Moreover ROS-induced cellular senescence may act as a tumor-suppressive barrier. However, the senescence-associated secretory phenotype (SASP) can paradoxically promote tumorigenesis. Targeting the key pathways involved in this process may suppress malignant progression, as suggested by Li et al. [43].

ROS and RNS regulate autophagy, particularly during nutrient deprivation. The p62/Keap1/Nrf2 axis plays a leading role in the relationship between oxidative stress and antioxidant response. Autophagy influences DNA repair mechanisms, with ROS and RNS functioning as upstream modulators that determine cellular fate under stressful conditions, according to Filomeni et al. [44].

Ferroptosis, a regulated, iron-dependent form of cell death marked by lipid ROS accumulation, plays a role in neurodegenerative diseases, such as Alzheimer's and Parkinson's [45]. Recent studies have explored redox regulation and ferroptosis in cancer, suggesting that targeting these pathways may provide therapeutic benefits, especially in resistant or metastatic tumors, as highlighted by Zeng et al. [46].

Altered energy metabolism has also been associated with oxidative stress. Dysregulated glycolysis and oxidative phosphorylation (OXPHOS) have been observed in several diseases. For instance, Jourdain et al. [47] showed that loss of LUC7L2, a component of the pre-mRNA splicing machinery, leads to enhanced OXPHOS and reduced glycolysis; this finding links aberrant splicing to oxidative stress and disease.

Mitochondrial dysfunction and ROS are key drivers of inflammatory myopathies such as inclusion body myositis (IBM), as reported by Danieli et al. [48]. Similarly, in muscular dystrophies (MDs), intracellular ROS accumulation causes contractile dysfunction. Monoamine oxidase (MAO), a major ROS source, is upregulated in dystrophic muscles, and its inhibition with pargyline shows therapeutic promise, as described by Canton et al. [49].

In the liver, oxidative stress plays a key role in hepatocellular injury, particularly during hypercholesterolemia, which increases ROS levels and apoptosis, according to Jadeja et al. [50].

Oxidative stress is a key factor in osteoporosis, especially in high-risk groups (e.g., postmenopausal women and patients with metabolic disorders). Oxidative stress disrupts bone remodeling, and mitochondria-targeted antioxidants are currently being investigated. Vitamin D deficiency worsens oxidative damage and is linked to osteoporosis, autoimmune diseases, and hematologic malignancies [51,52].

In cardiovascular diseases, oxidative stress impairs endothelial function, contributing to atherosclerosis, arrhythmias, and hypertension. As noted by Senoner and Dichtl [53], a Mediterranean diet rich in natural antioxidants reduces oxidative damage and cardiovascular risk.

4.2. Oxidative Stress and Mitochondrial Dysfunction in Cancer Biology and Therapy Response

In oncology, oxidative stress is an established mediator of both tumorigenesis and the treatment response. As described by Yamada et al. [54], various therapeutic strategies for regulating mitochondrial oxidative stress have been developed, including photodynamic therapy (PDT), photothermal therapy (PTT), and antioxidant therapy using a mitochondrial drug delivery system (DDS). The PDT effect arises from the dynamic interaction between a photosensitizer (PS), light, and molecular oxygen, resulting in the generation of lethal levels of ROS, primarily highly reactive singlet oxygen [54].

For example, PDT uses controlled oxidative damage to target skin cancer cells and is more effective than chemotherapy or surgery, as reported by Allegra et al. [55]. Cancer cells display the Warburg effect, relying on glycolysis despite oxygen availability, and they typically have high ROS levels. Their survival depends on enhanced antioxidant defenses, which can be selectively targeted for therapeutic purposes, as highlighted by Gorrini et al. [56].

A recent study by Allegra et al. [57] highlighted significant sex differences in cancer susceptibility, with males generally experiencing higher oxidative stress and cancer incidence than females. Young women are more protected from cancer due to hormonal regulation of the redox state and mitochondrial function. Gender differences in immunological responses and antioxidant enzyme activity influence cancer susceptibility and treatment outcomes.

ROS signaling also plays a key role in the regulation of mesenchymal stem cells (MSCs) by controlling their proliferation and differentiation through pathways such as p38-MAPK and glycolysis. SIRT1, a part of the NAD/SIRT axis, helps maintain stem cell function, and its loss accelerates aging phenotypes [58].

Cancer stem cells (CSCs) are particularly resilient, owing to their efficient ROS scavenging and DNA repair mechanisms. These features make them highly resistant to chemotherapy and radiotherapy [59].

In neoplastic myeloid diseases, including MDS, elevated ROS levels contribute to clonal evolution and progression. As shown by Hole et al. [60], the targeting of ROS pathways has dual potential: antioxidant approaches may reduce leukemic proliferation and protect normal cells from chemotherapy-induced damage, whereas pro-oxidant therapies can exploit ROS overload to selectively induce leukemic cell death.

Oxidative stress markers are also elevated in patients with multiple myeloma (MM). Gangemi et al. [61] reported that serum levels of advanced oxidation protein products (AOPPs) and S-nitrosylated proteins are significantly higher in MM patients than in MGUS patients and healthy controls, especially those MM patients with bone lesions.

Similarly, Hodgkin's lymphoma (HL) patients exhibit elevated levels of malondialdehyde (MDA), 4-HNE, and protein carbonyl groups, indicating increased lipid peroxidation and protein oxidation, compared to healthy individuals, as demonstrated by Morabito et al. [62]. These findings confirmed the role of oxidative stress in pathogenesis.

Further supporting the role of oxidative stress in cancer prognosis, Xie et al. [63] conducted a machine learning (ML) study on esophageal squamous cell carcinoma (ESCC) patients and found that oxidative stress markers, along with tumor and staging features, were among the strongest predictors of 3-year overall survival. The Random Forest (RF) model exhibited superior performance in both the training and validation sets.

On the other side, mitochondrial dysfunction is a common characteristic in cancer cells and contributes to cancer progression. Mitochondrial stress responses, including Mitochondrial Unfolded Protein Response (UPRmt) and Integrated Stress Response (ISR), play a role in cancer cell adaptation and growth, as discussed by Wang et al. [64].

A recent study by Winter et al. [65] identified the essential role of the electron transport chain (ETC) in generating aspartate in proliferating cells, which is a key finding in cancer cell metabolism. This finding describes how ETC dysfunction activates OMA1, a Zn^{2+}-dependent metalloendopeptidase, in the inner membrane of mitochondria, leading to the cleavage of DELE1 and activation of ISR, which is crucial for understanding how mitochondrial stress signals apoptosis. Prolonged stress activates a pro-apoptotic response through ISR, which converges on BCL2 family proteins to trigger mitochondrial outer membrane permeabilization (MOMP).

Finally, mitochondrial dysfunctions due to mtDNA mutations, Tricarboxylic Acid (TCA) cycle enzyme defects, and oxidative stress contribute to cancer development by disrupting metabolic pathways and redox balance. As noted by Luo et al. [66], this can lead to the accumulation of oncometabolites (D-2-hydroxyglutarate and succinate), inhibition of prolyl hydroxylases, and HIF1α stabilization. Additionally, enhanced NOX activity, increased ROS generation, and altered redox status play central roles.

5. Oxidative Stress in Myelodysplastic Syndromes

5.1. Oxidative Mechanisms Specific to MDS Pathogenesis

In the context of MDS, the association between oxidative stress and disease pathogenesis has become increasingly evident over the past few decades. HSC function is influenced by both intrinsic and extrinsic elements, with hypoxia playing a vital role in maintaining quiescence and metabolic dormancy. Leukemic stem cells exhibit distinct metabolic traits, relying more heavily on oxidative respiration and being more susceptible to oxidative stress than are normal HSCs. In AML cells, mitochondrial abnormalities, such as a shift to aerobic glycolysis, offer potential for therapeutic strategies, particularly through the use of IDH2 inhibitors, as discussed by Testa et al. [67].

Human hematopoietic progenitors and stem cells (HPSCs) exhibit a metabolic phenotype characterized by high glycolysis rates and low oxygen consumption. Cells with a low mitochondrial potential are enriched in HPSCs and have better repopulation abilities. The metabolic phenotype of HPSCs is regulated by Meis1 and its cofactors Pbx1 and HoxA9 through the transcriptional activation of Hif-1α, as shown by Kocabas et al. [68]. Moreover, a recent study revealed that in the initial phases of human red blood cell development, there is an increase in glutaminolysis and the production of α-ketoglutarate (αKG), which propels mitochondrial OXPHOS [68].

Furthermore, Gonzalez-Menendez et al. [69] highlighted that isocitrate dehydrogenase 1 (IDH1) is pivotal in managing the conversion between αKG and isocitrate, a process essential for the later stages of erythropoiesis. IDH mutations and their implications in cancer development have been reported previously. Specific IDH inhibitors, such as enasidenib and ivosidenib, have been approved and used in therapy [70].

Hypoxia-inducible factor 1-alpha (HIF-1α) is a central transcription factor that orchestrates the cellular adaptation to low oxygen availability [71]. Under normal oxygen conditions, HIF-1α is hydroxylated on conserved proline residues by prolyl hydroxylase domain (PHD) enzymes, which facilitates its recognition by the von Hippel–Lindau (VHL) E3 ubiquitin ligase complex, leading to proteasomal degradation, as first described by Jaakkola et al. [72]. In hypoxia, oxygen scarcity inhibits PHD activity, allowing HIF-1α to escape degradation, accumulate in the cytoplasm, translocate into the nucleus, and dimerize with HIF-1β. This heterodimer binds hypoxia response elements (HREs) in the promoter regions of target genes, activating transcriptional programs involved in glycolysis, angiogenesis (e.g., VEGF), and cell survival [73].

Importantly, these pathways have been implicated in the maintenance of leukemic stem cells and in the progression of hematologic malignancies such as MDS and AML, as reviewed by Deynoux et al. [74].

Beyond its role in oxygen sensing, HIF signaling exerts multifaceted effects on leukemogenesis by regulating energy metabolism, cell-cycle control, and immune modulation. The role of HIFs in leukemia is highly context-dependent, with evidence indicating that both oncogenic and tumor-suppressive activities are influenced by disease stage, microenvironmental factors, and genetic background [74].

Functional studies across various leukemia subtypes have shown that HIF overexpression promotes bone marrow neoangiogenesis, sustains LSC self-renewal, and contributes to chemotherapy resistance. Magliulo and Bernardi [75] further emphasized that HIF-1α has emerged as a critical regulator of LSC maintenance and dissemination, underscoring its role in leukemic propagation. In the context of MDS, aberrant activation of HIF-1 and pseudohypoxia signaling constitutes a hallmark of disease pathophysiology. These alterations are not merely bystanders, but actively contribute to ineffective hematopoiesis and disease progression. Notably, HIF-1α activity appears to correlate with disease severity, with therapeutic efficacy primarily in patients with lower blast counts, as noted by Stergiou et al. [76].

Disruption of the bone marrow microenvironment further exacerbates oxidative stress, leading to premature hematopoietic stem cell exhaustion or malignant transformation. The bone marrow microenvironment, particularly the endosteal niche, is crucial for maintaining quiescent hematopoietic stem cells through hypoxia. In hematologic malignancies, the bone marrow is highly hypoxic, and this hypoxia is associated with disease progression and stabilization of oncogenic factors like HIF-1α [77].

Moreover, constitutive HIF-1α activation has been linked to multiple genetic lesions in MDS and has been shown to be sufficient to initiate MDS-like phenotypes in murine models. According to Chen and Steidl [78], both the genetic and pharmacologic inhibition of HIF-1α suppress disease development while sparing normal hematopoietic function.

These data suggest that dysregulated HIF-1α signaling may actively drive clonal selection and leukemic progression by altering the metabolic and redox state of hematopoietic progenitors. In particular, HIF-1α promotes a shift toward glycolytic metabolism and suppresses mitochondrial respiration, thereby reducing the efficiency of DNA repair mechanisms and increasing the mutational burden under oxidative stress. This pseudohypoxic environment facilitates the expansion of preleukemic clones over healthy hematopoiesis and may synergize with additional oncogenic mutations to accelerate disease evolution from MDS to AML. Consequently, targeting HIF-1α or its downstream metabolic programs may represent a promising strategy for preventing or delaying malignant transformation in HR-MDS.

The evaluation of oxidative stress levels in MDS patients can be a useful tool. In fact, in a 2011 study, Saigo et al. [79] reported that a significant majority (85%) of MDS patients had higher oxidative stress levels than the reference range, with a positive correlation between ROS and serum ferritin levels and a negative correlation between ROS and hemoglobin levels. In addition, both iron accumulation and severe anemia contribute to oxidative stress in MDS patients.

Serological and molecular markers of oxidative stress are frequently observed in MDS patients. These include elevated levels of malondialdehyde, a lipid peroxidation byproduct, as well as increased oxidative DNA damage, such as the presence of oxidized bases in CD34+ hematopoietic progenitor cells [80].

The underlying mechanisms contributing to oxidative stress in MDS are multifactorial and include mitochondrial dysfunction, which is often driven by iron overload, mitochondrial DNA mutations, systemic inflammation, and abnormalities in the bone marrow stromal microenvironment [80].

In a 2014 study, Chung et al. [81] detected increased ROS levels in bone marrow nucleated cells from NHD13 mice, a transgenic mouse model that expresses a fusion gene consisting of NUP98 and HOXD13, which recapitulates key features of human MDS, including ineffective hematopoiesis, multilineage dysplasia, and progression to AML. These alterations were associated with increased DNA double-strand breaks and G2/M phase cell-cycle checkpoint activation. In addition, the study found an increased mutation frequency in NHD13 BMNC, suggesting that oxidative stress contributes to MDS progression to AML through ineffective DNA repair and oncogenic mutations. Mechanistically, the NUP98-HOXD13 fusion impairs genomic stability by altering the expression of genes involved in DNA repair and oxidative homeostasis, thereby promoting the accumulation of double-strand breaks. This is further exacerbated by mitochondrial dysfunction, as NHD13 cells exhibit elevated mitochondrial ROS and reduced antioxidant buffering capacity, linking fusion-induced transcriptional deregulation to redox imbalance and clonal evolution.

Furthermore, Gonçalves et al. [82] reported that MDS patients have lower glutathione (GSH) content and higher levels of peroxide and superoxide than controls, indicating increased oxidative stress. The correlation between GSH levels and transfusion dependency, as well as between peroxide levels and serum ferritin levels, indicates the potential clinical implications of oxidative stress.

Oxidative stress levels vary by MDS subtype and risk group, suggesting a complex relationship between oxidative stress and disease progression [82].

Novotna et al. [83] observed that patients with low-risk MDS exhibited a significant increase in oxidative DNA damage, compared to control subjects. This increase was observed in both erythroid and non-erythroid bone-marrow-cell populations, suggesting that oxidative DNA damage contributes to genomic instability and disease progression in low-risk MDS.

Additionally, Ghoti et al. [84] found that low-risk MDS patients have higher ROS and lower GSH levels in RBC and platelets, compared to standard controls, and there is a correlation between serum ferritin levels and ROS in RBC and platelets, suggesting that iron overload generates oxidative stress.

Finally, Jing et al. [85] highlighted that the NADPH oxidase (NOX) family is also involved in the pathogenesis of MDS, suggesting potential therapeutic targets. In a 2009 study, McCrann et al. [86] found that high expressions of Nox1 and weak expression of Nox4 were present in megakaryocytes, in addition to no significant expression of Nox2. The inhibition of Nox enzymes results in the accumulation of low-ploidy megakaryocytes and the reduction of high-ploidy cells. In addition, downregulation of cyclin E and D3 was observed with NOX inhibition, and upregulation of cyclin E partially restored ploidy levels. (Table 1).

Table 1. Key mechanisms linking oxidative stress to MDS.

Mechanism	Molecular Drivers	Cellular Impact	Therapeutic Strategies
DNA Damage	ROS, RNS	Genomic instability, mutations, apoptosis	Antioxidants, DNA repair enhancers
Mitochondrial Dysfunction	Iron overload, mtDNA mutations	Altered energy metabolism, increased ROS	Iron chelators (deferasirox), mitochondrial-targeted therapies
Epigenetic Alterations	TET2, DNMT3A, CEBPA methylation	Aberrant gene expression, impaired differentiation	HMAs, vitamin C (TET cofactor)
Redox Imbalance	Low GSH, high NOX activity	Sustained oxidative stress, ineffective hematopoiesis	GSH donors, NOX inhibitors
Immune Dysfunction	NK cells, inflammatory cytokines	Impaired immune surveillance	Immunomodulators, azacitidine

5.2. *The Dual Role of Reactive Oxygen Species in the Pathogenesis of Myelodysplastic Syndromes*

ROS exhibit a concentration- and context-dependent dual role in hematologic malignancies, including in MDS and acute AML. At low to moderate levels, ROS, particularly hydrogen peroxide (H_2O_2), function as essential second messengers that modulate signaling pathways involved in stem cell maintenance, proliferation, and survival. In both normal hematopoietic stem cells and leukemic stem cells, basal ROS levels regulate the activity of redox-sensitive transcription factors such as FOXO, HIF-1α, and NF-κB, sustaining quiescence and self-renewal capacity [58,87]. These mechanisms are hijacked by LSCs to promote resistance to apoptosis and chemotherapeutic agents, often through upregulation of antioxidant systems including NRF2, glutathione, and thioredoxin [88,89].

In contrast, elevated ROS levels, resulting from mitochondrial dysfunction, iron overload, inflammation, or oncogenic signaling, induce macromolecular damage that contributes to genomic instability and clonal evolution. DNA strand breaks, base modifications, lipid peroxidation, and protein oxidation have all been linked to disease progression in MDS and the transformation to AML [90,91]. Importantly, while LSCs maintain redox homeostasis under basal ROS levels, they become vulnerable when oxidative stress exceeds their buffering capacity. Emerging therapeutic approaches exploit this vulnerability by inducing oxidative overload or disrupting antioxidant defenses. For instance, ferroptosis-inducing compounds such as erastin and RSL3, as well as NRF2 pathway inhibitors, have shown selective cytotoxicity against leukemic cells in preclinical models [92,93].

These observations help explain the limited clinical success of broad-spectrum antioxidant therapies, which may indiscriminately suppress both damaging and physiologically beneficial ROS. Such non-specific interventions can impair normal hematopoietic function and blunt redox-dependent tumor-suppressive responses. A more effective strategy involves stratifying patients according to redox status and tailoring interventions accordingly, supporting antioxidant capacity in LR-MDS and addressing iron overload in MDS, while applying targeted pro-oxidant or redox-disruptive agents in HR-MDS or AML to selectively eliminate LSCs [94,95].

5.3. Impacts of Iron Dysregulation and Chelation Therapy on Oxidative Stress in Myelodysplastic Syndrome

Dysregulation of iron homeostasis in patients with MDS due to iron overload (IOL) plays a crucial role in oxidative stress activity in MDS. The interaction between hepcidin and ferroportin is fundamental for maintaining systemic iron homeostasis, as it regulates iron absorption and distribution. Changes in hepcidin levels can significantly affect iron export and plasma concentrations, particularly under conditions of iron deficiency or hemorrhage, as reviewed by Nemeth and Ganz [96] and further discussed by Roemhild et al. [97]. Hepcidin also has emerging importance in MDS pathophysiology and prognosis. Although high serum hepcidin levels are associated with MDS, they are not significantly different from those in healthy individuals; instead, the association appears to be influenced by MDS subtype, transfusion history, and genetic background [98].

Iron overload in hematological disorders typically arises from chronic blood transfusion and increased gastrointestinal absorption. Managing excess iron is critical, and iron chelation therapy (ICT) remains the primary approach for preventing tissue damage and organ dysfunction, as explained by Fibach and Rachmilewitz [99]. Indeed, chronic transfusion therapy is the leading cause of iron overload in MDS patients, as described by Gattermann and Rachmilewitz [100]. ICT has demonstrated effectiveness in restoring iron balance, lowering serum ferritin, and reducing hepatic and cardiac iron stores, all of which contribute to decreased morbidity and mortality [101,102].

In MDS-RS, ineffective erythropoiesis suppresses hepcidin synthesis, exacerbating the iron overload. In this context, ICT improves survival outcomes in transfusion-dependent patients by lowering the levels of toxic iron species and is considered the most accessible and effective chelation strategy [103]. Specifically, Liu et al. [104] reported that deferasirox (DFX) has been shown to improve hemoglobin, platelet, and neutrophil counts, potentially reducing mortality by minimizing hemorrhagic and infectious complications.

Beyond its systemic benefits, deferasirox also reduces oxidative stress markers at the cellular level. In fact, Rodríguez-García et al. [105] observed increased protein carbonylation, a marker of oxidative damage, in MDS bone marrow samples. Deferasirox treatment significantly reduced these levels. Four proteins with high carbonylation were identified: cytoplasmic actin, zinc finger protein 846, 14-3-3 protein zeta/delta, and l-lactate dehydrogenase A chain. Additionally, p21 expression, which was upregulated in patients with MDS, was downregulated after DFX treatment, suggesting a mechanistic link to its therapeutic effects.

Iron overload in MDS is driven by both transfusion practices and ineffective erythropoiesis. ICT not only reduces non-transferrin-bound iron (NTBI) and labile plasma iron (LPI) but may also directly improve overall survival, as discussed by Steensma and Gattermann [106].

The impact of iron overload on oxidative stress and disease progression has been well established. Excess iron catalyzes the production of ROS, disrupting cellular functions and leading to organ toxicity, cytopenia, and AML progression. Kim and Leitch [107] described how the resulting oxidative ROS damage to macromolecules, signaling pathways, and genomic integrity contributes to the further impairment of hematopoiesis and promotes clonal evolution. Therefore, ICT should be a critical consideration for improving both disease-free and overall survival in MDS.

Other iron chelators such as deferiprone have also demonstrated antioxidant effects. In a previous study conducted by Merkel et al. [108], deferiprone reduced ROS levels by 58.6%, 33.3%, and 39.8% in red blood cells, polymorphonuclear leukocytes (PMNs), and platelets, respectively. Additional improvements include reductions in phosphatidylserine exposure and lipid peroxidation, along with increased reductions in glutathione levels.

Interestingly, patients who responded positively to ICT had higher baseline expression levels of PI-PLCβ1, Cyclin D3, and PKCα, suggesting that these molecules may serve as biomarkers of treatment efficacy. According to Cappellini et al. [109], the expression of this pathway was downregulated following DFX treatment; this provides insight into the relevant potential mechanisms of action.

Moreover, iron overload-induced oxidative stress affects the self-renewal, proliferation, and differentiation capacities of hematopoietic stem cells, which are critical for maintaining effective hematopoiesis. ROS are implicated in clonal expansion, hematologic improvement, and recovery after hematopoietic stem cell transplantation (HSCT), as proposed by Pilo and Angelucci [110]. At diagnosis, patients with iron overload exhibited higher levels of superoxide anions than both healthy controls and patients with MDS without IOL. Additionally, Ivars et al. [111] reported significant alterations in the antioxidant defense system in IOL patients, including dysregulation of the catalase, glutathione peroxidase, and glutathione levels (Figure 1).

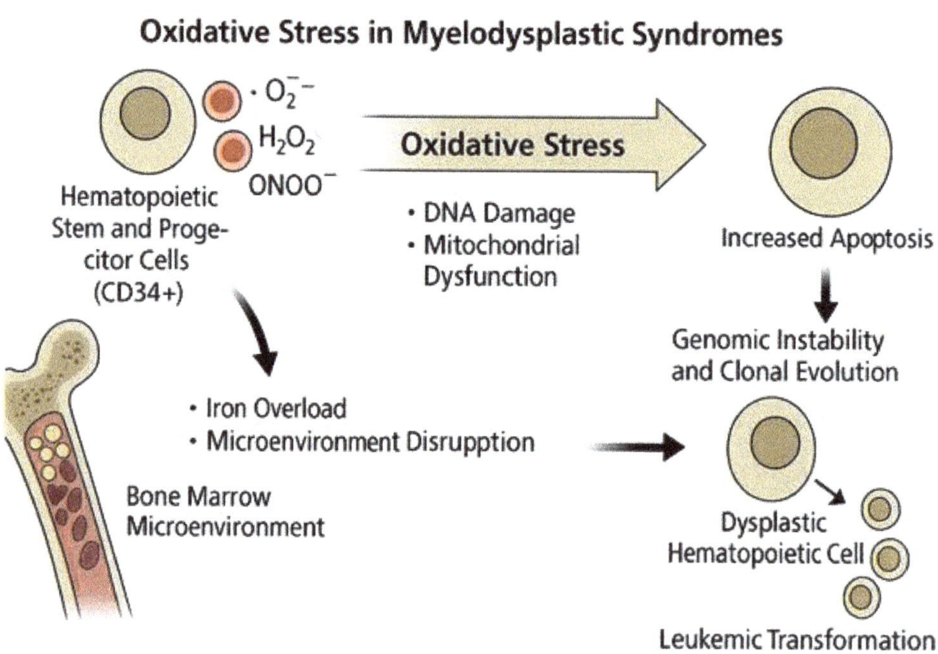

Figure 1. Effects of iron overload in MDS.

5.4. Mitochondrial Dynamics and Ferroptosis in the Metabolic Landscape of Myelodysplastic Syndromes

Ferroptosis is a regulated, iron-dependent form of cell death driven by the accumulation of lipid peroxides. It is distinct from apoptosis and is characterized by oxidative damage to cellular membranes, resulting from impaired antioxidant defenses, particularly glutathione peroxidase 4 (GPX4). This form of cell death has gained increasing relevance in cancer biology, especially in conditions involving metabolic reprogramming and iron overload, such as in myelodysplastic syndromes (MDS) [112].

In this context, ferroptosis is emerging as a novel therapeutic strategy, particularly for hematological malignancies that are resistant to conventional chemotherapy. These malignancies exhibit unique metabolic traits, including increased iron uptake and storage, which may enhance their sensitivity to ferroptotic triggers. As such, inducing ferroptosis represents a promising direction for the development of targeted therapies, provided that the molecular mechanisms of sensitivity and resistance are better understood [113].

Mitochondria play a central role in the regulation of ferroptosis, given their involvement in iron metabolism and reactive oxygen species (ROS) generation. Mitochondrial dynamics and interactions with other organelles also contribute significantly to the regulation of this death pathway [114]. In myeloid malignancies, including MDS, alterations in mitochondrial morphology—particularly excessive mitochondrial fragmentation—are associated with clonal evolution and disease progression. Notably, inhibition of the fission protein DRP1 has been shown to attenuate inflammatory signaling and improve survival in MDS preclinical models, highlighting a potential therapeutic avenue [115].

Moreover, metabolic rewiring in malignant cells, such as enhanced glycolysis, leads to a reorganization of mitochondrial tricarboxylic acid (TCA) cycle enzymes. This creates metabolic heterogeneity and alternative pathways that sustain increased cell proliferation. The Warburg effect, an "emergent property" of multiple integrated metabolic changes, further illustrates how altered energy metabolism supports tumor growth and contributes to the biology of leukemic transformation [116].

In normal hematopoietic stem cells (HSCs), anaerobic glycolysis is the predominant source of energy, and a high mitochondrial membrane potential is essential for maintaining quiescence and function. ROS regulation is critical in this setting, as oxidative stress impacts chromatin remodeling and cell fate decisions. Furthermore, nutrient pathways, including amino acid and fatty acid metabolism, contribute to acetyl-CoA production, which fuels the TCA cycle, despite the limited direct connection between glycolysis and mitochondrial respiration in HSCs [117].

Mitochondrial quality control (MQC) mechanisms are essential for preserving metabolic homeostasis in HSCs. Processes such as mitophagy remove dysfunctional mitochondria, thereby limiting ROS accumulation and preventing premature cellular aging. In parallel, mitochondrial biogenesis and intercellular mitochondrial transfer are crucial for maintaining energy balance and compensating for metabolic stress [118].

In fact, mitochondrial transfer has emerged as a therapeutic approach capable of restoring bioenergetic function by replacing damaged mitochondria with functional ones. This process plays a pivotal role not only in tissue repair and regeneration, but also in the pathogenesis, progression, and treatment resistance of hematologic malignancies, including AML and ALL [119].

Importantly, the oxidative stress and mitochondrial dynamics differ between low-risk and higher-risk MDS, with clear biological and clinical implications. Low-risk patients typically present with elevated basal ROS levels and reduced mitochondrial membrane potential ($\Delta\psi_m$), a profile that correlates with increased apoptosis and ineffective hematopoiesis1. In contrast, intermediate- and high-risk groups exhibit higher $\Delta\psi_m$ and enhanced OXPHOS capacity, features that support clonal proliferation and contribute to leukemic evolution [82]. Clinically, this divergence suggests that low-risk MDS may benefit from interventions targeting ROS accumulation or promoting ferroptosis, while high-risk MDS may be more vulnerable to therapies that disrupt mitochondrial potential or metabolic flexibility, offering a risk-adapted strategy to improve patient outcomes.

5.5. DNA Methylation and Epigenetic Regulation in Myelodysplastic Syndromes: Biomarkers and Functional Implications

Building on the connection between oxidative stress and disease mechanisms, epigenetic regulation, particularly DNA methylation, has emerged as a crucial factor in MDS pathophysiology. Changes in DNA methylation are considered potential biomarkers for diagnosis, prognosis, treatment response, and early toxicity prediction in both AML and MDS. As described by Dexheimer et al. [120], these alterations occur early during disease progression and can forecast myeloid or lymphoid transformation as well as therapeutic outcomes. Methylation profiling is currently being utilized for patient stratification, disease monitoring, and treatment optimization.

Furthermore, Gonçalves and colleagues [121] demonstrated a positive correlation between oxidative stress and DNA methylation levels in MDS patients. Higher global methylation was associated with poorer overall survival, highlighting the clinical significance of redox–epigenetic interactions. Specific oxidative stress markers—such as elevated peroxide levels and an increased peroxide/total antioxidant status (TAS) ratio—were found to be more prevalent in patients exhibiting promoter methylation of tumor suppressor genes, reinforcing a biochemical link between redox imbalance and epigenetic dysregulation [121]. In particular ROS were shown to correlate with the methylation status of the P15 and P16 gene promoters: patients with methylated genes had higher ROS levels, and parameters such as the peroxide/GSH ratio were proposed as potential discriminators between methylated and unmethylated gene profiles [122].

In addition to DNA methylation, transcriptional regulators play a pivotal role in MDS pathogenesis. One such factor is the myeloid lineage master regulator CCAAT enhancer-binding protein alpha (C/EBPα), encoded by the *CEBPA* gene. This transcription factor is essential for granulocytic lineage commitment and cell-cycle arrest. Its functional inhibition represents a leukemogenic event, as shown by Pulikkan, Tenen, and Behre [123], and restoration of C/EBPα levels can trigger granulocytic differentiation and prolong survival in leukemia models.

In MDS, CEBPA promoter methylation is significantly more frequent than in healthy controls, indicating its importance in disease development. As reported by Wen et al. [124], CEBPA mutations are rare and tend to occur mutually exclusively with respect to promoter methylation events. Despite its frequency, CEBPA methylation does not correlate strongly with transcriptional repression or patient outcome. Nevertheless, oxidative stress is hypothesized to contribute to aberrant CEBPA methylation, linking redox imbalance to defective granulocytic differentiation and disease progression in MDS.

Another key player in the epigenetic landscape is TET2, an Fe^{2+}- and α-ketoglutarate-dependent dioxygenase involved in active DNA demethylation. As discussed by Petzer et al. [125], TET2 mutations are common in MDS and have been shown to impair natural killer (NK) cell function by altering methylation patterns, leading to reduced expression of cytotoxic effector molecules such as KIRs, perforin, and TNF-α. These immune defects contribute to immune evasion and disease persistence. Importantly, Boy et al. [126] reported that treatment with hypomethylating agents (HMAs) like azacitidine can restore KIR expression and partially normalize NK cell function. Moreover, oxidative stress has been found to impair TET2 enzymatic activity, further reinforcing the connection between redox imbalance and the epigenetic alterations commonly observed in MDS.

5.6. Oxidative Stress in MDS and the Treatment Options Available

Oxidative stress in MDS can also serve as a valuable therapeutic target. In a recent study by Harris et al. [127], reduced expression of RPL22, a ribosomal protein, was found to be frequent in both MDS and AML patients and correlated with poorer clinical outcomes. The authors demonstrated that RPL22 deficiency enhances the self-renewal capacity of HSCs and impairs their differentiation by upregulating ALOX12, a key regulator of fatty acid oxidation (FAO). The resulting elevation of FAO supports leukemic cell survival, identifying a potential therapeutic vulnerability in RPL22-deficient MDS and AML.

Another promising axis involves arginine metabolism. Gonzalez-Menendez and colleagues [128] demonstrated that arginine uptake and its subsequent conversion to spermidine are crucial for the hypusination of eukaryotic initiation factor 5A (eIF5A), which plays a pivotal role in human erythroid differentiation. Notably, inhibition of hypusine synthesis selectively disrupts erythropoiesis while sparing myeloid differentiation, suggesting a lineage-specific function for eIF5A. These findings also highlight the regulatory role of ribosomal proteins in coupling the mitochondrial metabolism with red blood cell development.

Among the pharmacological agents, decitabine (DAC) is known to induce cell-cycle arrest and apoptosis in leukemia cells, triggering delayed ROS accumulation. This effect is independent of p53 and requires deoxycytidine kinase (DCK) activity [104]. DAC also upregulates ROS-generating enzymes, particularly NADPH oxidase isoforms, and increases Nox4 protein expression in an ATM-dependent manner, highlighting its link to DNA damage signaling and redox modulation [129].

Clinical evidence supports the therapeutic relevance of decitabine. In a multicenter phase II trial reported by Lübbert and colleagues [130], DAC was administered as a first-line treatment to elderly AML patients unfit for intensive chemotherapy. The study achieved a combined complete and partial remission rate of 26%, with a median overall survival of 5.5 months and a one-year survival rate of 28%, confirming its tolerability despite frequent myelosuppression.

Beyond decitabine, Montes et al. [131] explored the redox-modulatory effects of 5-azacitidine in patients with MDS. Their findings demonstrated that treatment with 5-azacitidine led to elevated oxidative stress markers, particularly increased ROS levels, without significantly affecting inflammatory parameters. Interestingly, prior to treatment, MDS patients showed a more favorable redox profile compared to healthy controls, as reflected by the lower ratio of oxidized glutathione (GSSG) to reduced glutathione (GSH), reduced lipid peroxidation, and higher catalase (CAT) activity.

In addition, upregulation of the HIF-1α signaling pathway has been associated with improved responses to 5-azacitidine in patients with high-risk MDS and AML. Elevated HIF-1α expression serves as an independent predictor of treatment response and correlates with better overall survival and a delayed progression to AML [132].

Vitamin C has also emerged as a promising redox-based therapeutic candidate. As reviewed by Gillberg et al. [133], vitamin C deficiency is commonly observed in cancer and may contribute to malignant transformation by impairing epigenetic regulation.

Notably, vitamin C levels are significantly lower in AML patients compared to healthy donors and show an inverse correlation with peripheral blast counts. These levels increase upon complete remission and decline further in cases of resistant disease. Additionally, the expression of vitamin C transporters is reduced in AML patients, although vitamin C concentration does not appear to predict survival or relapse [134].

At physiological levels, vitamin C synergizes with hypomethylating agents (HMAs) to enhance DNA demethylation via activation of TET and JHDM enzymes. At pharmacological doses, however, it promotes ROS production, selectively inducing cytotoxicity in neoplastic cells. In support of this dual mechanism, Cimmino et al. [135] demonstrated that vitamin C can mimic TET2 reactivation, reverse aberrant self-renewal in pre-leukemic stem cells, and restore normal DNA methylation dynamics, highlighting its therapeutic potential in MDS.

Furthermore, vitamin C has been shown to decrease cell proliferation and viability in a concentration-, time-, and administration-dependent manner, inducing apoptosis in F36P cells, a human erythroleukemia cell line commonly used to study erythroid differentiation and growth-factor responses. Its pro-oxidant effects, particularly the generation of superoxide and mitochondrial membrane depolarization, represent key mechanisms underlying its cytotoxic activity. Together, these findings support the exploration of vitamin C as a novel therapeutic strategy for MDS [136].

Natural compounds also contribute to the development of redox-targeted therapies. Among them, Withaferin A (WFA), a steroidal lactone derived from Withania somnifera (Ashwagandha), has shown antioxidant, anti-inflammatory, and anticancer properties through modulation of multiple oncogenic pathways [137]. A 2017 study demonstrated that WFA exerts selective cytotoxicity against MDS cells, particularly the MDS-L cell line, while sparing normal bone marrow cells. This selective effect is primarily mediated by the activation of the ROS-dependent JNK/AP-1 signaling pathway, ultimately leading to apoptosis. Thus, ROS generation is central to the therapeutic action of WFA in MDS [138].

In addition to its effects in MDS, WFA has demonstrated growth-suppressive activity in leukemia and lymphoma cell lines by inducing cell-cycle arrest at the G2/M phase. Although only partial apoptosis is observed in these models, its cytotoxicity can be significantly enhanced by combining WFA with autophagy inhibitors such as chloroquine. This combination strategy results in amplified apoptosis and tumor growth suppression, suggesting a promising redox-modulating approach in hematologic malignancies [139].

Finally, nicotinamide riboside (NR), another compound of interest, reduces the mitochondrial activity in HSCs by promoting mitochondrial clearance. This enhances asymmetric stem cell division, expands the progenitor pool, and improves survival and blood recovery after irradiation and transplantation. These findings link mitochondrial stress, mitophagy, and stem cell fate, highlighting the potential of NR in the treatment of hematological failure [140].

6. Future Perspectives in Oxidative Stress Research: The Role of Artificial Intelligence in Antioxidant Discovery in Myeloid Malignancies

Among these compounds, quercetin stands out for its multifunctional biological properties, including its antioxidant, antiproliferative, apoptotic, and autophagic effects. It has been shown to reduce the growth of various cancer cell lines, including AML and MDS cells. Through its multitarget activity, quercetin has demonstrated potential as a therapeutic agent in the treatment of AML and MDS by inducing cancer cell death [141].

Emerging technologies, particularly artificial intelligence (AI) and machine learning (ML), also contribute to our understanding of oxidative stress in hematological malignancies. A Korean study developed an ML model that accurately predicted oxidative stress levels in healthy individuals, using receiver operating characteristic (ROC) curves, and achieving high sensitivity and specificity [142].

AI and ML tools are being increasingly applied to evaluate antioxidant capacity by correlating the chemical structure (via molecular descriptors) with in vitro antioxidant activity. These models enhance compound screening efficiency, while supporting adherence to ethical research standards [143]. External validation using data from the BATMAN database confirmed the reliability of Random Forest (RF) and Support Vector Machines (SVM) models in predicting antioxidant potential [144].

In a recent GPT-based literature analysis, 1416 pro-oxidant and 1102 antioxidant compounds were identified and classified into chemical categories, such as flavonoids, thiols, pharmaceuticals, pesticides, and metals [145].

One promising area where these computational strategies are being applied is drug repurposing—the search for new therapeutic uses for existing or experimental compounds. This approach offers the advantage of reducing both the time and costs associated with drug development. Nevertheless, the field faces challenges such as legal uncertainties, intellectual property concerns, and regulatory barriers. Proposed strategies aim to address these obstacles and fully leverage the potential of repurposed drugs [146]. ML and AI enhance this process by offering cost-effective methods for identifying new applications of approved drugs. These supervised techniques often rely on publicly available databases, although their effectiveness is limited by the scarcity of clinical patient data and an overreliance on genomics-based information. Functional assays on patient-derived cancer cells can provide additional insight, complement in silico predictions, and help to mitigate the financial and developmental risks inherent in drug discovery [147].

Computational tools, including ML and deep learning models, are also being applied to uncover novel drug-target relationships in oncology. Among the therapeutic strategies under investigation, microRNA modulation has emerged as a key approach. Advances in Next Generation Sequencing (NGS) have significantly expanded our understanding of cancer biology, providing the high-quality data essential for the accuracy of ML-based drug repurposing models. Despite these advances, the clinical potential of drug repurposing in oncology remains largely untapped [148].

Finally, AI and ML are also revolutionizing traditional drug discovery by addressing longstanding challenges such as high development costs and lengthy timelines. Sophisticated AI frameworks, including deep neural networks (DNNs), convolutional neural networks (CNNs), and deep reinforcement learning (DRL), are being used to identify drug targets and enhance delivery systems. Personalized treatment strategies are also being refined through models like CURATE.AI and the Hartung algorithm, which aim to optimize therapeutic efficacy and predict toxicological risks [149].

7. Conclusions

Myelodysplastic syndromes represent a heterogeneous group of clonal hematopoietic disorders driven by complex genetic, epigenetic, and metabolic alterations. Among the emerging contributors to the pathophysiology of MDS, oxidative stress has gained increasing recognition with respect to its roles in promoting genomic instability, disrupting hematopoietic stem cell function, and influencing disease progression. Elevated ROS levels, often exacerbated by iron overload, mitochondrial dysfunction, and impaired antioxidant defenses, are associated with the key clinical features of MDS, including ineffective erythropoiesis and increased leukemic transformation risk. Therapeutically, redox-modulating strategies, such as iron chelation, antioxidant supplementation, and agents that influence ROS-mediated signaling pathways (e.g., decitabine, vitamin C, and Withaferin A), offer promising adjuncts to conventional treatment regimens. These approaches may reduce oxidative damage, restore redox balance, and enhance hematologic responses, particularly in transfusion-dependent or lower-risk MDS patients. From a clinical perspective, the integration of oxidative stress markers (e.g., malondialdehyde, protein carbonylation, glutathione levels, and ROS/GSH ratios) into existing risk stratification models could refine prognostic assessments and personalize treatment choices. Measuring these parameters routinely may help identify the patients more likely to benefit from iron chelation or redox-targeted therapies. Future research should focus on validating oxidative stress biomarkers in prospective clinical trials and exploring their predictive value for treatment response and disease evolution. In parallel, further mechanistic studies are needed to clarify the interactions between redox imbalance, clonal hematopoiesis, immune dysfunction, and epigenetic deregulation. The application of artificial intelligence and machine learning to large genomic and biochemical datasets may facilitate the discovery of new therapeutic targets and support drug repurposing strategies. Ultimately, a more comprehensive integration of redox biology into MDS management could pave the way for precision medicine approaches that optimize outcomes based on molecular and metabolic patient profiles.

Author Contributions: Conceptualization, A.A. and F.P.; Data Curation, G.M., F.S. and S.G.; Formal Analysis, F.P. and M.F.; Investigation, F.P. and F.S.; Methodology, G.M. and M.F.; Supervision, A.A., F.S. and S.G.; Validation, A.A.; Writing—Original Draft Preparation, F.P. and A.A.; Writing—Review and Editing, all the authors. All authors have read and agreed to the published version of the manuscript.

Funding: This research received no external funding.

Conflicts of Interest: The authors declare no conflicts of interest.

References

1. Jacobs, A. The pathogenesis and classification of the myelodysplastic syndromes. *Br. J. Haematol.* **1990**, *75* (Suppl. 1), 7–11.
2. Hofmann, W.-K.; Koeffler, H.P. Important features of myelodysplastic syndrome. *Int. J. Hematol.* **2002**, *76* (Suppl. 2), 222–227. [CrossRef]
3. Hasserjian, R.P. Myelodysplastic Syndrome Updated. *Pathobiology* **2019**, *86*, 7–13. [CrossRef] [PubMed]
4. Khoury, J.D.; Solary, E.; Abla, O.; Akkari, Y.; Alaggio, R.; Apperley, J.F.; Bejar, R.; Berti, E.; Busque, L.; Chan, J.K.C.; et al. The 5th edition of the World Health Organization Classification of Haematolymphoid Tumours: Myeloid and Histiocytic/Dendritic Neoplasms. *Leukemia* **2022**, *36*, 1703–1719. [CrossRef] [PubMed]
5. Zhang, Y.; Wu, J.; Qin, T.; Xu, Z.; Qu, S.; Pan, L.; Li, B.; Wang, H.; Zhang, P.; Yan, X.; et al. Comparison of the revised 4th (2016) and 5th (2022) editions of the World Health Organization classification of myelodysplastic neoplasms. *Leukemia* **2022**, *36*, 2875–2882. [CrossRef]
6. Tanaka, T.N.; Bejar, R. MDS overlap disorders and diagnostic boundaries. *Blood* **2019**, *133*, 1086–1095. [CrossRef] [PubMed]
7. Hosono, N. Genetic abnormalities and pathophysiology of MDS. *Int. J. Clin. Oncol.* **2019**, *24*, 885–892. [CrossRef]
8. Pellagatti, A.; Boultwood, J. The molecular pathogenesis of the myelodysplastic syndromes. *Eur. J. Haematol.* **2015**, *95*, 3–15. [CrossRef]
9. Chiereghin, C.; Travaglino, E.; Zampini, M.; Saba, E.; Saitta, C.; Riva, E.; Bersanelli, M.; Della Porta, M.G. The Genetics of Myelodysplastic Syndromes: Clinical Relevance. *Genes* **2021**, *12*, 1144. [CrossRef]
10. Haferlach, T. The Molecular Pathology of Myelodysplastic Syndrome. *Pathobiology* **2019**, *86*, 24–29. [CrossRef]
11. Peng, X.; Zhu, X.; Di, T.; Tang, F.; Guo, X.; Liu, Y.; Bai, J.; Li, Y.; Li, L.; Zhang, L. The yin-yang of immunity: Immune dysregulation in myelodysplastic syndrome with different risk stratification. *Front. Immunol.* **2022**, *13*, 994053. [CrossRef]
12. Glenthøj, A.; Ørskov, A.D.; Hansen, J.W.; Hadrup, S.R.; O'Connell, C.; Grønbæk, K. Immune Mechanisms in Myelodysplastic Syndrome. *Int. J. Mol. Sci.* **2016**, *17*, 944. [CrossRef]
13. Giannouli, S.; Kanellopoulou, T.; Voulgarelis, M. Myelodysplasia and autoimmunity. *Curr. Opin. Rheumatol.* **2012**, *24*, 97–102. [CrossRef]
14. Grignano, E.; Jachiet, V.; Fenaux, P.; Adès, L.; Fain, O.; Mekinian, A. Autoimmune manifestations associated with myelodysplastic syndromes. *Ann. Hematol.* **2018**, *97*, 2015–2023. [CrossRef] [PubMed]
15. Greenberg, P.L.; Tuechler, H.; Schanz, J.; Sanz, G.; Garcia-Manero, G.; Solé, F.; Bennett, J.M.; Bowen, D.; Fenaux, P.; Dreyfus, F.; et al. Revised International Prognostic Scoring System for Myelodysplastic Syndromes. *Blood* **2012**, *120*, 2454–2465. [CrossRef]
16. Bernard, E.; Tuechler, H.; Greenberg, P.L.; Hasserjian, R.P.; Ossa, J.E.A.; Nannya, Y.; Devlin, S.M.; Creignou, M.; Pinel, P.; Monnier, L.; et al. Molecular International Prognostic Scoring System for Myelodysplastic Syndromes. *NEJM Evid.* **2022**, *1*, EVIDoa2200008. [CrossRef] [PubMed]
17. Tobiasson, M.; Kittang, A.O. Treatment of myelodysplastic syndrome in the era of next-generation sequencing. *J. Intern. Med.* **2019**, *286*, 41–62. [CrossRef] [PubMed]
18. Fenaux, P.; Platzbecker, U.; Adès, L. How we manage adults with myelodysplastic syndrome. *Br. J. Haematol.* **2020**, *189*, 1016–1027. [CrossRef]
19. Carraway, H.E.; Saygin, C. Therapy for lower-risk MDS. *Hematology* **2020**, *2020*, 426–433. [CrossRef]

20. DeFilipp, Z.; Ciurea, S.O.; Cutler, C.; Robin, M.; Warlick, E.D.; Nakamura, R.; Brunner, A.M.; Dholaria, B.; Walker, A.R.; Kröger, N.; et al. Hematopoietic Cell Transplantation in the Management of Myelodysplastic Syndrome. *Transplant. Cell. Ther.* **2023**, *29*, 71–81. [CrossRef]
21. Saygin, C.; Carraway, H.E. Current and emerging strategies for management of myelodysplastic syndromes. *Blood Rev.* **2021**, *48*, 100791. [CrossRef]
22. Fenaux, P.; Platzbecker, U.; Mufti, G.J.; Garcia-Manero, G.; Buckstein, R.; Santini, V.; Díez-Campelo, M.; Finelli, C.; Cazzola, M.; Ilhan, O.; et al. Luspatercept in Patients with Lower-Risk Myelodysplastic Syndromes. *N. Engl. J. Med.* **2020**, *382*, 140–151. [CrossRef]
23. List, A.; Dewald, G.; Bennett, J.; Giagounidis, A.; Raza, A.; Feldman, E.; Powell, B.; Greenberg, P.; Thomas, D.; Stone, R.; et al. Lenalidomide in the Myelodysplastic Syndrome with Chromosome 5q Deletion. *N. Engl. J. Med.* **2006**, *355*, 1456–1465. [CrossRef] [PubMed]
24. Fenaux, P.; Santini, V.; Spiriti, M.A.A.; Giagounidis, A.; Schlag, R.; Radinoff, A.; Gercheva-Kyuchukova, L.; Anagnostopoulos, A.; Oliva, E.N.; Symeonidis, A.; et al. A phase 3 randomized, placebo-controlled study assessing the efficacy and safety of epoetin-α in anemic patients with low-risk MDS. *Leukemia* **2018**, *32*, 2648–2658. [CrossRef] [PubMed]
25. Fenaux, P.; Mufti, G.J.; Hellstrom-Lindberg, E.; Santini, V.; Finelli, C.; Giagounidis, A.; Schoch, R.; Gattermann, N.; Sanz, G.; List, A.; et al. Efficacy of azacitidine compared with that of conventional care regimens in the treatment of higher-risk myelodysplastic syndromes: A randomised, open-label, phase III study. *Lancet Oncol.* **2009**, *10*, 223–232. [CrossRef] [PubMed]
26. Garcia-Manero, G.; Santini, V.; Almeida, A.; Platzbecker, U.; Jonasova, A.; Silverman, L.R.; Falantes, J.; Reda, G.; Buccisano, F.; Fenaux, P.; et al. Phase III, Randomized, Placebo-Controlled Trial of CC-486 (Oral Azacitidine) in Patients With Lower-Risk Myelodysplastic Syndromes. *J. Clin. Oncol.* **2021**, *39*, 1426–1436. [CrossRef]
27. Wei, A.H.; Döhner, H.; Pocock, C.; Montesinos, P.; Afanasyev, B.; Dombret, H.; Ravandi, F.; Sayar, H.; Jang, J.-H.; Porkka, K.; et al. Oral Azacitidine Maintenance Therapy for Acute Myeloid Leukemia in First Remission. *N. Engl. J. Med.* **2020**, *383*, 2526–2537. [CrossRef]
28. Zeidan, A.M.; Jayade, S.; Schmier, J.; Botteman, M.; Hassan, A.; Ruiters, D.; Hill, K.; Joshi, N. Injectable Hypomethylating Agents for Management of Myelodysplastic Syndromes: Patients' Perspectives on Treatment. *Clin. Lymphoma Myeloma Leuk.* **2022**, *22*, e185–e198. [CrossRef]
29. Şenel, P.; Agar, S.; Yurtsever, M.; Gölcü, A. Voltammetric quantification, spectroscopic, and DFT studies on the binding of the antineoplastic drug Azacitidine with DNA. *J. Pharm. Biomed. Anal.* **2024**, *237*, 115746. [CrossRef]
30. Teodorescu, P.; Pasca, S.; Dima, D.; Tomuleasa, C.; Ghiaur, G. Targeting the Microenvironment in MDS: The Final Frontier. *Front. Pharmacol.* **2020**, *11*, 1044. [CrossRef]
31. Syed, K.; Naguib, S.; Liu, Z.-J.; Cimmino, L.; Yang, F.-C. Novel combinations to improve hematopoiesis in myelodysplastic syndrome. *Stem Cell Res. Ther.* **2020**, *11*, 132. [CrossRef] [PubMed]
32. Velegraki, M.; Stiff, A.; Papadaki, H.A.; Li, Z. Myeloid-Derived Suppressor Cells: New Insights into the Pathogenesis and Therapy of MDS. *J. Clin. Med.* **2022**, *11*, 4908. [CrossRef] [PubMed]
33. Trivedi, G.; Inoue, D.; Zhang, L. Targeting low-risk myelodysplastic syndrome with novel therapeutic strategies. *Trends Mol. Med.* **2021**, *27*, 990–999. [CrossRef]
34. Henry, D.H.; Glaspy, J.; Harrup, R.; Mittelman, M.; Zhou, A.; Carraway, H.E.; Bradley, C.; Saha, G.; Modelska, K.; Bartels, P.; et al. Roxadustat for the treatment of anemia in patients with LOWER-RISK myelodysplastic syndrome: Open-label, dose-selection, lead-in stage of a phase 3 study. *Am. J. Hematol.* **2022**, *97*, 174–184. [CrossRef]
35. Hara, R.; Goto, N.; Furuya, D.; Kitahara, T.; Numata, H.; Watanabe, S.; Kawada, H.; Ando, K. The Effect of Roxadustat on Transfusion-Dependent Myelodysplastic Syndrome Complicated by Chronic Kidney Disease. *Case Rep. Oncol.* **2021**, *14*, 1574–1579. [CrossRef]
36. Lennox, A.L.; Huang, F.; Behrs, M.K.; González-Sales, M.; Bhise, N.; Wan, Y.; Sun, L.; Berry, T.; Feller, F.; Morcos, P.N. Imetelstat, a novel, first-in-class telomerase inhibitor: Mechanism of action, clinical, and translational science. *Clin. Transl. Sci.* **2024**, *17*, e70076. [CrossRef]
37. Platzbecker, U.; Santini, V.; Fenaux, P.; Sekeres, M.A.; Savona, M.R.; Madanat, Y.F.; Díez-Campelo, M.; Valcárcel, D.; Illmer, T.; Jonášová, A.; et al. Imetelstat in patients with lower-risk myelodysplastic syndromes who have relapsed or are refractory to erythropoiesis-stimulating agents (IMerge): A multinational, randomised, double-blind, placebo-controlled, phase 3 trial. *Lancet* **2024**, *403*, 249–260. [CrossRef] [PubMed]
38. Abaza, Y.; Zeidan, A.M. Immune Checkpoint Inhibition in Acute Myeloid Leukemia and Myelodysplastic Syndromes. *Cells* **2022**, *11*, 2249. [CrossRef]
39. Sallman, D.A.; Al Malki, M.M.; Asch, A.S.; Wang, E.S.; Jurcic, J.G.; Bradley, T.J.; Flinn, I.W.; Pollyea, D.A.; Kambhampati, S.; Tanaka, T.N.; et al. Magrolimab in Combination With Azacitidine in Patients With Higher-Risk Myelodysplastic Syndromes: Final Results of a Phase Ib Study. *J. Clin. Oncol.* **2023**, *41*, 2815–2826. [CrossRef]

40. Valko, M.; Leibfritz, D.; Moncol, J.; Cronin, M.T.D.; Mazur, M.; Telser, J. Free radicals and antioxidants in normal physiological functions and human disease. *Int. J. Biochem. Cell Biol.* **2007**, *39*, 44–84. [CrossRef]
41. Cabello-Verrugio, C.; Simon, F.; Trollet, C.; Santibañez, J.F. Oxidative Stress in Disease and Aging: Mechanisms and Therapies Oxid. *Oxidative Med. Cell. Longev.* **2017**, *2017*, 4310469. [CrossRef] [PubMed]
42. Kudryavtseva, A.V.; Krasnov, G.S.; Dmitriev, A.A.; Alekseev, B.Y.; Kardymon, O.L.; Sadritdinova, A.F.; Fedorova, M.S.; Pokrovsky, A.V.; Melnikova, N.V.; Kaprin, A.D.; et al. Mitochondrial dysfunction and oxidative stress in aging and cancer. *Oncotarget* **2016**, *7*, 44879–44905. [CrossRef] [PubMed]
43. Li, D.; Yu, Q.; Wu, R.; Tuo, Z.; Wang, J.; Ye, L.; Shao, F.; Chaipanichkul, P.; Yoo, K.H.; Wei, W.; et al. Interactions between oxidative stress and senescence in cancer: Mechanisms, therapeutic implications, and future perspectives. *Redox Biol.* **2024**, *73*, 103208. [CrossRef]
44. Filomeni, G.; De Zio, D.; Cecconi, F. Oxidative stress and autophagy: The clash between damage and metabolic needs. *Cell Death Differ.* **2015**, *22*, 377–388. [CrossRef] [PubMed]
45. Li, J.; Jia, B.; Cheng, Y.; Song, Y.; Li, Q.; Luo, C.; Birla, H. Targeting Molecular Mediators of Ferroptosis and Oxidative Stress for Neurological Disorders. *Oxidative Med. Cell. Longev.* **2022**, *2022*, 3999083. [CrossRef]
46. Zeng, W.; Long, X.; Liu, P.; Xie, X. Interplay of oncogenic signaling, oxidative stress, and ferroptosis in cancer. *Int. J. Cancer* **2023**, *153*, 918–931. [CrossRef]
47. Jourdain, A.A.; Begg, B.E.; Mick, E.; Shah, H.; Calvo, S.E.; Skinner, O.S.; Sharma, R.; Blue, S.M.; Yeo, G.W.; Burge, C.B.; et al. Loss of LUC7L2 and U1 snRNP subunits shifts energy metabolism from glycolysis to OXPHOS. *Mol. Cell* **2021**, *81*, 1905–1919.e12. [CrossRef]
48. Danieli, M.G.; Antonelli, E.; Piga, M.A.; Cozzi, M.F.; Allegra, A.; Gangemi, S. Oxidative stress, mitochondrial dysfunction, and respiratory chain enzyme defects in inflammatory myopathies. *Autoimmun. Rev.* **2023**, *22*, 103308. [CrossRef]
49. Canton, M.; Menazza, S.; Di Lisa, F. Oxidative stress in muscular dystrophy: From generic evidence to specific sources and targets. *J. Muscle Res. Cell Motil.* **2014**, *35*, 23–36. [CrossRef]
50. Jadeja, R.N.; Devkar, R.V.; Nammi, S. Oxidative Stress in Liver Diseases: Pathogenesis, Prevention, and Therapeutics. *Oxidative Med. Cell. Longev.* **2017**, *2017*, 8341286. [CrossRef]
51. Zhang, C.; Li, H.; Li, J.; Hu, J.; Yang, K.; Tao, L. Oxidative stress: A common pathological state in a high-risk population for osteoporosis. *Biomed. Pharmacother.* **2023**, *163*, 114834. [CrossRef]
52. De Martinis, M.; Allegra, A.; Sirufo, M.M.; Tonacci, A.; Pioggia, G.; Raggiunti, M.; Ginaldi, L.; Gangemi, S. Vitamin D Deficiency, Osteoporosis and Effect on Autoimmune Diseases and Hematopoiesis: A Review. *Int. J. Mol. Sci.* **2021**, *22*, 8855. [CrossRef] [PubMed]
53. Senoner, T.; Dichtl, W. Oxidative Stress in Cardiovascular Diseases: Still a Therapeutic Target? *Nutrients* **2019**, *11*, 2090. [CrossRef] [PubMed]
54. Yamada, Y.; Takano, Y.; Satrialdi; Abe, J.; Hibino, M.; Harashima, H. Therapeutic strategies for regulating mitochondrial oxidative stress. *Biomolecules* **2020**, *10*, 83. [CrossRef]
55. Allegra, A.; Pioggia, G.; Tonacci, A.; Musolino, C.; Gangemi, S. Oxidative Stress and Photodynamic Therapy of Skin Cancers: Mechanisms, Challenges and Promising Developments. *Antioxidants* **2020**, *9*, 448. [CrossRef] [PubMed]
56. Gorrini, C.; Harris, I.S.; Mak, T.W. Modulation of oxidative stress as an anticancer strategy. *Nat. Rev. Drug Discov.* **2013**, *12*, 931–947. [CrossRef]
57. Allegra, A.; Caserta, S.; Genovese, S.; Pioggia, G.; Gangemi, S. Gender differences in oxidative stress in relation to cancer susceptibility and survival. *Antioxidants* **2023**, *12*, 1255. [CrossRef]
58. Bigarella, C.L.; Liang, R.; Ghaffari, S. Stem cells and the impact of ROS signaling. *Development* **2014**, *141*, 4206–4218. [CrossRef]
59. Soundararajan, L.; Warrier, S.; Dharmarajan, A.; Bhaskaran, N. Predominant factors influencing reactive oxygen species in cancer stem cells. *J. Cell. Biochem.* **2024**, *125*, 3–21. [CrossRef]
60. Hole, P.S.; Darley, R.L.; Tonks, A. Do reactive oxygen species play a role in myeloid leukemias? *Blood* **2011**, *117*, 5816–5826. [CrossRef]
61. Gangemi, S.; Allegra, A.; Alonci, A.; Cristani, M.; Russo, S.; Speciale, A.; Penna, G.; Spatari, G.; Cannavò, A.; Bellomo, G.; et al. Increase of novel biomarkers for oxidative stress in patients with plasma cell disorders and in multiple myeloma patients with bone lesions. *Inflamm. Res.* **2012**, *61*, 1063–1067. [CrossRef] [PubMed]
62. Morabito, F.; Cristani, M.; Saija, A.; Stelitano, C.; Callea, V.; Tomaino, A.; Minciullo, P.L.; Gangemi, S. Lipid peroxidation and protein oxidation in patients affected by Hodgkin's lymphoma. *Mediat. Inflamm.* **2004**, *13*, 381–383. [CrossRef] [PubMed]
63. Xie, J.-B.; Huang, S.-J.; Yang, T.-B.; Wang, W.; Chen, B.-Y.; Guo, L. Comparison of machine learning methods for Predicting 3-Year survival in elderly esophageal squamous cancer patients based on oxidative stress. *BMC Cancer* **2024**, *24*, 1432. [CrossRef] [PubMed]
64. Wang, S.-F.; Chen, S.; Tseng, L.-M.; Lee, H.-C. Role of the mitochondrial stress response in human cancer progression. *Exp. Biol. Med.* **2020**, *245*, 861–878. [CrossRef] [PubMed]

65. Winter, J.M.; Yadav, T.; Rutter, J. Stressed to death: Mitochondrial stress responses connect respiration and apoptosis in cancer. *Mol. Cell* **2022**, *82*, 3321–3332. [CrossRef]
66. Luo, Y.; Ma, J.; Lu, W. The significance of mitochondrial dysfunction in cancer. *Int. J. Mol. Sci.* **2020**, *21*, 5598. [CrossRef]
67. Testa, U.; Labbaye, C.; Castelli, G.; Pelosi, E. Oxidative stress and hypoxia in normal and leukemic stem cells. *Exp. Hematol.* **2016**, *44*, 540–560. [CrossRef]
68. Kocabas, F.; Xie, L.; Xie, J.; Yu, Z.; DeBerardinis, R.J.; Kimura, W.; Thet, S.; Elshamy, A.F.; Abouellail, H.; Muralidhar, S.; et al. Hypoxic metabolism in human hematopoietic stem cells. *Cell Biosci.* **2015**, *5*, 39. [CrossRef]
69. Gonzalez-Menendez, P.; Romano, M.; Yan, H.; Deshmukh, R.; Papoin, J.; Oburoglu, L.; Daumur, M.; Dumé, A.-S.; Phadke, I.; Mongellaz, C.; et al. An IDH1-vitamin C crosstalk drives human erythroid development by inhibiting pro-oxidant mitochondrial metabolism. *Cell Rep.* **2021**, *34*, 108723. [CrossRef]
70. Ivanov, S.; Nano, O.; Hana, C.; Bonano-Rios, A.; Hussein, A. Molecular Targeting of the Isocitrate Dehydrogenase Pathway and the Implications for Cancer Therapy. *Int. J. Mol. Sci.* **2024**, *25*, 7337. [CrossRef]
71. Semenza, G.L. Hypoxia-inducible factors in physiology and medicine. *Cell* **2012**, *148*, 399–408. [CrossRef] [PubMed]
72. Jaakkola, P.; Mole, D.R.; Tian, Y.M.; Wilson, M.I.; Gielbert, J.; Gaskell, S.J.; Kriegsheim, A.V.; Hebestreit, H.F.; Mukherji, M.; Schofield, C.J.; et al. Targeting of HIF-α to the von Hippel–Lindau ubiquitylation complex by O2-regulated prolyl hydroxylation. *Science* **2001**, *292*, 468–472. [CrossRef] [PubMed]
73. Kaelin, W.G., Jr.; Ratcliffe, P.J. Oxygen sensing by metazoans: The central role of the HIF hydroxylase pathway. *Mol. Cell* **2008**, *30*, 393–402. [CrossRef]
74. Deynoux, M.; Sunter, N.; Hérault, O.; Mazurier, F. Hypoxia and hypoxia-inducible factors in leukemias. *Front. Oncol.* **2016**, *6*, 41. [CrossRef]
75. Magliulo, D.; Bernardi, R. Hypoxic stress and hypoxia-inducible factors in leukemias. *Front. Oncol.* **2022**, *12*, 973978. [CrossRef]
76. Stergiou, I.E.; Kambas, K.; Poulaki, A.; Giannouli, S.; Katsila, T.; Dimitrakopoulou, A.; Vidali, V.; Mouchtouris, V.; Kloukina, I.; Xingi, E.; et al. Exploiting the role of hypoxia-inducible factor 1 and pseudohypoxia in the myelodysplastic syndrome pathophysiology. *Int. J. Mol. Sci.* **2021**, *22*, 4099. [CrossRef]
77. Benito, J.; Zeng, Z.; Konopleva, M.; Wilson, W.R. Targeting hypoxia in the leukemia microenvironment. *Int. J. Hematol. Oncol.* **2013**, *2*, 279–288. [CrossRef] [PubMed]
78. Chen, J.; Steidl, U. Inhibition of HIF1α signaling: A grand slam for MDS therapy? *Cancer Discov.* **2018**, *8*, 1355–1357. [CrossRef]
79. Saigo, K.; Takenokuchi, M.; Hiramatsu, Y.; Tada, H.; Hishita, T.; Takata, M.; Misawa, M.; Imoto, S.; Imashuku, S. Oxidative Stress Levels in Myelodysplastic Syndrome Patients: Their Relationship to Serum Ferritin and Haemoglobin Values. *J. Int. Med. Res.* **2011**, *39*, 1941–1945. [CrossRef]
80. Farquhar, M.J.; Bowen, D.T. Oxidative Stress and the Myelodysplastic Syndromes. *Int. J. Hematol.* **2003**, *77*, 342–350. [CrossRef]
81. Chung, Y.J.; Robert, C.; Gough, S.M.; Rassool, F.V.; Aplan, P.D. Oxidative stress leads to increased mutation frequency in a murine model of myelodysplastic syndrome. *Leuk. Res.* **2014**, *38*, 95–102. [CrossRef]
82. Gonçalves, A.C.; Cortesão, E.; Oliveiros, B.; Alves, V.; Espadana, A.I.; Rito, L.; Magalhães, E.; Lobão, M.J.; Pereira, A.; Costa, J.M.N.; et al. Oxidative stress and mitochondrial dysfunction play a role in myelodysplastic syndrome development, diagnosis, and prognosis: A pilot study. *Free. Radic. Res.* **2015**, *49*, 1081–1094. [CrossRef]
83. Novotna, B.; Bagryantseva, Y.; Siskova, M.; Neuwirtova, R. Oxidative DNA damage in bone marrow cells of patients with low-risk myelodysplastic syndrome. *Leuk. Res.* **2009**, *33*, 340–343. [CrossRef] [PubMed]
84. Ghoti, H.; Amer, J.; Winder, A.; Rachmilewitz, E.; Fibach, E. Oxidative stress in red blood cells, platelets and polymorphonuclear leukocytes from patients with myelodysplastic syndrome. *Eur. J. Haematol.* **2007**, *79*, 463–467. [CrossRef]
85. Jing, Q.; Zhou, C.; Zhang, J.; Zhang, P.; Wu, Y.; Zhou, J.; Tong, X.; Li, Y.; Du, J.; Wang, Y. Role of reactive oxygen species in myelodysplastic syndromes. *Cell. Mol. Biol. Lett.* **2024**, *29*, 53. [CrossRef]
86. McCrann, D.J.; Eliades, A.; Makitalo, M.; Matsuno, K.; Ravid, K. Differential expression of NADPH oxidases in megakaryocytes and their role in polyploidy. *Blood* **2009**, *114*, 1243–1249. [CrossRef] [PubMed]
87. Schieber, M.; Chandel, N.S. ROS Function in Redox Signaling and Oxidative Stress. *Curr. Biol.* **2014**, *24*, R453–R462. [CrossRef] [PubMed]
88. Hammad, M.; Raftari, M.; Cesário, R.; Salma, R.; Godoy, P.; Emami, S.N.; Haghdoost, S. Roles of Oxidative Stress and Nrf2 Signaling in Pathogenic and Non-Pathogenic Cells: A Possible General Mechanism of Resistance to Therapy. *Antioxidants* **2023**, *12*, 1371. [CrossRef]
89. Dodson, M.; de la Vega, M.R.; Cholanians, A.B.; Schmidlin, C.J.; Chapman, E.; Zhang, D.D. Modulating NRF2 in Disease: Timing Is Everything. *Annu. Rev. Pharmacol. Toxicol.* **2019**, *59*, 555–575. [CrossRef]
90. Zhao, Y.; Ye, X.; Xiong, Z.; Ihsan, A.; Ares, I.; Martínez, M.; Lopez-Torres, B.; Martínez-Larrañaga, M.-R.; Anadón, A.; Wang, X.; et al. Cancer Metabolism: The Role of ROS in DNA Damage and Induction of Apoptosis in Cancer Cells. *Metabolites* **2023**, *13*, 796. [CrossRef]

91. Boura-Theodorou, A.; Psatha, K.; Maniatsi, S.; Kourti, A.; Kaiafa, G.; Aivaliotis, M.; Makedou, K. Oxidative Stress and Its Role in the Emergence and Progression of Myelodysplastic Syndromes: Insights from Proteomic Analysis and Other Methodologies. *Proteomes* **2025**, *13*, 21. [CrossRef] [PubMed]
92. Stockwell, B.R.; Angeli, J.P.F.; Bayir, H.; Bush, A.I.; Conrad, M.; Dixon, S.J.; Fulda, S.; Gascón, S.; Hatzios, S.K.; Kagan, V.E.; et al. Ferroptosis: A Regulated Cell Death Nexus Linking Metabolism, Redox Biology, and Disease. *Cell* **2017**, *171*, 273–285. [CrossRef]
93. Viswanathan, V.S.; Ryan, M.J.; Dhruv, H.D.; Gill, S.; Eichhoff, O.M.; Seashore-Ludlow, B.; Kaffenberger, S.D.; Eaton, J.K.; Shimada, K.; Aguirre, A.J.; et al. Dependency of a therapy-resistant state of cancer cells on a lipid peroxidase pathway. *Nature* **2017**, *547*, 453–457. [CrossRef] [PubMed]
94. Hole, P.S.; Zabkiewicz, J.; Munje, C.; Newton, Z.; Pearn, L.; White, P.; Marquez, N.; Hills, R.K.; Burnett, A.K.; Tonks, A.; et al. Overproduction of NOX-derived ROS in AML promotes proliferation and is associated with defective oxidative stress signaling. *Blood* **2013**, *122*, 3322–3330. [CrossRef]
95. Trachootham, D.; Alexandre, J.; Huang, P. Targeting cancer cells by ROS-mediated mechanisms: A radical therapeutic approach? *Nat. Rev. Drug Discov.* **2009**, *8*, 579–591. [CrossRef] [PubMed]
96. Nemeth, E.; Ganz, T. Hepcidin-Ferroportin Interaction Controls Systemic Iron Homeostasis. *Int. J. Mol. Sci.* **2021**, *22*, 6493. [CrossRef]
97. Roemhild, K.; von Maltzahn, F.; Weiskirchen, R.; Knüchel, R.; von Stillfried, S.; Lammers, T. Iron metabolism: Pathophysiology and pharmacology. *Trends Pharmacol. Sci.* **2021**, *42*, 640–656. [CrossRef]
98. Słomka, A.; Pokrzywa, A.; Strzała, D.; Kubiaczyk, M.; Wesolowska, O.; Denkiewicz, K.; Styczyński, J. The Role of Hepcidin in Myelodysplastic Syndromes (MDS): A Systematic Review of Observational Studies. *Cancers* **2024**, *16*, 332. [CrossRef]
99. Fibach, E.; Rachmilewitz, E.A. Iron overload in hematological disorders. *Presse Méd.* **2017**, *46*, e296–e305. [CrossRef]
100. Gattermann, N.; Rachmilewitz, E.A. Iron overload in MDS—Pathophysiology, diagnosis, and complications. *Ann. Hematol.* **2011**, *90*, 1–10. [CrossRef]
101. Bruzzese, A.; Martino, E.A.; Mendicino, F.; Lucia, E.; Olivito, V.; Bova, C.; Filippelli, G.; Capodanno, I.; Neri, A.; Morabito, F.; et al. Iron chelation therapy. *Eur. J. Haematol.* **2023**, *110*, 490–497. [CrossRef] [PubMed]
102. Leitch, H.A.; Buckstein, R.; Zhu, N.; Nevill, T.J.; Yee, K.W.L.; Leber, B.; Keating, M.-M.; Hilaire, E.S.; Kumar, R.; Delage, R.; et al. Iron overload in myelodysplastic syndromes: Evidence based guidelines from the Canadian consortium on MDS. *Leuk. Res.* **2018**, *74*, 21–41. [CrossRef]
103. Gattermann, N. Iron overload in acquired sideroblastic anemias and MDS: Pathophysiology and role of chelation and luspatercept. *Hematology* **2024**, *2024*, 443–449. [CrossRef]
104. Liu, H.; Yang, N.; Meng, S.; Zhang, Y.; Zhang, H.; Zhang, W. Iron chelation therapy for myelodysplastic syndrome: A systematic review and meta-analysis. *Clin. Exp. Med.* **2020**, *20*, 1–9. [CrossRef] [PubMed]
105. Rodríguez-García, A.; Morales, M.L.; Garrido-García, V.; García-Baquero, I.; Leivas, A.; Carreño-Tarragona, G.; Sánchez, R.; Arenas, A.; Cedena, T.; Ayala, R.M.; et al. Protein Carbonylation in Patients with Myelodysplastic Syndrome: An Opportunity for Deferasirox Therapy. *Antioxidants* **2019**, *8*, 508. [CrossRef] [PubMed]
106. Steensma, D.P.; Gattermann, N. When is iron overload deleterious, and when and how should iron chelation therapy be administered in myelodysplastic syndromes? *Best Pract. Res. Clin. Haematol.* **2013**, *26*, 431–444. [CrossRef]
107. Kim, C.H.; Leitch, H.A. Iron overload-induced oxidative stress in myelodysplastic syndromes and its cellular sequelae. *Crit. Rev. Oncol. Hematol.* **2021**, *163*, 103367. [CrossRef] [PubMed]
108. Merkel, D.; Soffer, S.; Filanovsky, K.; Braester, A.; Fibach, E.; Dana, M.; Ofran, Y.; Greenbaum, U.; Nagler, A.; Amitai, I.; et al. The Effect of Oral Iron Chelator Deferiprone on Iron Overload and Oxidative Stress in Patients with Myelodysplastic Syndromes: A Study by the Israeli MDS Working Group. *Acta Haematol.* **2024**, *147*, 427–434. [CrossRef]
109. Cappellini, A.; Mongiorgi, S.; Finelli, C.; Fazio, A.; Ratti, S.; Marvi, M.V.; Curti, A.; Salvestrini, V.; Pellagatti, A.; Billi, A.M.; et al. Phospholipase C beta1 (PI-PLCβ1)/Cyclin D3/protein kinase C (PKC) alpha signaling modulation during iron-induced oxidative stress in myelodysplastic syndromes (MDS). *FASEB J.* **2020**, *34*, 15400–15416. [CrossRef]
110. Pilo, F.; Angelucci, E. A storm in the niche: Iron, oxidative stress and haemopoiesis. *Blood Rev.* **2018**, *32*, 29–35. [CrossRef]
111. Ivars, D.; Orero, M.T.; Javier, K.; Díaz-Vico, L.; García-Giménez, J.L.; Mena, S.; Tormos, C.; Egea, M.; Pérez, P.L.; Arrizabalaga, B.; et al. Oxidative imbalance in low/intermediate-1-risk myelodysplastic syndrome patients: The influence of iron overload. *Clin. Biochem.* **2017**, *50*, 911–917. [CrossRef] [PubMed]
112. Dixon, S.J.; Lemberg, K.M.; Lamprecht, M.R.; Skouta, R.; Zaitsev, E.M.; Gleason, C.E.; Patel, D.N.; Bauer, A.J.; Cantley, A.M.; Yang, W.S.; et al. Ferroptosis: An Iron-Dependent Form of Nonapoptotic Cell Death. *Cell* **2012**, *149*, 1060–1072. [CrossRef]
113. Zhang, J.; Liu, Y.; Li, Q.; Xu, A.; Hu, Y.; Sun, C. Ferroptosis in hematological malignancies and its potential network with abnormal tumor metabolism. *Biomed. Pharmacother.* **2022**, *148*, 112747. [CrossRef] [PubMed]
114. Guo, J.; Zhou, Y.; Liu, D.; Wang, M.; Wu, Y.; Tang, D.; Liu, X. Mitochondria as multifaceted regulators of ferroptosis. *Life Metab.* **2022**, *1*, 134–148. [CrossRef]

115. Hayashi, Y.; Harada, H. Mitochondrial dynamics as a pathobiological mediator of clonal myeloid disorders. *Cancer Sci.* **2023**, *114*, 2722–2728. [CrossRef] [PubMed]
116. Alberghina, L. The Warburg Effect Explained: Integration of Enhanced Glycolysis with Heterogeneous Mitochondria to Promote Cancer Cell Proliferation. *Int. J. Mol. Sci.* **2023**, *24*, 15787. [CrossRef]
117. Morganti, C.; Cabezas-Wallscheid, N.; Ito, K. Metabolic Regulation of Hematopoietic Stem Cells. *HemaSphere* **2022**, *6*, e740. [CrossRef]
118. Liao, Y.; Octaviani, S.; Tian, Z.; Wang, S.R.; Huang, C.; Huang, J. Mitochondrial quality control in hematopoietic stem cells: Mechanisms, implications, and therapeutic opportunities. *Stem Cell Res. Ther.* **2025**, *16*, 180. [CrossRef]
119. Guo, X.; Can, C.; Liu, W.; Wei, Y.; Yang, X.; Liu, J.; Jia, H.; Jia, W.; Wu, H.; Ma, D. Mitochondrial transfer in hematological malignancies. *Biomark. Res.* **2023**, *11*, 29. [CrossRef]
120. Dexheimer, G.M.; Alves, J.; Reckziegel, L.; Lazzaretti, G.; Abujamra, A.L. DNA methylation events as markers for diagnosis and management of acute myeloid leukemia and myelodysplastic syndrome. *Dis. Markers* **2017**, *2017*, 5472893. [CrossRef]
121. Gonçalves, A.C.; Alves, R.; Baldeiras, I.; Marques, B.; Oliveiros, B.; Pereira, A.; Costa, J.M.N.; Cortesão, E.; Vieira, L.M.; Ribeiro, A.B.S. DNA Methylation Is Correlated with Oxidative Stress in Myelodysplastic Syndrome—Relevance as Complementary Prognostic Biomarkers. *Cancers* **2021**, *13*, 3138. [CrossRef]
122. Gonçalves, A.C.; Cortesão, E.; Oliveiros, B.; Alves, V.; Espadana, A.I.; Rito, L.; Magalhães, E.; Pereira, S.; Pereira, A.; Costa, J.M.N.; et al. Oxidative stress levels are correlated with P15 and P16 gene promoter methylation in myelodysplastic syndrome patients. *Clin. Exp. Med.* **2016**, *16*, 333–343. [CrossRef] [PubMed]
123. Pulikkan, J.A.; Tenen, D.G.; Behre, G. C/EBPα deregulation as a paradigm for leukemogenesis. *Leukemia* **2017**, *31*, 2279–2285. [CrossRef] [PubMed]
124. Wen, X.-M.; Hu, J.-B.; Yang, J.; Qian, W.; Yao, D.-M.; Deng, Z.-Q.; Zhang, Y.-Y.; Zhu, X.-W.; Guo, H.; Lin, J.; et al. CEBPA methylation and mutation in myelodysplastic syndrome. *Med. Oncol.* **2015**, *32*, 192. [CrossRef]
125. Petzer, V.; Theurl, I.; Weiss, G.; Wolf, D. EnvIRONmental Aspects in Myelodysplastic Syndrome. *Int. J. Mol. Sci.* **2021**, *22*, 5202. [CrossRef]
126. Boy, M.; Bisio, V.; Zhao, L.-P.; Guidez, F.; Schell, B.; Lereclus, E.; Henry, G.; Villemonteix, J.; Rodrigues-Lima, F.; Gagne, K.; et al. Myelodysplastic syndrome associated TET2 mutations affect NK cell function and genome methylation. *Nat. Commun.* **2023**, *14*, 588. [CrossRef] [PubMed]
127. Harris, B.; Singh, D.K.; Verma, M.; Fahl, S.P.; Rhodes, M.; Sprinkle, S.R.; Wang, M.; Zhang, Y.; Perrigoue, J.; Kessel, R.; et al. Ribosomal protein control of hematopoietic stem cell transformation through direct, non-canonical regulation of metabolism. *bioRxiv* **2023**. [CrossRef]
128. Gonzalez-Menendez, P.; Phadke, I.; Olive, M.E.; Joly, A.; Papoin, J.; Yan, H.; Galtier, J.; Platon, J.; Kang, S.W.S.; McGraw, K.L.; et al. Arginine metabolism regulates human erythroid differentiation through hypusination of eIF5A. *Blood* **2023**, *141*, 2520–2536. [CrossRef]
129. Fandy, T.E.; Jiemjit, A.; Thakar, M.; Rhoden, P.; Suarez, L.; Gore, S.D. Decitabine Induces Delayed Reactive Oxygen Species (ROS) Accumulation in Leukemia Cells and Induces the Expression of ROS Generating Enzymes. *Clin. Cancer Res.* **2014**, *20*, 1249–1258. [CrossRef]
130. Lübbert, M.; Rüter, B.H.; Claus, R.; Schmoor, C.; Schmid, M.; Germing, U.; Kuendgen, A.; Rethwisch, V.; Ganser, A.; Platzbecker, U.; et al. A multicenter phase II trial of decitabine as first-line treatment for older patients with acute myeloid leukemia judged unfit for induction chemotherapy. *Haematologica* **2012**, *97*, 393–401. [CrossRef]
131. Montes, P.; Guerra-Librero, A.; García, P.; Cornejo-Calvo, M.E.; López, M.d.S.; de Haro, T.; Martínez-Ruiz, L.; Escames, G.; Acuña-Castroviejo, D. Effect of 5-Azacitidine Treatment on Redox Status and Inflammatory Condition in MDS Patients. *Antioxidants* **2022**, *11*, 139. [CrossRef] [PubMed]
132. Mpakou, V.; Spathis, A.; Bouchla, A.; Tsakiraki, Z.; Kontsioti, F.; Papageorgiou, S.; Bazani, E.; Gkontopoulos, K.; Thomopoulos, T.; Glezou, I.; et al. Upregulated hypoxia inducible factor 1α sig-naling pathway in high risk myelodysplastic syndrome and acute myeloid leukemia patients is associated with better response to 5-azacytidine—Data from the Hellenic myelodysplastic syndrome study group. *Hematol. Oncol.* **2021**, *39*, 231–242. [CrossRef] [PubMed]
133. Gillberg, L.; Ørskov, A.D.; Liu, M.; Harsløf, L.B.; Jones, P.A.; Grønbæk, K. Vitamin C—A new player in regulation of the cancer epigenome. *Semin. Cancer Biol.* **2018**, *51*, 59–67. [CrossRef] [PubMed]
134. Ottone, T.; Faraoni, I.; Fucci, G.; Divona, M.; Travaglini, S.; De Bellis, E.; Marchesi, F.; Angelini, D.F.; Palmieri, R.; Gurnari, C.; et al. Vitamin C Deficiency in Patients With Acute Myeloid Leukemia. *Front. Oncol.* **2022**, *12*, 890344. [CrossRef]
135. Cimmino, L.; Dolgalev, I.; Wang, Y.; Yoshimi, A.; Martin, G.H.; Wang, J.; Ng, V.; Xia, B.; Witkowski, M.T.; Mitchell-Flack, M.; et al. Restoration of TET2 Function Blocks Aberrant Self-Renewal and Leukemia Progression. *Cell* **2017**, *170*, 1079–1095.e20. [CrossRef]
136. Gonçalves, A.C.; Alves, V.; Silva, T.; Carvalho, C.; de Oliveira, C.R.; Sarmento-Ribeiro, A.B. Oxidative stress mediates apoptotic effects of ascorbate and dehydroascorbate in human Myelodysplasia cells in vitro. *Toxicol. Vitr.* **2013**, *27*, 1542–1549. [CrossRef]

137. Kumar, S.; Mathew, S.O.; Aharwal, R.P.; Tulli, H.S.; Mohan, C.D.; Sethi, G.; Ahn, K.-S.; Webber, K.; Sandhu, S.S.; Bishayee, A. Withaferin A: A Pleiotropic Anticancer Agent from the Indian Medicinal Plant *Withania somnifera* (L.) Dunal. *Pharmaceuticals* **2023**, *16*, 160. [CrossRef] [PubMed]
138. Oben, K.Z.; Alhakeem, S.S.; McKenna, M.K.; Brandon, J.A.; Mani, R.; Noothi, S.K.; Jinpeng, L.; Akunuru, S.; Dhar, S.K.; Singh, I.P.; et al. Oxidative stress-induced JNK/AP-1 signaling is a major pathway involved in selective apoptosis of myelodysplastic syndrome cells by Withaferin-A. *Oncotarget* **2017**, *8*, 77436–77452. [CrossRef]
139. Okamoto, S.; Tsujioka, T.; Suemori, S.; Kida, J.; Kondo, T.; Tohyama, Y.; Tohyama, K. Withaferin A suppresses the growth of myelodysplasia and leukemia cell lines by inhibiting cell cycle progression. *Cancer Sci.* **2016**, *107*, 1302–1314. [CrossRef]
140. Vannini, N.; Campos, V.; Girotra, M.; Trachsel, V.; Rojas-Sutterlin, S.; Tratwal, J.; Ragusa, S.; Stefanidis, E.; Ryu, D.; Rainer, P.Y.; et al. The NAD-booster nicotinamide riboside potently stimulates hematopoiesis through increased mitochondrial clearance. *Cell Stem Cell* **2019**, *24*, 405–418.e7. [CrossRef]
141. Torello, C.O.; Alvarez, M.C.; Saad, S.T.O. Polyphenolic flavonoid compound quercetin effects in the treatment of acute my-eloid leukemia and myelodysplastic syndromes. *Molecules* **2021**, *26*, 5781. [CrossRef] [PubMed]
142. Kim, Y.; Kim, Y.; Hwang, J.; Van Den Broek, T.J.; Oh, B.; Kim, J.Y.; Wopereis, S.; Bouwman, J.; Kwon, O. A Machine Learning Algorithm for Quantitatively Diag-nosing Oxidative Stress Risks in Healthy Adult Individuals Based on Health Space Methodology: A Proof-of-Concept Study Using Korean Cross-Sectional Cohort Data. *Antioxidants* **2021**, *10*, 1132. [CrossRef]
143. Idowu, S.O.; Fatokun, A.A. Artificial Intelligence (AI) to the Rescue: Deploying Machine Learning to Bridge the Biorelevance Gap in Antioxidant Assays. *SLAS Technol. Transl. Life Sci. Innov.* **2021**, *26*, 16–25. [CrossRef] [PubMed]
144. Jung, J.; Moon, J.-O.; Ahn, S.I.; Lee, H. Predicting antioxidant activity of compounds based on chemical structure using machine learning methods. *Korean J. Physiol. Pharmacol.* **2024**, *28*, 527–537. [CrossRef] [PubMed]
145. Liang, W.; Su, W.; Zhong, L.; Yang, Z.; Li, T.; Liang, Y.; Ruan, T.; Jiang, G. Comprehensive Characterization of Oxidative Stress-Modulating Chemicals Using GPT-Based Text Mining. *Environ. Sci. Technol.* **2024**, *58*, 20540–20552. [CrossRef]
146. Pushpakom, S.; Iorio, F.; Eyers, P.A.; Escott, K.J.; Hopper, S.; Wells, A.; Doig, A.; Guilliams, T.; Latimer, J.; McNamee, C.; et al. Drug repurposing: Progress, challenges and recom-mendations. *Nat. Rev. Drug Discov.* **2019**, *18*, 41–58. [CrossRef]
147. Tanoli, Z.; Vähä-Koskela, M.; Aittokallio, T. Artificial intelligence, machine learning, and drug repurposing in cancer. *Expert Opin. Drug Discov.* **2021**, *16*, 977–989. [CrossRef]
148. Issa, N.T.; Stathias, V.; Schürer, S.; Dakshanamurthy, S. Machine and deep learning approaches for cancer drug repurposing. *Semin. Cancer Biol.* **2021**, *68*, 132–142. [CrossRef]
149. Ambreen, S.; Umar, M.; Noor, A.; Jain, H.; Ali, R. Advanced AI and ML frameworks for transforming drug discovery and opti-mization: With innovative insights in polypharmacology, drug repurposing, combination therapy and nanomedicine. *Eur. J. Med. Chem.* **2025**, *284*, 117164. [CrossRef]

Disclaimer/Publisher's Note: The statements, opinions and data contained in all publications are solely those of the individual author(s) and contributor(s) and not of MDPI and/or the editor(s). MDPI and/or the editor(s) disclaim responsibility for any injury to people or property resulting from any ideas, methods, instructions or products referred to in the content.

International Journal of
Molecular Sciences

MDPI

Review

Oxidative Stress and Cerebral Vascular Tone: The Role of Reactive Oxygen and Nitrogen Species

Michele Salvagno [1,*], Elda Diletta Sterchele [1], Mario Zaccarelli [1], Simona Mrakic-Sposta [2], Ian James Welsby [3], Costantino Balestra [4,5,6,7] and Fabio Silvio Taccone [1]

1 Department of Intensive Care, Hôpital Universitaire de Bruxelles (HUB), 1000 Brussels, Belgium
2 Institute of Clinical Physiology—National Research Council (CNR-IFC), 20133 Milan, Italy
3 Department of Anesthesiology, Duke University Medical Center, Durham, NC 27710, USA
4 Environmental, Occupational, Aging (Integrative) Physiology Laboratory, Haute Ecole Bruxelles-Brabant (HE2B), 1160 Brussels, Belgium
5 Anatomical Research and Clinical Studies, Vrije Universiteit Brussels (VUB), 1050 Elsene, Belgium
6 DAN Europe Research Division (Roseto-Brussels), 1160 Brussels, Belgium
7 Motor Sciences Department, Physical Activity Teaching Unit, Université Libre de Bruxelles (ULB), 1050 Brussels, Belgium
* Correspondence: michele.salvagno@ulb.be

Abstract: The brain's unique characteristics make it exceptionally susceptible to oxidative stress, which arises from an imbalance between reactive oxygen species (ROS) production, reactive nitrogen species (RNS) production, and antioxidant defense mechanisms. This review explores the factors contributing to the brain's vascular tone's vulnerability in the presence of oxidative damage, which can be of clinical interest in critically ill patients or those presenting acute brain injuries. The brain's high metabolic rate and inefficient electron transport chain in mitochondria lead to significant ROS generation. Moreover, non-replicating neuronal cells and low repair capacity increase susceptibility to oxidative insult. ROS can influence cerebral vascular tone and permeability, potentially impacting cerebral autoregulation. Different ROS species, including superoxide and hydrogen peroxide, exhibit vasodilatory or vasoconstrictive effects on cerebral blood vessels. RNS, particularly NO and peroxynitrite, also exert vasoactive effects. This review further investigates the neuroprotective effects of antioxidants, including superoxide dismutase (SOD), vitamin C, vitamin E, and the glutathione redox system. Various studies suggest that these antioxidants could be used as adjunct therapies to protect the cerebral vascular tone under conditions of high oxidative stress. Nevertheless, more extensive research is required to comprehensively grasp the relationship between oxidative stress and cerebrovascular tone, and explore the potential benefits of antioxidants as adjunctive therapies in critical illnesses and acute brain injuries.

Keywords: oxidants; reactive oxygen species; reactive nitrogen species; antioxidants; cerebral vascular tone

1. Introduction

Brain tissue is exceptionally susceptible to the harmful effects of oxidative stress due to its unique characteristics. Despite accounting for only 2% of the body weight, the brain consumes approximately 20% of the total basal oxygen [1,2]. This heightened oxygen consumption is essential for ATP production, which is necessary to maintain the brain's high metabolic rate. Unfortunately, the electron transport chain in the mitochondria, responsible for ATP synthesis, leads to the leakage of reactive oxygen species (ROS) [3]. Consequently, the brain cells ceaselessly generate a significant amount of ROS. Additionally, the brain comprises non-replicating neuronal cells, possesses a high cell surface-to-cytoplasm ratio, and has a weak antioxidant capacity and a relatively low repair capacity. These structural and functional features further contribute to its high susceptibility and vulnerability to oxidative damage [4].

The regulation of vascular tone in cerebral vessels is controlled by both muscular and endothelial mechanisms [5]. The former is regulated by myogenic mechanisms originating from vascular smooth muscle. The latter is regulated by endothelial factors, such as nitric oxide and endothelin, which can decrease or increase the vascular tone, respectively. In addition, local hormones, metabolic by-products, ROS, reactive nitrogen species (RNS), and medications can influence and contribute to cerebral vascular tone. Notably, ROS can arise from all the layers of the vascular wall and adjacent tissues through several mechanisms, and, among these, the NADPH-oxidase enzyme may be the primary source of ROS production from the vascular cells [6].

This widespread existence of ROS within and surrounding cerebral blood vessels aligns with their ability to influence the vascular tone and vascular permeability [7–10], and their effects may be greater in the cerebral vasculature than in any other areas [11,12]. Even cerebral autoregulation (CAR), a complex physiological mechanism that adjusts cerebrovascular tone to maintain cerebral blood flow within desired ranges in response to changes in cerebral perfusion pressure, may be altered by ROS [13]. All these vascular effects may primarily come from the direct activity of ROS on ion channels [14,15], through their interrelation with RNS, particularly nitric oxide (NO), or other unknown vasoactive mechanisms. The balance of redox reactions, given by ROS and RNS, may be of clinical interest, especially in critically ill settings when high oxygen levels are frequently given to the patients (thus increasing reactive species production), or in acute brain injuries when these species are more frequently produced [16,17].

In the last few years, there has been an increasing interest in the physiology of ROS and RNS and how they can impact a patient's clinical status. Similarly, antioxidants have been applied as an adjunctive therapy in several clinical conditions. A thorough understanding of the mechanisms that regulate cerebrovascular tone is essential for further improving our knowledge of various brain injuries' pathophysiology. This narrative review offers a comprehensive understanding of ROS and RNS, and delivering a contemporary summary of research on how oxidants and antioxidants affect cerebrovascular tone modulation. It facilitates more knowledgeable investigations into this field, aiming to improve therapies for brain injury patients, for whom slight alterations in vascular tone may result in worsened outcomes.

2. Experimental Approach and Methodology

A comprehensive search was performed to gather relevant literature from PubMed, Scopus, and Google Scholar databases. The search covered studies published up to August 2023, utilizing combinations of keywords including "oxidative stress", "reactive oxygen species", "reactive nitrogen species", "cerebral vascular tone", and "antioxidants". Both text words and, where applicable, medical subject headings (MeSH) were employed to ensure a broad retrieval of pertinent studies. The search was limited to articles published in English. The selection criteria were designed to include studies contributing to understanding the interplay between oxidative stress and cerebral vascular tone, including original research articles, comprehensive review articles, and meta-analyses. The articles' references were also reviewed for additional papers to further explore relevant aspects.

3. Cerebral Vascular Tone

The vascular tone is defined by the contractile state of the vascular smooth muscle cells lining the blood vessels [18]. The cerebral vascular tone contributes to modulating cerebral blood flow (CBF) [19], ensuring sufficient oxygen and nutrients reach the brain tissue. In physiological situations where intracranial hypertension is absent, cerebrovascular tone predominantly defines the effective downstream pressure in the cerebral circulation, highlighting its significance as the principal factor in regulating this pressure [20]. For this reason, the maintenance of cerebrovascular tone plays a key role in the proper functioning of the cerebral vasculature, contributing to balancing the needs of the brain's metabolic demands with the systemic blood pressure and preventing conditions such as ischemia or hemorrhage, which can occur when CBF is either too low or too high, respectively. Disruptions in cerebrovascular tone regulation can contribute to insults in cerebrovascular diseases [21], such as stroke or brain injury.

The regulation of cerebrovascular tone involves neural, endothelial, and myogenic mechanisms [5]. Neural control is mediated primarily through the autonomic nervous system, with sympathetic, parasympathetic, and non-adrenergic non-cholinergic (NANC) pathways modulating vessel diameter. Myogenic mechanisms respond to changes in intravascular pressure to maintain constant CBF during fluctuations in systemic blood pressure, a phenomenon known as autoregulation. The endothelium contributes to cerebrovascular tone by producing vasodilators such as nitric oxide (NO) and prostacyclin, and vasoconstrictors like endothelin 1. Furthermore, cerebrovascular tone is influenced by metabolic factors, including CO_2 and O_2 levels [22,23]. Hypercapnia leads to vasodilation, increasing CBF, while hypocapnia causes vasoconstriction, reducing CBF. Similarly, hypoxia can induce vasodilation to enhance blood flow to oxygen-deprived areas of the brain [24]. Therefore, the regulation of cerebrovascular tone involves a complex interaction of multiple factors, including oxidative status, and is vital for preserving cerebral homeostasis, as its disruption can result in neurological deficits. To investigate the effects of oxidative stress in cerebral vasculature, a variety of experimental models and techniques have been explored in the literature and research, as outlined also in this review. These methods are summarized in Table 1.

Table 1. Experimental models and techniques for studying oxidative stress in cerebral vasculature. Overview of the various experimental approaches employed or that could be utilized to investigate the impacts of oxidative stress on cerebral vasculature. Each method offers a different point of view of the mechanisms by which ROS, RNS, and antioxidants may affect cerebral vascular tone and blood flow.

Model/Technique	Investigations on Cerebral Vasculature
Animal models (e.g., rats, rabbits, etc.) [25–27]	ROS/RNS effects on cerebral blood flow, microperfusion and autoregulation
In vitro studies [28–30]	Molecular mechanisms modulating the endothelial and smooth muscle cell response
Use of antioxidants [31–33]	Therapeutic neuroprotective therapies and modulation of vascular tone in oxidative stress conditions
Diagnostic tools	Non-invasive measurement of the effects of ROS/RNS on cerebral blood flow and metabolism
Pharmacological interventions	Investigation of the causal relationship among ROS, RNS, antioxidants, and vascular tone

4. Reactive Oxygen Species

The term Reactive Oxygen Species (ROS) refers to oxygen-containing chemical species that are unstable and highly reactive, capable of causing damage to various biological molecules. These species arise from the uptake of electrons from molecular oxygen, O_2.

The main mechanisms of the formation of ROS are depicted in Figure 1. Several mechanisms contribute to the generation of reactive oxygen species (ROS). Initially, during cellular respiration in mitochondria, electrons pass through protein complexes in the electron transport chain: when an electron leaks or is prematurely transferred to molecular oxygen, a superoxide anion (O_2^-) is created. Ionizing radiation, such as X-rays and gamma rays, can also ionize water molecules to produce hydroxyl radicals. Moreover, enzymatic reactions can inadvertently generate ROS, as can the Fenton Reaction (which can be simplified as $Fe^{2+} + H_2O_2 \rightarrow Fe^{3+} + OH^- + HO^\bullet$), where iron ($Fe^{2+}$) and hydrogen peroxide react to form hydroxyl radical ($HO^•$), and hydroxyl ion (OH^-) which is not a radical. Peroxisomes, which play roles in metabolism and detoxification, produce ROS and rely on catalase to break down hydrogen peroxide into water and oxygen. This process can lead to an excess of ROS if catalase is overwhelmed. Additionally, the enzyme NOX produces superoxide ions by transferring electrons from NADPH to oxygen. Endoplasmic Reticulum (ER) stress and the Unfolded Protein Response also contribute to ROS production. Indeed, the ER, responsible for protein synthesis, folding, and modification, can become stressed by an overload of misfolded proteins due to factors like nutrient deprivation, hypoxia, and calcium level changes. This stress can induce oxidative stress, while the cell's response, aimed at restoring ER homeostasis, increases mitochondrial activity, and thereby ROS production. Lastly, xenobiotics subjected to metabolization and microbes, either during their metabolism or as a defense mechanism, can generate ROS.

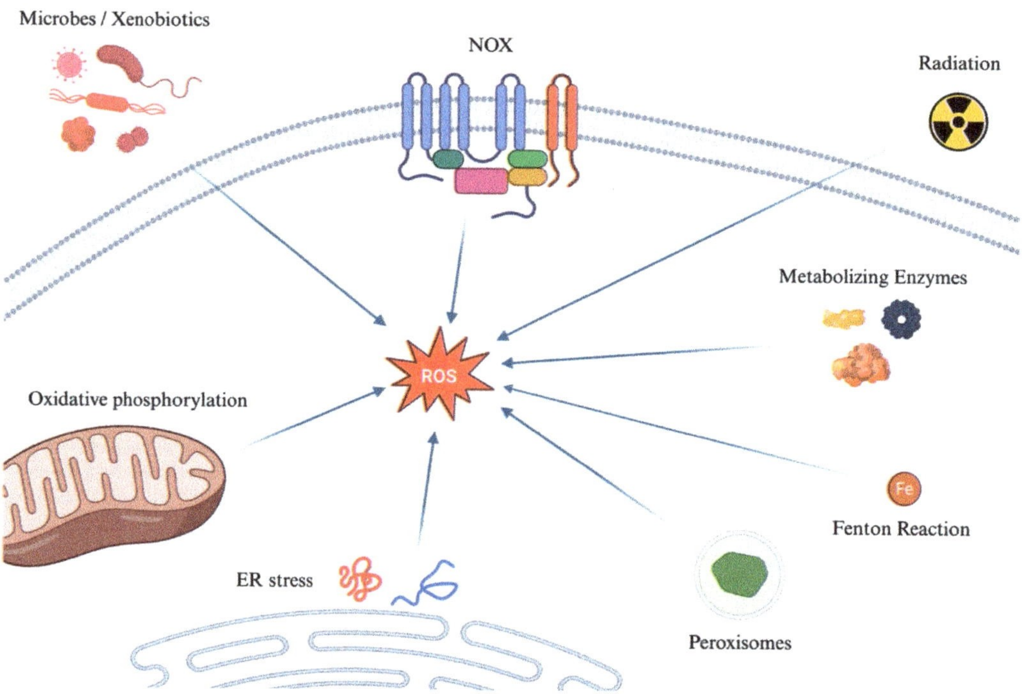

Figure 1. A graphical summary of the main pathways of the formation of ROS. Reactive oxygen species (ROS) are generated through various mechanisms, impacting cellular functions positively and negatively. They originate from microbes and xenobiotics metabolism, NOX enzyme activity, ionizing radiation effects, and metabolic enzymes, leading to superoxide, hydroxyl radicals, and other ROS forms. The Fenton reaction, peroxisomes' metabolic activities, and the breakdown of fatty acids further contribute to ROS accumulation. Endoplasmic reticulum stress and the unfolded protein response enhance oxidative stress by increasing mitochondrial activity and oxidative phosphorylation, where electron leakage can form superoxide. ROS: Reactive Oxygen Species. NOX: NADPH oxidase. ER: Endoplasmic Reticulum.

Given their strong ability to react chemically with their environment, ROS are well known to lead to several pathological consequences [34]. Surprisingly, depending on the specific context, ROS can exhibit both protective and deleterious effects on the organism, with the same molecule exerting opposing effects on biological processes [35]. The impact of these effects relies on the interplay between the production of ROS and their clearance rates, wherein antioxidants and scavengers assume a critical role [36]. When this balance is disrupted, these reactive molecules can interact unopposed with, and damage, vital cellular components such as DNA, proteins, and lipids. This molecular damage can compromise the normal functions of cells, leading to tissue injury. This harmful state, characterized by the overwhelming presence of oxidative species and the resultant cellular and tissue damage, is termed "oxidative stress" [34].

4.1. Generation Pathways of Reactive Oxygen Species

As previously mentioned, ROS originate from O_2, a diradical, meaning it has two unpaired electrons in its molecular orbital. Despite being relatively stable under standard conditions, its diradical nature makes O_2 more reactive than if it were a closed-shell molecule, and prone to participate in various chemical reactions, especially those involving electron transfer.

When O_2 acquires an electron, primarily from the mitochondrial electron transport chain as earlier described, it gives rise to superoxide anion (O_2^-). This species carries both a negative electric charge and an unpaired electron, making it both an anion and a radical. It can be seen as the precursor to ROS and it also plays a role in the formation of RNS. It is a free radical, i.e., a molecule that contains one free unpaired electron in its outer orbital. However, O_2^- does not seem to act as a potent oxidizing agent despite its name. Instead, its detrimental effects stem from its secondary interactions, particularly when it reacts with nitric oxide (NO). Due to its low permeability, the actions of superoxide are primarily related to the compartment in which it is produced; however, it can also influence the surrounding cellular environment by crossing the cell's ion channels, exerting its effects at a distance from the production point, even with a half-life, at normal pH, of about 5 s [37].

Hydrogen peroxide (H_2O_2) is generated from O_2^- through a reaction called dismutation (i.e., a reaction in which the same species is both reduced and oxidized), in which two superoxide molecules are transformed in H_2O_2 and O_2, catalyzed by the enzyme superoxide dismutase (SOD). H_2O_2 is not a free radical, and therefore it does not directly oxidize other molecules. However, it can move quickly through the cell membranes and, transforming into a potent compound (hydroxyl radical, described further in the text), it can exert the effects of ROS at different sites instead of its production site. Indeed, due to a non-enzymatic reaction that requires iron in its reduced state (Fe^{2+}), known as the Fenton reaction, the most reactive compound known, hydroxyl radical ($HO^\bullet$), can be generated from H_2O_2. The $OH^\bullet$ can also be formed through the reaction between O_2^- and nitric oxide (NO), and the Haber–Weiss reaction (which can be simplified as $O_2^- + H_2O_2 \rightarrow HO^\bullet + OH^- + O_2$) [13,38]. Due to its tendency to react quickly with the first available molecule, this radical has a short half-life [36]. To prevent the continuation of the reaction chain, catalases can decompose H_2O_2 into water and O_2, thereby preventing the formation of $HO^\bullet$. Because of this cooperative capability, both SOD and catalase are classified as antioxidants.

The main ROS described and their formation mechanisms are schematically depicted in Figure 2.

4.2. The Effects of ROS on Cerebral Vascular Tone

In the brain, whose metabolism relies almost exclusively on the presence of oxygen, ROS appear to have a decisive influence on cerebral flow [13,39]. Indeed, the brain has a unique neurovascular coupling structure, facilitating functional and anatomical interactions among neurons, astrocytes, pericytes, microglia, and blood vessels, known as the neurovascular unit [40]. This unit allows the selective adaptation of blood flow in different brain regions, influenced by ROS and NO, which act on smooth muscle cells and pericytes [13,41]. For example, in animal models, ROS have been shown to have a role in microvascular reperfusion disturbances [25].

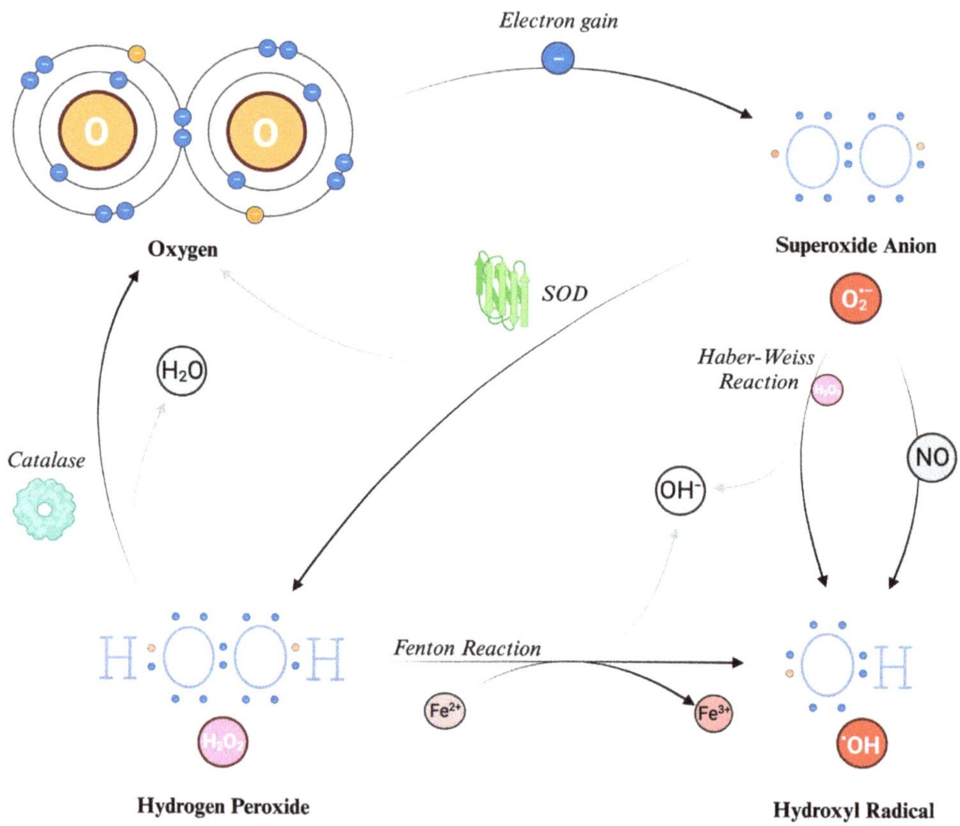

Figure 2. Reactive Oxygen Species (ROS): their structure and formation. The process begins with molecular oxygen (O_2), which has two unpaired electrons in the outer orbital. Thus, it can acquire an electron to form the superoxide anion (O_2^-), which is a radical (i.e., with an unpaired electron). Superoxide dismutase (SOD) converts superoxide into hydrogen peroxide (H_2O_2) and oxygen. Catalases can further break down H_2O_2 into water and oxygen. The Haber–Weiss reaction generates hydroxyl radicals ($HO^\bullet$) and hydroxyl ions (OH^-) from superoxide and H_2O_2. The Fenton reaction also produces hydroxyl radicals and hydroxyl ions by reducing H_2O_2 in the presence of iron ions. O: oxygen atom. H: hydrogen atom. H_2O: water molecule. O_2^-: superoxide anion. H_2O_2: hydrogen peroxide. $HO^\bullet$: hydroxyl radical. OH^-: hydroxyl ion. NO: nitric oxide. Fe^{2+}: iron in reduced state. Fe^{3+}: iron in oxidized state. SOD: superoxide dismutase.

ROS can affect cerebral vascular smooth muscle tone in several biochemical pathways [42], potentially in a more pronounced way in the presence of cerebrovascular diseases [43]. The overall vasoactive effect varies based on (1) the specific type of molecule involved and (2) its concentration. For example, O_2^- can act as a direct endothelium-dependent vasodilator and a smooth muscle vasoconstrictor through the inactivation of NO [44,45]. Indeed, O_2^-, as well as H_2O_2, can affect the vascular tone, causing vasodilation, by activating calcium-dependent potassium channels (K_{ca}), which are the most common K^+ channel expressed on cerebral arteriolar musculature, and which are sensitive to the redox state of the environment [13]. By contrast, O_2^- leads to vasoconstriction through a powerful inhibition of endothelial NO-mediated dilation. The equilibrium between these two opposite results depends on the net concentration of the reactive species. Indeed, findings from numerous in vitro and in vivo animal studies confirm that both O_2^- and H_2O_2 exhibit a biphasic impact on cerebral blood vessels, contingent upon their concentration.

At low concentrations, O_2^- leads to vasodilation, while at high concentrations, it causes vasoconstriction. Similarly, H_2O_2, when present in very high concentrations, may initially induce vasoconstriction, and later lead to vasodilation [44].

In addition to the aforementioned mechanisms, the modulation of cerebral arteriolar tone through chloride channels has also been suggested [46]. Moreover, O_2^- can react with arachidonic acid and other unsaturated fatty acids to form isoprostanes. These are known as strong vasoconstrictors that can cause a reduction in cerebral blood flow. Thus, O_2^- can indirectly further affect vascular tone, and may be of pathological interest in traumatic brain injuries [13,44]. Finally, H_2O_2 would also act in some cases as a membrane depolarizer, exerting, with hyperpolarization, a vasodilatory effect [13,44,45].

Lastly, the production rates of ROS and antioxidants vary according to different oxygenation levels, each following unique kinetic patterns [35,47]. Therefore, it is conceivable to assume that the vasoactive activity of ROS, as well as RNS and antioxidants, may depend not only on the types of ROS and their concentration, but also on a third feature, i.e., the kinetics of their production and degradation. Indeed, compensatory mechanisms might come into play when a stimulus enters a new steady state. This can occur especially in pathological conditions, such as in acute brain injury or in critically ill patients, where elevated ROS levels may increase acutely, and persist for an extended period.

The vascular impacts of ROS on cerebrovascular tone are diverse and involve complex mechanisms. These also include interactions with NO and RNS, which will be further discussed later.

4.3. NADPH Oxidases

The nicotinamide adenine dinucleotide (phosphate) oxidases (NADH/NADPH oxidases, or Nox) are prominently involved in the enzymatic generation of ROS [48]. These membrane-bound enzymes produce superoxide radicals by utilizing NADH or NADPH as electron donors. In mammals, there exist seven isoforms of Nox. Among them, Nox1, Nox2, Nox4, and Nox5 are expressed in various tissues, such as the endothelium, vascular smooth muscle cells, fibroblasts, and perivascular adipocytes [49]. Under normal physiological conditions, vascular Nox exhibits a relatively low baseline activity. However, in response to various stimuli, like cytokines, the enzyme activity can be augmented both in the short term and over an extended period. This response to stimuli disrupts vascular homeostasis, leading to pathological changes and associated health issues, such as increased blood pressure [50].

The involvement of NADH and NADPH reinforces the notion that the redox state is critical in influencing the tone of cerebral circulation. Indeed, interestingly, studies have shown that NADPH oxidase activity occurs at a significantly higher magnitude in cerebral arteries than in systemic arteries [12]. As electron acceptors, both NADH and NADPH facilitate the activity of Nox enzymes, leading to the production of O_2^- [26,39], which is, in the end, responsible for the impact on the vascular tone. Thus, ROS production derived from NADPH oxidase may contribute both to maintaining normal physiological vascular tone and to vascular pathology.

4.4. ROS as Signaling Molecules in HIF-1α Regulation

ROS have more effects than expected, and they could work as signal molecules. In this way, it is thought that ROS play a role in the degradation of Hypoxia Inducible Factor HIF-1α, as there is evidence of a negative correlation between HIF-1α and ROS [41]. HIF-1α is a cytosolic transcription factor that moves to the nucleus during hypoxia. It binds to HIF-β and activates the expression of genes containing hypoxia-responsive elements (HRE), producing hypoxia-related proteins such as erythropoietin (EPO). The production of ROS is implicated in the proposed "normobaric oxygen paradox" [51], whereby intermittent hyperoxic stimulation could paradoxically mimic a hypoxic-like condition, leading to the activation of HIF-1α [52]. Moreover, ROS production via NADPH oxidase, especially Nox2, may intervene in the evoked HIF-1α synthesis and stability [53]. These mechanisms may be especially relevant in brain cells, as they tend to increase ROS production under injured conditions. However, the existence of this phenomenon and its potential effects on brain tissue have not yet been thoroughly investigated.

4.5. Regional Variability in Oxidative Stress Responses within Brain Vasculature

It has been observed that the mechanisms that intervene in oxidative equilibrium may show differences between the contexts of cerebral and systemic circulation [12,54]. Indeed, differences may be seen in susceptibility to oxidative stress among the cerebral microvessels in various brain regions [55]. Additionally, neurons situated in particular areas of the brain, such as the hippocampus and the cerebellar granule cell layer, are more prone to oxidative stress [56]. These regional differences may also be influenced by the local availability of NO during brain injuries, which has been demonstrated in experimental animal models [27]. Therefore, it appears conceivable that even small changes in ROS and RNS concentrations can lead to clinical changes via their effect on the brain vasculature, especially during brain injuries and cerebrovascular diseases. Nevertheless, further human research is required to gain data and a deeper comprehension of these aspects, moving beyond theoretical discourses.

5. Reactive Nitrogen Species

Reactive Nitrogen Species (RNS) are a group of highly reactive nitrogen-containing molecules that are generated as by-products of nitrogen metabolism. These molecules are crucial in various physiological and pathological processes, including vascular control [57].

5.1. Generation Pathways of the Main Reactive Nitrogen Species

Nitric oxide (NO) is the most well-known and significant member of the RNS family. Also formerly known as endothelium-derived relaxing factor (EDRF), it is constantly generated in the body through the enzymatic action of nitric oxide synthases (NOS) on L-arginine and oxygen. There are three distinct isoforms of NOS present in the body: iNOS (inducible), eNOS (endothelial), and nNOS (neuronal) [58,59]. NOS generates in loco NO, which readily exerts its biological activity. Although its half-life is limited to a few seconds, NO can react with hemoglobin, forming S-nitroso hemoglobin, or be converted to nitrite. S-nitroso hemoglobin (SNO-Hb) is a derivative of hemoglobin modified by adding a NO group to a cysteine thiol group, in a reaction called S-nitrosylation.

Nitrite (NO_2^-) is a chemical compound that consists of one nitrogen atom and two oxygen atoms. It is an anion that can form salts such as sodium nitrite ($NaNO_2$) or potassium nitrite (KNO_2). SNO-Hb and NO_2^- salts act as NO reservoirs, which can be transported through systemic circulation and released under certain conditions to promote vasodilation and increase blood flow to tissues distant from the site of origin [60,61].

Other molecules can be categorized into RNS, produced as metabolites in NO decomposition or by reactions between other compounds such as CO_2 and ROS. For example, peroxynitrite ($ONOO^-$) is formed from the reaction between NO and superoxide ions, thus reducing NO concentrations [62]. Although evidence suggests that NOS is responsible for nitroxyl (HNO) production, it is still unclear how this compound is synthesized in vivo [63,64]. Indeed, HNO can also be generated after the reduction in NO levels by mitochondrial cytochrome C, xanthine oxidase, ubiquinol, hemoglobin, and manganese superoxide dismutase (SOD) [64].

Nitrate (NO_3^-) is a chemical compound that consists of one nitrogen atom and three oxygen atoms. Similarly to NO_2^-, it carries a negative charge and is thus found in salt chemical form. A significant amount of nitrate comes from leafy green vegetables. Salivary glands actively take up nitrate from circulation, resulting in a saliva concentration 10-fold higher than in plasma [65]. A certain quantity of NO_3^- is converted to NO_2^- by reductase enzymes in the salivary glands [65]. Finally, some nitrites are absorbed when ingested and become part of the "nitrate–nitrite–nitric oxide pathway" [66]. Kapil et al. have demonstrated how nitrate supplementation can lower blood pressure, and that depleting oral microbiomes can jeopardize endogenous nitrate production, leading to hypertension [67]. There are other endogenous ways to synthesize nitrate and nitrite [66]. Over the years, many trials have established the conversion of NO to nitrite as occurring naturally in vivo. This reaction has been linked to hypoxia, deoxyhemoglobin, and lower pH [68–72]. Furthermore, a significant increase in plasma nitrite was displayed during the administration of 80 ppm iNO in a murine model [73]. Given all these observations, nitrates and nitrites can be considered a NO reservoir [74]. Indeed, while NO has a half-life limited to 2 ms, that of nitrite is much longer, and can quickly spread all over the organism [66].

The formation of the main RNS described is schematically depicted in Figure 3.

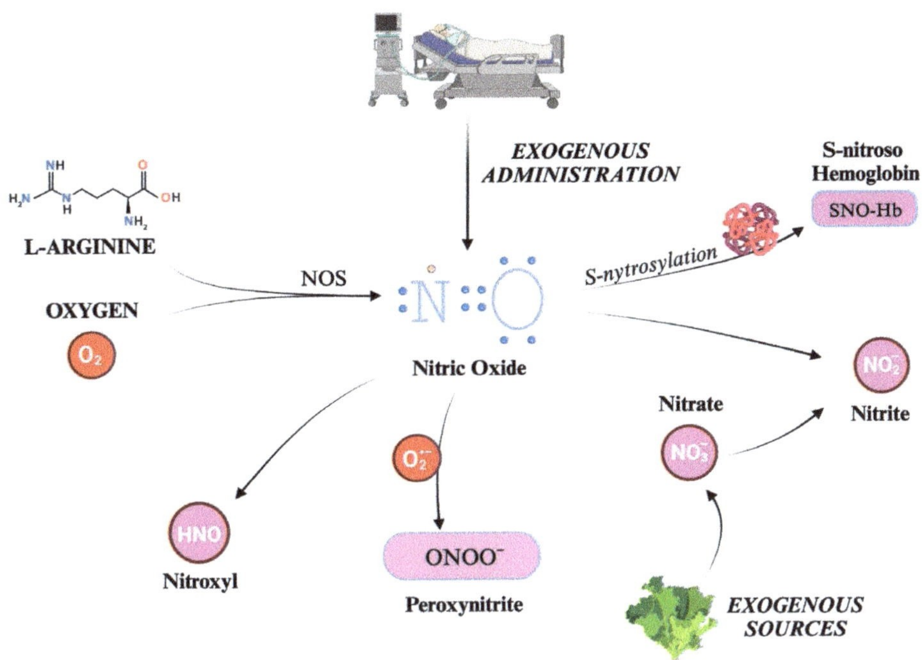

Figure 3. Overview of the main reactive nitrogen species (RNS) and their formation pathways. The figure illustrates the generation of nitric oxide (NO), a small, gaseous molecule that acts as a signaling molecule in the body. It is produced by the enzyme nitric oxide synthase (NOS) from the amino acid L-arginine and molecular oxygen. S-nitrosylation adds a NO group to the thiol group of a cysteine residue, for example, Hb. Otherwise, NO can be transformed into salts or esters of nitrous acid, containing the anion nitrite (NO_2^-), which can be converted back to NO under certain conditions. Nitrates are taken into the body from external sources, such as food or supplements. They can be converted into nitrites (and thus potentially into NO). This process is known as the nitrate–nitrite–NO pathway and is an alternative source of NO, especially when the enzymatic production of NO is impaired. Peroxynitrite is a highly reactive nitrogen species formed by NO with O^{2-}. Finally, nitroxyl (HNO) is an isoelectronic reactive nitrogen species with NO, formed by the reduction of NO or the decomposition of certain NO donors. O_2: molecular oxygen. NO: nitric oxide. NOS: nitric oxide synthase. N: nitrogen atom. Hb: hemoglobin. NO_2^-: nitrite. NO_3^-: nitrate. $ONOO^-$: peroxynitrite. HNO: nitroxyl.

5.2. The Effects of RNS on Cerebral Vascular Tone

5.2.1. Nitric Oxide

Since its recognition as an endothelium-derived relaxing factor [75,76], several studies have described NO as a strong vasodilator agent [58]. After being synthesized in the endothelium, NO increases the levels of cyclic guanosine monophosphate (cGMP) in smooth muscles by stimulating soluble guanylyl cyclase. cGMP finally inhibits the proteins responsible for contraction, causing vasorelaxation [58,77]. In adjunct to this mechanism, NO induces a reduction in intracellular calcium, mediated by ATPases that actively transport calcium inside the sarcoplasmic/endoplasmic reticulum [58,77]. Other pathways toward vasodilation include the reduction in 20-hydroxyeicosatetraenoic acid [78] and prostaglandins [79]. NO may be key in regulating cerebral blood flow (CBF) [80]. Indeed, in hyperoxia [81–83], hypoxia [81,82], and hypercapnia [84], it was found to be an essential mediator of CBF in animal models. Moreover, NO also plays a leading role in coupling CBF and neuronal activity [85].

Interestingly, CO_2 may act as a regulator of NO. Indeed, the process of adjusting cerebral vascular tone in response to changes in arterial carbon dioxide partial pressure ($PaCO_2$) is known as chemoregulation, which could be the main trigger of endothelial NO-release [86]. In humans, hypocapnia leads to vasoconstriction and reduced CBF, while hypercapnia and changes in perivascular pH result in vasodilation and increased CBF [86]. Cerebral endothelial cells and astrocytes have been shown to release NO under normocapnic conditions, while NO production increases during hypercapnia and decreases during hypocapnia, regardless of pH levels [87]. It has been proposed that these NO variations in response to $PaCO_2$ are specific to NOS regulation, and that administering exogenous NO may influence the CO_2-dependent chemoregulation mechanism [87].

Several studies have explored the role of NO in critical neurologic illnesses. Indeed, early stages of severe brain injuries recognize a depletion of NO, probably contributing to secondary brain damage [88]. By contrast, when present, NO reduces injuries and has neuroprotective properties in ischemia/reperfusion animal models, both in relation to stroke and cardiac arrest [88]. For this reason, a prospective trial has been performed, proving the feasibility of iNO administration in cardiac arrest, and showing promising results in terms of survival [89]. In subarachnoid hemorrhage, NOS inactivation is associated with alterations in microvascular density and hemostasis, leading to rebleeding, intracranial hypertension, and larger hemorrhage volume [90]. Conversely, NO reduction is also correlated with a lower grade of neuroinflammation and better neurobehavioral function in rats [91]. Studies in humans have showed a correlation between elevated asymmetric dimethylarginine (which is an inhibitor of iNOS, and thus of the vasodilator molecule NO) and vasospasm and worse outcomes [92]. Another small human study found elevated levels of NO metabolites, especially in subjects with poorer outcomes [93]. Although the results may be controversial, the literature suggests deleterious effects of NO depletion, supported by increased microthrombi formation and reduced cortical activity [88]. A pilot human trial established the safety of iNO administration and showed promising results in treating delayed cerebral ischemia [94].

Pathways in traumatic brain injury (TBI) appear more complex. Mechanical insults may induce the upregulation of iNOS and the over-production of NO and $ONOO^-$. The RNS stimulate the production of glutamate, which triggers nNOS. Nevertheless, NO plays an uncertain role in this disease, and its implications are still unknown [95]. Studies in newborn animal models are also contradictory. Some reports showed protective properties of NO related to vasodilation, reducing ROS concentrations and scavenging radicals; others linked it to deleterious effects and greater brain injuries. These discrepancies might depend on the production timing and NO concentrations [96]. The brain controls blood flow by interacting with vessel diameter. Autoregulation ensures constant blood supply; changes in systemic blood pressure induce vasodilation or vasoconstriction. Additionally, the brain increases blood flow in areas where neurons are more active through a mechanism named neurovascular coupling. Although other pathways and elements participate, NO plays a significant role in both of them. NOS inhibition (and thus the lowering of NO production) increases the lower limit of mean arterial blood pressure where autoregulation acts, reducing its efficiency. Through neurovascular coupling, blood flow is directed to more active areas, where glutamate (the main excitatory neurotransmitter) induces calcium entry in neurons and the activation of neuronal nNOS, finally resulting in NO production and vasodilation [79].

Finally, as a NO reservoir, the vasodilating effects of nitrites have long been investigated. Although some studies failed to find any vasoactive activity [97], most studies confirmed that nitrite has vasorelaxant effects through the activation of guanylate cyclase [60,98–101].

In summary, NO is a potent vasodilator, playing diverse roles in regulating blood flow and brain protection. Its mechanism is intricate and involves numerous interactions. When it comes to brain injuries, a deficiency in NO could contribute to secondary brain damage, while NO possesses neuroprotective qualities in animal models of ischemia/reperfusion, including stroke. Interestingly, NO inhalation has been suggested as a neuroprotective intervention during cardiopulmonary resuscitation [102]. Consequently, extensive research is needed to better understand its mechanisms and potential therapeutic effects.

5.2.2. Peroxynitrite

Peroxynitrite ($ONOO^-$) has shown vasoactive properties, producing vasorelaxation in arterioles in vitro [28] and in vivo [36], although its potency seems very low, and is up to 50-fold less than that of NO [103]. The effect does not appear to involve the endothelium [104], and the vasoactive mechanism remains unclear. Some authors have proposed that the effect is linked to the opening of ATP-sensitive potassium channels [36,105], directly activating the channels or reducing ATP concentration by interfering with cellular metabolism [36,105,106]. Other mechanisms proposed to explain this vasodilating activity include the elevation of cGMP levels, membrane hyperpolarization via K^+ channel activation, the activation of myosin phosphatase activity, and interference with cytosolic calcium movement and cellular membrane Ca^{2+} entry [28].

However, in contrast with all the above results, Daneva et al. induced an increase in $ONOO^-$ by upregulating iNOS in mice, reporting an increase in pulmonary arterial pressure by impeding calcium entry in smooth muscle cells of pulmonary arteries [107]. Similarly, Ottolini et al. investigated the same pathway in diet-induced obese mice, finding a link between obese hypertension and high $ONOO^-$ levels [108]. Finally, in vitro studies [29, 30] have observed that peroxynitrite may induce vasoconstriction in cerebral arteries. This effect is likely due to the inhibition of the cerebral K^+-dependent calcium channel. Interestingly, the addition of glutathione inhibited this cerebral vasoconstrictive effect.

Therefore, the net effects of peroxynitrite appear conflicting, and are not completely understood, but are probably dose- and time-dependent [109].

5.2.3. Nitroxyl

HNO has been proven to act as an endothelium-derived vasorelaxant [110–113] that is not susceptible to tolerance [111]. Moreover, HNO has multiple effects, including inhibiting platelet aggregation, limiting vascular smooth muscle proliferation, and interacting with metallo and thiol-containing proteins.

Although we failed to find in the literature any research focused on the impact of this molecule on cerebral tone, we have reported its effects on the general vasculature. Indeed, HNO promotes vasodilation by activating several molecular pathways [64,112–114]. These pathways include the stimulation of soluble guanylyl cyclase (sGC), leading to an increase in cGMP. From animal studies, it has been inferred that the sGC-cGMP pathway may be necessary and sufficient for HNO-induced vasodilation in vivo [115]. Others proposed that HNO may activate ATP-sensitive potassium (K_{ATP}) channels and voltage-dependent potassium (K_V) channels, resulting in the outflow of potassium ions. This causes the cell membrane to become hyperpolarized and leads to a reduction in intracellular calcium levels. Finally, following an elegant animal study, Eberhardt et al. suggested HNO-mediated vasodilation via the transient receptor potential channel A1 (TRPA1) and calcitonin gene-related peptide (CGRP) [116]. This HNO–TRPA1–CGRP signaling pathway could be a crucial component in the neuroendocrine regulation of vascular tone, mediated by HNO.

Figure 4 presents a visual abstract illustrating how ROS and RNS might influence the cerebrovascular tone.

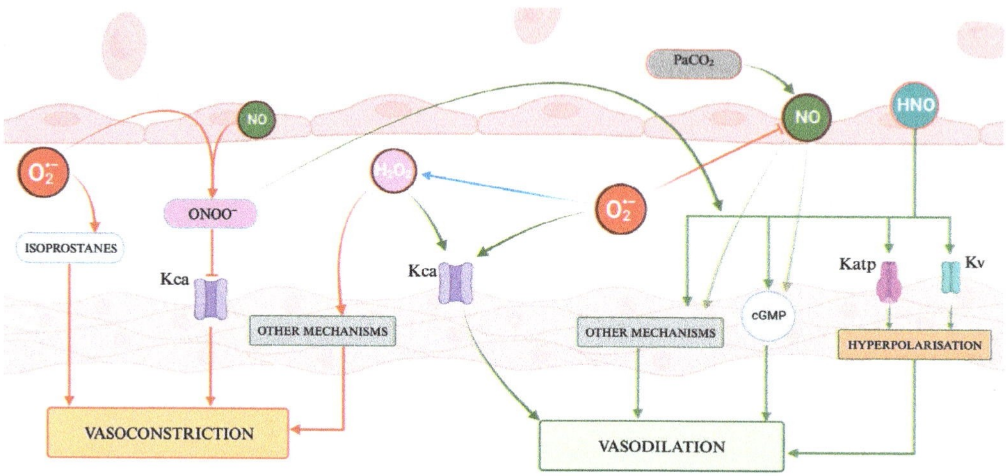

Figure 4. A representation of the regulation of vascular tone by Reactive Oxygen Species and nitric species. ROS presents a dual role, with hydrogen peroxide acting as a signaling molecule inducing vasodilation through the activation of potassium channels and vasoconstriction through other mechanisms, while superoxide contributes to vasodilation by affecting K_{ca} channels and vasoconstriction by generating isoprostanes. Nitric oxide and the other RNS mainly promote vasodilation via cGMP and several mechanisms. The balance of vasoactive molecules and their net effect on vascular smooth muscle contribute to determining the cerebral vascular tone.

6. Antioxidants

Antioxidants are substances that protect from the deleterious effects of free radicals. Their action, which can be enzymatic and non-enzymatic, can be further divided into two groups: (1) preventing the generation of ROS and blocking the generated ROS, and (2) repairing the damages the free radicals have caused.

Reducing the level of antioxidants leads to an increase in oxidative stress, thus indirectly influencing the cerebrovascular tone. Indeed, a more oxidative cellular environment can contribute to an increase in vascular tone by reducing the activity of NO [117,118]. For this reason, antioxidant mechanisms are widely expressed in vascular cells and brain tissue.

6.1. Superoxide Dismutase

Superoxide dismutase (SOD) is an enzymatic defense system catalyzing O_2^- into H_2O_2. It exists in three different forms: copper–zinc SOD (SOD1 or Cu-Zn SODI), manganese SOD (SOD2 or MnSOD), and extracellular SOD (SOD3 or ecSOD). These are some of the most important protective mechanisms against oxidative stress in the body, and decreased SOD levels may be associated with a worse outcome in acute ischemic stroke (AIS) patients, faster vascular damage, and blood–brain barrier breakdown [119]. SOD has been proposed as a marker of cardiovascular alterations in hypertensive and diabetic patients, as fluctuations in serum levels are linked to alterations in vascular structure and function [120].

SOD1 is predominantly found in the cytoplasm and nucleus of cells, where it helps neutralize superoxide radicals generated during normal metabolic processes. The copper and zinc ions are essential to its enzymatic activity. SOD2 is usually located in the mitochondria, thus representing a critical defense mechanism against oxidative damage to mitochondrial components. Finally, SOD3 is primarily found in the extracellular matrix and fluids, acting as a defense outside the cells, protecting from oxidative stress caused by superoxide radicals released from inflammatory cells. Moreover, it is active in the arterial wall, strategically between the endothelium and smooth muscle, thus controlling reactivity to oxygen levels and vascular tone [83] by regulating nitric oxide. Indeed, from animal studies, we can infer that SOD regulates in vivo both the basal tone and the vascular response to different pressures of oxygen [83]. In TBI patients, SOD levels may be reduced already during the first day, and may remain low for 7 days [121]. Indeed, exogenous SOD has been proposed as a therapeutic adjunct in several conditions [122], and it may reduce vasospasm after SAH [123]. The reduction in cerebral vasospasm in experimental SAH animal models obtained by administering SOD [31] underscores the significant involvement of superoxide anions and redox equilibrium in vascular regulation, particularly under pathological conditions.

6.2. Glutathione Redox System

Glutathione peroxidase (GPx) is an enzyme that reduces hydrogen peroxide to water via a tripeptide called glutathione (GSH). GSH is the most common thiol, i.e., a molecule that contains a sulfhydryl group (SH), and is present in the cytosol and its organelles. Composed of glutamine, cysteine, and glycine, glutathione works as an electron donor, passing from its reduced state (GSH), the active form, to an oxidized state (GSSG). The enzyme glutathione reductase converts GSSG back into GSH, using NADPH as an electron donor. GPx plays a central role in reducing hydrogen peroxide to water, keeping it away from the production of hydroxyl radicals. Moreover, GSH can directly and independently neutralize free radicals, acting as a non-enzymatic antioxidant. Indeed, it can donate electrons to free radicals, an activity called "scavenging", oxidizing them to form GSSG.

This mechanism is one of the most important antioxidant processes in the body. Indeed, GSH is the most abundant intracellular antioxidant, as its concentration within the cytoplasm where it is produced is in the mmol range, where the ratio GSH:GSSG is normally maintained around 100:1 (but it can fall lower than 10:1 during oxidative stress). It can move into the extracellular fluids, but plasma levels are 1000 times less concentrated than intracellular levels. An exception is in the lining fluid in the lungs, where the concentration is 140 times higher than in the plasma.

Other molecules can also intervene in this system. For example, as already described, NADPH serves to keep GSH reduced. The pentose phosphate pathway generates NADPH, and glucose-6-phosphate dehydrogenase (G6PD) is one of the enzymes in the pathway. Deficiency of this enzyme, which affects millions of people worldwide, can result in GSH deficiency, predisposing one to oxidative injury. Thiamine is a cofactor inhibiting the pentose phosphate. Indeed, evidence has been found that thiamine administration may alleviate oxidative stress, even in cases where it is not attributable to thiamine deficiency [124,125]. Finally, selenium is necessary to glutathione peroxidase activity. Indeed, this enzyme contains selenium in the active site [126]. In sepsis and septic shock, selenium is abnormally low and, when infused, has been shown to reduce mortality [127]. This has also been reported by a recent meta-analysis, even if with a low quality of evidence [128].

Glutathione deficiency is a common finding in neurological disorders [129], and it may be related to several cardiovascular diseases [130]. Even in the brain vasculature, GSH may have protective effects. Despite apparently being the most convenient and safe method of GSH administration, oral GSH is not frequently utilized in clinical trials due to its limited effectiveness [131].

An alternative approach to increasing GSH production involves employing N-acetylcysteine (NAC). NAC is smaller than GSH, can move into the cells, and acts as a cysteine precursor, a crucial factor in limiting GSH synthesis [127]. NAC administration presents various neuroprotective effects, such as a reduction in the size of cerebral stroke [132] and better outcomes in neurological deficits and disability [133]. Moreover, NAC can potentially reduce ischemia–reperfusion injury [134,135], and may enhance the vasodilator effects of other compounds, such as acetylcholine [136]. As shown with other antioxidants, NAC treatment may effectively reduce cerebral vasospasm in SAH animal models [32], potentially carrying significant clinical implications that will require clinical trials to determine efficacy, despite promising pre-clinical data.

6.3. Vitamin C (Ascorbic Acid)

Vitamin C, also known as ascorbic acid (AA), is a crucial water-soluble antioxidant that plays multiple roles in the body, including acting as a cofactor for various enzymes and inhibiting the generation of ROS. Additionally, it directly scavenges ROS and RNS while repairing other oxidized scavengers. One fascinating aspect of ascorbic acid is its neuroprotective activity, and AA has been proposed as a therapeutical adjunct in several neurological conditions [137].

Indeed, the brain exhibits one of the highest ascorbic acid concentrations in the body, thanks to an active uptake from the bloodstream. The brain concentration of AA varies from 200–400 μM in the extracellular space to 10 mM intracellular, i.e., almost 100 times the concentration in the plasma [138,139].

The effect of AA on vessels started to be investigated more than forty years ago [140]. It has demonstrated that it has the potential to enhance impaired endothelium-dependent vasodilation in peripheral arteries in various conditions characterized by endothelial dysfunction [141]. However, the impacts of vitamin C on peripheral and cerebral circulations may differ [142].

Although blood hyperoxia does not appear to be convincingly associated with cerebral vasospasm following a subarachnoid hemorrhage [143], animal studies have shown that intracisternal injected Oxy-Hb (oxyhemoglobin) may result in a concentration-dependent contraction of cerebral artery strips. However, the presence of ascorbic acid significantly modifies the biological activity of Oxy-Hb, suppressing its vasoconstrictor activity and minimizing its ability to reduce vasodilator actions [144].

The cerebrovascular effects of AA were recently evaluated in an elegant study by Mattos et al. [33], investigating the effects of isocapnic hyperoxia (IH) on CBF and metabolism. Ten male participants underwent a 10 min IH trial with intravenous saline and AA infusion (3 g). AA infusion inhibited ROS production and preserved NO bioavailability, as indicated by the reduced ROS biomarkers and unchanged nitrite levels. The infusion also prevented regional and total CBF decline, and restored the cerebral metabolic rate of oxygen ($CMRO_2$) during IH. This study further confirms that ROS play a role in CBF regulation and metabolism, and antioxidants such as AA can have indirect vasoactive effects.

Considering all this, the use of ascorbic acid in protecting the cerebral vascular tone during high oxidative stress conditions, like those seen in critically ill patients or those with acute brain injuries, requires further study, as there are a few adverse reactions [145].

6.4. Vitamin E (Tocopherols and Tocotrienols)

Vitamin E is not a single molecule, but rather a group of fat-soluble substances with similar vitamin activity, which includes four tocopherols (alpha, beta, gamma, delta) and four tocotrienols (alpha, beta, gamma, delta). The most biologically active isoform among them is alpha-tocopherol [146]. These compounds protect the integrity of cellular membranes by shielding them from the free radicals that can generate and by directly neutralizing superoxide and hydroxyl radicals. Vitamin E may have potential neuroprotective effects, particularly in neurodegenerative diseases, stemming from its activity in reducing neuroinflammation [147].

Besides its role as an antioxidant, vitamin E plays a significant role in various cellular processes, such as in the vascular vessels. For example, in patients with coronary spastic angina, administering alpha-tocopherol acetate at 300 mg/day restored flow-dependent vasodilation [148]. This improvement was accompanied by a reduction in levels of plasma lipid peroxidation substances and a decrease in anginal attacks.

Endothelial cells, when replete with vitamin E, are better equipped to prevent blood cell components from adhering to their interior surface in blood vessels. Moreover, vitamin E enhances the expression of two enzymes that suppress arachidonic acid metabolism, leading to the increased release of prostacyclin from the endothelium, promoting blood vessel dilation and inhibiting platelet aggregation [6]. Its administration can improve arteriolar compliance [149] and endothelium-dependent relaxation [150]. Furthermore, a meta-analysis has indicated that vitamin E might provide protection in preventing ischemic stroke [151], but another recent one failed to show a benefit [152], suggesting that further well-designed randomized controlled trials are required to reach a conclusive result.

6.5. Other Antioxidants

Other antioxidants can be used as promising adjunct therapies in critically ill patients or those with brain injuries. For instance, catalase, which degrades hydrogen peroxide when administered intracisternally in meningitis models, caused a reduction in the elevation of rCBF (regional cerebral blood flow), ICP (intracranial pressure), and brain water content, primarily caused by superoxide or its derivatives [153]. Indeed, hydrogen peroxide induced relaxation in cerebral arteries, regardless of the presence of intact endothelial cells. However, these relaxations were suppressed by catalase, while SOD (superoxide dismutase) had no impact, suggesting that the relaxations resulted from the direct effect of hydrogen peroxide [154]. Likewise, other than improving endothelial function [155], flavonoids may elicit favorable impacts on the vascular system, resulting in ameliorating cerebrovascular blood flow [156], potentially preventing vasospasm in SAH [157], and with therapeutic effects on ischemic stroke-induced models [158].

Vitamin D has demonstrated the potential to improve neurological outcomes in brain-injured patients with significant vitamin D deficiency [159]. Interestingly, its levels have shown a correlation with intracranial aneurysm rupture in patients with SAH [160]. Furthermore, it has been suggested that the vasoprotective effects induced by vitamin D may be attributed to a reduction in oxidative stress [161]. Nevertheless, its ability to effectively prevent oxidative stress remains inconclusive, and its role as an antioxidant cannot currently be definitively established [162].

Vitamin A may have both antioxidant and oxidant activity [163]. It is a fat-soluble vitamin that exists in two primary forms: retinol, a directly absorbable form found in animal products, and carotenoids, which the body can convert into Vitamin A. Its use in TBI patients has been shown to have potential neuroprotective effects, reducing brain lesion sizes [164]. Although it seems to play a key role in the development of cerebral vasculature [165], we failed to find specific studies evaluating its effects on cerebrovascular tone.

Finally, circulating uric acid may act as a significant water-soluble antioxidant, particularly against peroxynitrites in hydrophilic settings. However, within the cells, uric acid may turn into a potent pro-oxidant, triggering oxidative stress cells and mitochondria and promoting the production of inflammatory cytokines [35], in a paradoxical dualism [166]. This exemplifies the difficulties in evaluating these data and underscores the need for high-quality clinical studies.

7. Discussion

The regulation of vascular tone in cerebral vessels is a complex process that involves multiple factors and mechanisms [167], which include pressure-induced regulation, shear stress, local metabolism, and the control of vascular diameter by neuronal activity. As previously described, the presence of ROS, RNS, and antioxidants can result in vasodilatory and vasoconstrictive effects in cerebral blood vessels, with a complex interplay activity [168]. The main effects of the various oxidative and nitrosative species involved in modulating the cerebral vascular tone are reported in Table 2.

Table 2. Mechanisms of oxidative stress-mediated modulation of cerebral vascular tone. This table outlines the various oxidative and nitrosative species involved in modulating cerebral vascular tone, and their mechanisms and effects (either vasodilation or vasoconstriction).

Mechanisms	ROS/RNS Involved	Effect on Cerebral Vascular Tone
Interaction with ion channels	O_2^-, H_2O_2, HNO, $ONOO^-$	Modulation of K^+ channels, leading to vasodilation or vasoconstriction [13,36,105,116]
Interaction with nitric oxide	O_2^-	Inactivation of NO, leading to vasoconstriction [44,45]
Other endothelial and myogenic mechanisms	O_2^-, H_2O_2, NO, $ONOO^-$	Vasodilation/vasoconstriction [28,46,60]

In situations of intense hyperoxia, where there is a significant rise in O_2^-, the existing NO can be neutralized by O_2^-. The rate of this reaction matches the combined rates of other known superoxide degradation reactions [169]. The chemistry of NO suggests that its half-life is likely controlled by ROS, which increases in proportion to the partial pressure of oxygen in the brain, leading to an increase in arterial tone. Interestingly, during hyperbaric oxygenation in animal models, the vasodilating effect of superoxide dismutase when animals were pre-treated with a NO-synthase inhibitor was not seen [170], suggesting that one cause of vasoconstriction in the brain during hyperoxia might be the neutralization of NO by O_2^-, impacting its natural ability to relax blood vessels.

Besides playing a role in regulating the tone of cerebral vessels under physiological conditions, the equilibrium between ROS, RNS, and antioxidants becomes crucial under pathological conditions. Indeed, the brain is especially susceptible to oxidative injury due to its rapid metabolic rate and proneness to ischemic damage. Oxidative stress occurs due to an imbalance between the generation and detoxification of free radicals, increasing reactive species [34]. This equilibrium is disrupted in several acute brain injuries, including TBI and stroke [121,171,172], and chronic neurodegenerative diseases [173]. For instance, studies have demonstrated that SOD activity decreases 24 h following a TBI and continues to be reduced 7 days after a severe TBI [121]. Similarly, there appears to be a disruption in cerebrovascular tone, involving mechanisms that may encompass both nitrogen [174] and oxygen-reactive species [175]. The SOD activity also resulted in reductions in the serum of stroke patients for several days [176]. Therefore, the injured brain may suffer secondary damage resulting not only from the well-known direct oxidative activities of ROS, but also from the lesser-explored impacts these molecules have on blood vessels.

In these patients, the balance of redox reactions becomes essential, making antioxidants potential therapeutic agents to counteract oxidative damage. Antioxidants have been considered as a potential adjunctive treatment for various critical illnesses and have notably been suggested as a potential therapeutic option for patients with sepsis [177]. Nevertheless, they have been shown to be ineffective in a clinical study of sepsis [178]. Antioxidants can neutralize ROS and RNS, prevent their generation, and repair the damage caused by free radicals. For this reason, they have been proposed and tested to reduce the effects of reactive species on cerebral blood flow [33]. Indeed, even the mildest reduction in the regional cerebral blood may lead to cognitive dysfunction [179]. Therefore, utilizing antioxidants may potentially serve as a relatively safe supplementary therapy for specific critically ill patients or those with brain injuries. This may mitigate cognitive impairments in the former group and reduce secondary brain damage in the latter. For example, ascorbic acid has demonstrated its ability to preserve NO bioavailability, prevent CBF decline, and protect the cerebral metabolic rate of oxygen during conditions of high oxidative stress [33]. NAC administration has shown neuroprotective effects in reducing the size of cerebral stroke and improving neurological deficits [133]. In the context of patient-tailored therapy, it is plausible that antioxidant therapy should also be targeted toward those who truly require it, and it is conceivable that antioxidant levels should be evaluated in the intensive care unit, as most ICU patients experienced swift and severe deficiencies in antioxidants [180].

While antioxidants hold promise for offering potential benefits to brain injuries and the control of cerebrovascular tone, there is currently limited human evidence available. To our knowledge, as of now, there are no approved antioxidant therapies for TBI and stroke. Thus, further research is required to elucidate their precise mechanisms of action, effects on the vascular tone, optimal dosages, combinations of antioxidants, and potential interactions with other treatment modalities.

8. Conclusions

ROS, RNS and antioxidants contribute to regulate the tone of the cerebral vessels in different ways. Understanding the complex interplay between ROS, RNS, antioxidants and their impacts on cerebral vascular tone is essential for deepening our comprehension of brain physiology and mechanisms of secondary damage in brain injuries. This knowledge holds the potential to pave the way for the development of effective therapeutic approaches to neurological disorders, with antioxidants emerging as promising supplementary treatments. These treatments aim to counteract the detrimental effects of oxidative stress and maintain cerebral blood flow, particularly in individuals with acute brain injuries or those in critical conditions. As the field of study progresses, it may reveal novel avenues to enhance outcomes and the quality of life for individuals suffering from neurological injuries.

Author Contributions: Conceptualization, M.S.; methodology, M.S., C.B. and F.S.T.; writing—original draft preparation, M.S., E.D.S., M.Z., S.M.-S., I.J.W., C.B. and F.S.T.; writing—review and editing, M.S., S.M.-S., I.J.W., C.B. and F.S.T.; visualization, M.S.; supervision, I.J.W., C.B. and F.S.T. All authors have read and agreed to the published version of the manuscript.

Funding: This research received no external funding.

Institutional Review Board Statement: Not applicable.

Informed Consent Statement: Not applicable.

Data Availability Statement: Not applicable.

Acknowledgments: The figures have been created with biorender.com.

Conflicts of Interest: The authors declare no conflicts of interest.

Abbreviations

AA	Ascorbic Acid
AIS	Acute Ischemic Stroke
ATP	Adenosine Triphosphate
CAR	Cerebral Autoregulation
CBF	Cerebral Blood Flow
CGRP	Calcitonin Gene-Related Peptide
$CMRO_2$	Cerebral Metabolic Rate of Oxygen
cGMP	cyclic Guanosine Monophosphate
Cu-Zn SOD	Copper Zinc Superoxide Dismutase
EDRF	Endothelium-Derived Relaxing Factor
ER	Endoplasmic Reticulum
G6PD	Glucose-6-Phosphate Dehydrogenase
GGS	Glutathione Disulfide
GSH	Glutathione
GPx	Glutathione Peroxidase
Hb	Hemoglobin
HIF-1α	Hypoxia Inducible Factor 1 alpha

HNO	Nitroxyl
HRE	Hypoxia Responsive Elements
IH	Isocapnic Hyperoxia
iNOS	inducible Nitric Oxide Synthase
ICP	Intracranial Pressure
K_{ATP}	ATP–Sensitive Potassium
K_{ca}	Calcium–Dependent Potassium Channels
K_v	Voltage–Dependent Potassium
MnSOD	Manganese Superoxide Dismutase
$NaNO_2$	Sodium Nitrite
NAC	N-acetylcysteine
NADH	Nicotinamide Adenine Dinucleotide
NADPH	Nicotinamide Adenine Dinucleotide Phosphate
NO	Nitric Oxide
NO_2^-	Nitrite
NO_3^-	Nitrate
NOX	NADPH Oxidase
NOS	Nitric Oxide Synthase
$ONOO^-$	Peroxynitrite
Oxy-Hb	Oxyhemoglobin
$PaCO_2$	Partial Pressure of Arterial Carbon Dioxide
ROS	Reactive Oxygen Species
RNS	Reactive Nitrogen Species
SNO-Hb	S-nitroso Hemoglobin
SOD	Superoxide Dismutase
SOD1	Copper-Zinc Superoxide Dismutase
SOD2	Manganese Superoxide Dismutase
SOD3	Extracellular Superoxide Dismutase
TBI	Traumatic Brain Injury
TRPA1	Transient Receptor Potential Channel A1

References

1. Rink, C.; Khanna, S. Significance of Brain Tissue Oxygenation and the Arachidonic Acid Cascade in Stroke. *Antioxid. Redox Signal.* **2011**, *14*, 1889–1903. [CrossRef] [PubMed]
2. Clarke, D.D.; Sokoloff, L. Regulation of Cerebral Metabolic Rate. In *Basic Neurochemistry: Molecular, Cellular and Medical Aspects*, 6th ed.; American Society for Neurochemistry: Windermere, FL, USA, 1999.
3. Turrens, J.F. Mitochondrial Formation of Reactive Oxygen Species. *J. Physiol.* **2003**, *552*, 335–344. [CrossRef] [PubMed]
4. Salim, S. Oxidative Stress and the Central Nervous System. *J. Pharmacol. Exp. Ther.* **2017**, *360*, 201–205. [CrossRef] [PubMed]
5. Cipolla, M.J. Regulation of Cerebrovascular Tone. In *The Cerebral Circulation;* Morgan & Claypool Life Sciences: San Rafael, CA, USA, 2009.
6. Griendling, K.K.; Sorescu, D.; Ushio-Fukai, M. NAD(P)H Oxidase: Role in Cardiovascular Biology and Disease. *Circ. Res.* **2000**, *86*, 494–501. [CrossRef]
7. Staiculescu, M.C.; Foote, C.; Meininger, G.A.; Martinez-Lemus, L.A. The Role of Reactive Oxygen Species in Microvascular Remodeling. *Int. J. Mol. Sci.* **2014**, *15*, 23792–23835. [CrossRef]
8. Lee, K.S.; Kim, S.R.; Park, S.J.; Park, H.S.; Min, K.H.; Lee, M.H.; Jin, S.M.; Jin, G.Y.; Yoo, W.H.; Lee, Y.C. Hydrogen Peroxide Induces Vascular Permeability via Regulation of Vascular Endothelial Growth Factor. *Am. J. Respir. Cell Mol. Biol.* **2006**, *35*, 190–197. [CrossRef] [PubMed]
9. Li, H.; Horke, S.; Förstermann, U. Oxidative Stress in Vascular Disease and Its Pharmacological Prevention. *Trends Pharmacol. Sci.* **2013**, *34*, 313–319. [CrossRef]
10. Montezano, A.C.; Touyz, R.M. Reactive Oxygen Species, Vascular Noxs, and Hypertension: Focus on Translational and Clinical Research. *Antioxid. Redox Signal.* **2014**, *20*, 164–182. [CrossRef]
11. Miller, A.A.; Drummond, G.R.; De Silva, T.M.; Mast, A.E.; Hickey, H.; Williams, J.P.; Broughton, B.R.S.; Sobey, C.G. NADPH Oxidase Activity Is Higher in Cerebral versus Systemic Arteries of Four Animal Species: Role of Nox2. *Am. J. Physiol. Heart Circ. Physiol.* **2009**, *296*, 220–225. [CrossRef]
12. Miller, A.A.; Drummond, G.R.; Schmidt, H.H.H.W.; Sobey, C.G. NADPH Oxidase Activity and Function Are Profoundly Greater in Cerebral versus Systemic Arteries. *Circ. Res.* **2005**, *97*, 1055–1062. [CrossRef]
13. Terashvili, M.; Pratt, P.F.; Gebremedhin, D.; Narayanan, J.; Harder, D.R. Reactive Oxygen Species Cerebral Autoregulation in Health and Disease. *Pediatr. Clin. N. Am.* **2006**, *53*, 1029–1037. [CrossRef]

14. Kitazono, T.; Faraci, F.M.; Taguchi, H.; Heistad, D.D. Role of Potassium Channels in Cerebral Blood Vessels. *Stroke* **1995**, *26*, 1713–1723. [CrossRef]
15. Gutterman, D.D.; Miura, H.; Liu, Y. Redox Modulation of Vascular Tone: Focus of Potassium Channel Mechanisms of Dilation. *Arterioscler. Thromb. Vasc. Biol.* **2005**, *25*, 671–678. [CrossRef]
16. Yang, J. The Role of Reactive Oxygen Species in Angiogenesis and Preventing Tissue Injury after Brain Ischemia. *Microvasc. Res.* **2019**, *123*, 62–67. [CrossRef] [PubMed]
17. Khatri, N.; Thakur, M.; Pareek, V.; Kumar, S.; Sharma, S.; Datusalia, A.K. Oxidative Stress: Major Threat in Traumatic Brain Injury. *CNS Neurol. Disord. Drug Targets* **2018**, *17*, 689–695. [CrossRef]
18. Jackson, W.F. Ion Channels and Vascular Tone. *Hypertension* **2000**, *35*, 173–178. [CrossRef]
19. Claassen, J.A.H.R.; Thijssen, D.H.J.; Panerai, R.B.; Faraci, F.M. Regulation of Cerebral Blood Flow in Humans: Physiology and Clinical Implications of Autoregulation. *Physiol. Rev.* **2021**, *101*, 1487–1559. [CrossRef]
20. Weyland, A.; Buhre, W.; Grund, S.; Ludwig, H.; Kazmaier, S.; Weyland, W.; Sonntag, H. Cerebrovascular Tone Rather than Intracranial Pressure Determines the Effective Downstream Pressure of the Cerebral Circulation in the Absence of Intracranial Hypertension. *J. Neurosurg. Anesthesiol.* **2000**, *12*, 210–216. [CrossRef] [PubMed]
21. Hu, X.; Michael De Silva, T.; Chen, J.; Faraci, F.M. Cerebral Vascular Disease and Neurovascular Injury in Ischemic Stroke. *Circ. Res.* **2017**, *120*, 449–471. [CrossRef]
22. Battisti-Charbonney, A.; Fisher, J.; Duffin, J. The Cerebrovascular Response to Carbon Dioxide in Humans. *J. Physiol.* **2011**, *589*, 3039–3048. [CrossRef] [PubMed]
23. Hoiland, R.L.; Bain, A.R.; Rieger, M.G.; Bailey, D.M.; Ainslie, P.N. Oxygen as a Regulator of Biological Systems: Hypoxemia, Oxygen Content, and the Regulation of Cerebral Blood Flow. *Am. J. Physiol. Regul. Integr. Comp. Physiol.* **2016**, *310*, R398–R413. [CrossRef]
24. Pearce, W.J. Mechanisms of Hypoxic Cerebral Vasodilatation. *Pharmacol. Ther.* **1995**, *65*, 75–91. [CrossRef]
25. Xu, Y.; Liachenko, S.M.; Tang, P.; Chan, P.H. Faster Recovery of Cerebral Perfusion in SOD1-Overexpressed Rats after Cardiac Arrest and Resuscitation. *Stroke* **2009**, *40*, 2512–2518. [CrossRef]
26. Didion, S.P.; Hathaway, C.A.; Faraci, F.M. Superoxide Levels and Function of Cerebral Blood Vessels after Inhibition of CuZn-SOD. *Am. J. Physiol. Heart Circ. Physiol.* **2001**, *281*, H1697–H1703. [CrossRef]
27. Shibata, M.; Araki, N.; Hamada, J.; Sasaki, T.; Ohta, K.; Shimazu, K.; Fukuuchi, Y. Regional Difference in Nitric Oxide Production during Forebrain Ischemia. *Microchem. J.* **1997**, *56*, 188–191. [CrossRef]
28. Li, J.; Li, W.; Altura, B.T.; Altura, B.M. Peroxynitrite-Induced Relaxation in Isolated Canine Cerebral Arteries and Mechanisms of Action. *Toxicol. Appl. Pharmacol.* **2004**, *196*, 176–182. [CrossRef]
29. Brzezinska, A.K.; Gebremedhin, D.; Chilian, W.M.; Kalyanaraman, B.; Elliott, S.J. Peroxynitrite Reversibly Inhibits Ca(2+)-Activated K(+) Channels in Rat Cerebral Artery Smooth Muscle Cells. *Am. J. Physiol. Heart Circ. Physiol.* **2000**, *278*, H1883–H1890. [CrossRef]
30. Elliott, S.J.; Lacey, D.J.; Chilian, W.M.; Brzezinska, A.K. Peroxynitrite Is a Contractile Agonist of Cerebral Artery Smooth Muscle Cells. *Am. J. Physiol.* **1998**, *275*, H1585–H1591. [CrossRef] [PubMed]
31. Aladag, M.A.; Turkoz, Y.; Sahna, E.; Parlakpinar, H.; Gul, M. The Attenuation of Vasospasm by Using a Sod Mimetic after Experimental Subarachnoidal Haemorrhage in Rats. *Acta Neurochir.* **2003**, *145*, 673–677. [CrossRef] [PubMed]
32. Güney, O.; Erdi, F.; Esen, H.; Kiyici, A.; Kocaogullar, Y. N-Acetylcysteine Prevents Vasospasm after Subarachnoid Hemorrhage. *World Neurosurg.* **2010**, *73*, 42–49. [CrossRef] [PubMed]
33. Mattos, J.D.; Campos, M.O.; Rocha, M.P.; Mansur, D.E.; Rocha, H.N.M.; Garcia, V.P.; Batista, G.; Alvares, T.S.; Oliveira, G.V.; Souza, M.V.; et al. Human Brain Blood Flow and Metabolism during Isocapnic Hyperoxia: The Role of Reactive Oxygen Species. *J. Physiol.* **2019**, *597*, 741–755. [CrossRef]
34. Pizzino, G.; Irrera, N.; Cucinotta, M.; Pallio, G.; Mannino, F.; Arcoraci, V.; Squadrito, F.; Altavilla, D.; Bitto, A. Oxidative Stress: Harms and Benefits for Human Health. *Oxid. Med. Cell. Longev.* **2017**, *2017*, 8416763. [CrossRef]
35. Leveque, C.; Mrakic-Sposta, S.; Lafère, P.; Vezzoli, A.; Germonpré, P.; Beer, A.; Mievis, S.; Virgili, F.; Lambrechts, K.; Theunissen, S.; et al. Oxidative Stress Response's Kinetics after 60 Minutes at Different (30% or 100%) Normobaric Hyperoxia Exposures. *Int. J. Mol. Sci.* **2023**, *24*, 664. [CrossRef] [PubMed]
36. Wei, E.P.; Kontos, H.A.; Beckman, J.S. Mechanisms of Cerebral Vasodilation by Superoxide, Hydrogen Peroxide, and Peroxynitrite. *Am. J. Physiol.* **1996**, *271*, H1262–H1266. [CrossRef] [PubMed]
37. Marklund, S. Spectrophotometric Study of Spontaneous Disproportionation of Superoxide Anion Radical and Sensitive Direct Assay for Superoxide Dismutase. *J. Biol. Chem.* **1976**, *251*, 7504–7507. [CrossRef] [PubMed]
38. Beckman, J.S.; Beckman, T.W.; Chen, J.; Marshall, P.A.; Freeman, B.A. Apparent Hydroxyl Radical Production by Peroxynitrite: Implications for Endothelial Injury from Nitric Oxide and Superoxide. *Proc. Natl. Acad. Sci. USA* **1990**, *87*, 1620–1624. [CrossRef] [PubMed]
39. Miller, A.A.; Drummond, G.R.; Sobey, C.G. Reactive Oxygen Species in the Cerebral Circulation: Are They All Bad? *Antioxid. Redox Signal.* **2006**, *8*, 1113–1120. [CrossRef] [PubMed]
40. Roy, C.S.; Sherrington, C.S. On the Regulation of the Blood-Supply of the Brain. *J. Physiol.* **1890**, *11*, 85–158. [CrossRef] [PubMed]
41. Watts, M.E.; Pocock, R.; Claudianos, C. Brain Energy and Oxygen Metabolism: Emerging Role in Normal Function and Disease. *Front. Mol. Neurosci.* **2018**, *11*, 216. [CrossRef]

42. Faraci, F.M. Oxidative Stress: The Curse That Underlies Cerebral Vascular Dysfunction? *Stroke* **2005**, *36*, 186–188. [CrossRef]
43. De Silva, T.M.; Faraci, F.M. Reactive Oxygen Species and the Regulation of Cerebral Vascular Tone. In *Oxidative Stress in Applied Basic Research and Clinical Practice*; Humana Press: Boston, MA, USA, 2017; pp. 89–112. [CrossRef]
44. Faraci, F.M. Reactive Oxygen Species: Influence on Cerebral Vascular Tone. *J. Appl. Physiol.* **2006**, *100*, 739–743. [CrossRef] [PubMed]
45. Kontos, H.A. Oxygen Radicals in Cerebral Ischemia. *Stroke* **2001**, *32*, 2712–2716. [CrossRef] [PubMed]
46. Nelson, M.T.; Conway, M.A.; Knot, H.J.; Brayden, J.E. Chloride Channel Blockers Inhibit Myogenic Tone in Rat Cerebral Arteries. *J. Physiol.* **1997**, *502 Pt 2*, 259–264. [CrossRef] [PubMed]
47. Balestra, C.; Mrakic-Sposta, S.; Virgili, F. Oxygen Variations—Insights into Hypoxia, Hyperoxia and Hyperbaric Hyperoxia—Is the Dose the Clue? *Int. J. Mol. Sci.* **2023**, *24*, 13472. [CrossRef] [PubMed]
48. Paravicini, T.M.; Chrissobolis, S.; Drummond, G.R.; Sobey, C.G. Increased NADPH-Oxidase Activity and Nox4 Expression During Chronic Hypertension Is Associated With Enhanced Cerebral Vasodilatation to NADPH In Vivo. *Stroke* **2004**, *35*, 584–589. [CrossRef] [PubMed]
49. Lassègue, B.; Clempus, R.E. Vascular NAD(P)H Oxidases: Specific Features, Expression, and Regulation. *Am. J. Physiol. Regul. Integr. Comp. Physiol.* **2003**, *285*, R277–R297. [CrossRef] [PubMed]
50. Konior, A.; Schramm, A.; Czesnikiewicz-Guzik, M.; Guzik, T.J. NADPH Oxidases in Vascular Pathology. *Antioxid. Redox Signal.* **2014**, *20*, 2794–2814. [CrossRef] [PubMed]
51. Balestra, C.; Germonpré, P. Hypoxia, a Multifaceted Phenomenon: The Example of the Normobaric Oxygen Paradox. *Eur. J. Appl. Physiol.* **2012**, *112*, 4173–4175. [CrossRef]
52. Salvagno, M.; Coppalini, G.; Taccone, F.S.; Strapazzon, G.; Mrakic-Sposta, S.; Rocco, M.; Khalife, M.; Balestra, C. The Normobaric Oxygen Paradox-Hyperoxic Hypoxic Paradox: A Novel Expedient Strategy in Hematopoiesis Clinical Issues. *Int. J. Mol. Sci.* **2022**, *24*, 82. [CrossRef]
53. Nanduri, J.; Vaddi, D.R.; Khan, S.A.; Wang, N.; Makarenko, V.; Semenza, G.L.; Prabhakar, N.R. HIF-1α Activation by Intermittent Hypoxia Requires NADPH Oxidase Stimulation by Xanthine Oxidase. *PLoS ONE* **2015**, *10*, e0119762. [CrossRef]
54. Mattos, J.D.; Campos, M.O.; Rocha, M.P.; Daniel, X.; Mansur, E.; Rocha, H.N.M.; Vinicius, X.; Garcia, P.; Rocha, N.G.; Thiago, X.; et al. Differential Vasomotor Responses to Isocapnic Hyperoxia: Cerebral versus Peripheral Circulation. *Am. J. Physiol. Regul. Integr. Comp. Physiol.* **2020**, *318*, 182–187. [CrossRef]
55. Austin, S.A.; Santhanam, A.V.R.; D'Uscio, L.V.; Katusic, Z.S. Regional Heterogeneity of Cerebral Microvessels and Brain Susceptibility to Oxidative Stress. *PLoS ONE* **2015**, *10*, e0144062. [CrossRef]
56. Wang, X.; Michaelis, E.K. Selective Neuronal Vulnerability to Oxidative Stress in the Brain. *Front. Aging Neurosci.* **2010**, *2*, 12. [CrossRef] [PubMed]
57. Nathan, C. Specificity of a Third Kind: Reactive Oxygen and Nitrogen Intermediates in Cell Signaling. *J. Clin. Investig.* **2003**, *111*, 769–778. [CrossRef] [PubMed]
58. Tousoulis, D.; Kampoli, A.-M.; Tentolouris Nikolaos Papageorgiou, C.; Stefanadis, C. The Role of Nitric Oxide on Endothelial Function. *Curr. Vasc. Pharmacol.* **2012**, *10*, 4–18. [CrossRef] [PubMed]
59. Tejero, J.; Shiva, S.; Gladwin, M.T. Sources of Vascular Nitric Oxide and Reactive Oxygen Species and Their Regulation. *Physiol. Rev.* **2019**, *99*, 311–379. [CrossRef]
60. Gladwin, M.T.; Raat, N.J.H.; Shiva, S.; Dezfulian, C.; Hogg, N.; Kim-Shapiro, D.B.; Patel, R.P. Nitrite as a Vascular Endocrine Nitric Oxide Reservoir That Contributes to Hypoxic Signaling, Cytoprotection, and Vasodilation. *Am. J. Physiol. Heart Circ. Physiol.* **2006**, *291*, H2026–H2035. [CrossRef]
61. Premont, R.T.; Reynolds, J.D.; Zhang, R.; Stamler, J.S. Role of Nitric Oxide Carried by Hemoglobin in Cardiovascular Physiology: Developments on a Three-Gas Respiratory Cycle. *Circ. Res.* **2020**, *126*, 129–158. [CrossRef]
62. Piacenza, L.; Zeida, A.; Trujillo, M.; Radi, R. The Superoxide Radical Switch in the Biology of Nitric Oxide and Peroxynitrite. *Physiol. Rev.* **2022**, *102*, 1881–1906. [CrossRef]
63. Fukuda, S.; Koga, Y.; Fujita, M.; Suehiro, E.; Kaneda, K.; Oda, Y.; Ishihara, H.; Suzuki, M.; Tsuruta, R. Hyperoxemia during the Hyperacute Phase of Aneurysmal Subarachnoid Hemorrhage Is Associated with Delayed Cerebral Ischemia and Poor Outcome: A Retrospective Observational Study. *J. Neurosurg.* **2019**, *134*, 25–32. [CrossRef]
64. Irvine, J.C.; Ritchie, R.H.; Favaloro, J.L.; Andrews, K.L.; Widdop, R.E.; Kemp-Harper, B.K. Nitroxyl (HNO): The Cinderella of the Nitric Oxide Story. *Trends Pharmacol. Sci.* **2008**, *29*, 601–608. [CrossRef] [PubMed]
65. Ahluwalia, A.; Gladwin, M.; Coleman, G.D.; Hord, N.; Howard, G.; Kim-Shapiro, D.B.; Lajous, M.; Larsen, F.J.; Lefer, D.J.; McClure, L.A.; et al. Dietary Nitrate and the Epidemiology of Cardiovascular Disease: Report from a National Heart, Lung, and Blood Institute Workshop. *J. Am. Heart Assoc.* **2016**, *5*, e003402. [CrossRef]
66. DeMartino, A.W.; Kim-Shapiro, D.B.; Patel, R.P.; Gladwin, M.T. Nitrite and Nitrate Chemical Biology and Signalling. *Br. J. Pharmacol.* **2019**, *176*, 228–245. [CrossRef]
67. Kapil, V.; Haydar, S.M.A.; Pearl, V.; Lundberg, J.O.; Weitzberg, E.; Ahluwalia, A. Physiological Role for Nitrate-Reducing Oral Bacteria in Blood Pressure Control. *Free Radic. Biol. Med.* **2013**, *55*, 93–100. [CrossRef]
68. Cosby, K.; Partovi, K.S.; Crawford, J.H.; Patel, R.P.; Reiter, C.D.; Martyr, S.; Yang, B.K.; Waclawiw, M.A.; Zalos, G.; Xu, X.; et al. Nitrite Reduction to Nitric Oxide by Deoxyhemoglobin Vasodilates the Human Circulation. *Nat. Med.* **2003**, *9*, 1498–1505. [CrossRef]

69. Crawford, J.H.; Isbell, T.S.; Huang, Z.; Shiva, S.; Chacko, B.K.; Schechter, A.N.; Darley-Usmar, V.M.; Kerby, J.D.; Lang, J.D.; Kraus, D.; et al. Hypoxia, Red Blood Cells, and Nitrite Regulate NO-Dependent Hypoxic Vasodilation. *Blood* **2006**, *107*, 566–574. [CrossRef] [PubMed]
70. Dalsgaard, T.; Simonsen, U.; Fago, A. Nitrite-Dependent Vasodilation Is Facilitated by Hypoxia and Is Independent of Known NO-Generating Nitrite Reductase Activities. *Am. J. Physiol. Heart Circ. Physiol.* **2007**, *292*, H3072–H3078. [CrossRef]
71. Maher, A.R.; Milsom, A.B.; Gunaruwan, P.; Abozguia, K.; Ahmed, I.; Weaver, R.A.; Thomas, P.; Ashrafian, H.; Born, G.V.R.; James, P.E.; et al. Hypoxic Modulation of Exogenous Nitrite-Induced Vasodilation in Humans. *Circulation* **2008**, *117*, 670–677. [CrossRef]
72. Pinder, A.G.; Pittaway, E.; Morris, K.; James, P.E. Nitrite Directly Vasodilates Hypoxic Vasculature via Nitric Oxide-Dependent and -Independent Pathways. *Br. J. Pharmacol.* **2009**, *157*, 1523–1530. [CrossRef] [PubMed]
73. Hataishi, R.; Rodrigues, A.C.; Neilan, T.G.; Morgan, J.G.; Buys, E.; Shiva, S.; Tambouret, R.; Jassal, D.S.; Raher, M.J.; Furutani, E.; et al. Inhaled Nitric Oxide Decreases Infarction Size and Improves Left Ventricular Function in a Murine Model of Myocardial Ischemia-Reperfusion Injury. *Am. J. Physiol. Heart Circ. Physiol.* **2006**, *291*, H379–H384. [CrossRef]
74. Ma, L.; Hu, L.; Feng, X.; Wang, S. Nitrate and Nitrite in Health and Disease. *Aging Dis.* **2018**, *9*, 938–945. [CrossRef]
75. Stamler, J.S.; Singel, D.J.; Loscalzo, J. Biochemistry of Nitric Oxide and Its Redox-Activated Forms. *Science* **1992**, *258*, 1898–1902. [CrossRef]
76. Palmer, R.M.J.; Ferrige, A.G.; Moncada, S. Nitric Oxide Release Accounts for the Biological Activity of Endothelium-Derived Relaxing Factor. *Nature* **1987**, *327*, 524–526. [CrossRef] [PubMed]
77. Cohen, R.A.; Adachi, T. Nitric-Oxide-Induced Vasodilatation: Regulation by Physiologic s-Glutathiolation and Pathologic Oxidation of the Sarcoplasmic Endoplasmic Reticulum Calcium ATPase. *Trends Cardiovasc. Med.* **2006**, *16*, 109–114. [CrossRef]
78. Sun, C.W.; Falck, J.R.; Okamoto, H.; Harder, D.R.; Roman, R.J. Role of CGMP versus 20-HETE in the Vasodilator Response to Nitric Oxide in Rat Cerebral Arteries. *Am. J. Physiol. Heart Circ. Physiol.* **2000**, *279*, H339–H350. [CrossRef]
79. Attwell, D.; Buchan, A.M.; Charpak, S.; Lauritzen, M.; MacVicar, B.A.; Newman, E.A. Glial and Neuronal Control of Brain Blood Flow. *Nature* **2010**, *468*, 232–243. [CrossRef]
80. Iadecola, C.; Pelligrino, D.A.; Moskowitz, M.A.; Lassen, N.A. Nitric Oxide Synthase Inhibition and Cerebrovascular Regulation. *J. Cereb. Blood Flow Metab.* **1994**, *14*, 175–192. [CrossRef]
81. Matsuura, T.; Kanno, I. Effect of Nitric Oxide Synthase Inhibitor on the Local Cerebral Blood Flow Evoked by Rat Somatosensory Stimulation under Hyperoxia. *Comp. Biochem. Physiol. A Mol. Integr. Physiol.* **2002**, *131*, 267–274. [CrossRef]
82. Takuwa, H.; Matsuura, T.; Bakalova, R.; Obata, T.; Kanno, I. Contribution of Nitric Oxide to Cerebral Blood Flow Regulation under Hypoxia in Rats. *J. Physiol. Sci.* **2010**, *60*, 399–406. [CrossRef] [PubMed]
83. Demchenko, I.T.; Oury, T.D.; Crapo, J.D.; Piantadosi, C.A. Regulation of the Brain's Vascular Responses to Oxygen. *Circ. Res.* **2002**, *91*, 1031–1037. [CrossRef]
84. Iadecola, C. Does Nitric Oxide Mediate the Increases in Cerebral Blood Flow Elicited by Hypercapnia? *Proc. Natl. Acad. Sci. USA* **1992**, *89*, 3913–3916. [CrossRef]
85. Hoiland, R.L.; Macleod, D.B.; Stacey, B.S.; Caldwell, H.G.; Howe, C.A.; Carr, J.M.J.R.; Tymko, M.M.; Nowak-flu, D.; Coombs, G.B.; Patrician, A.; et al. Hemoglobin and Cerebral Hypoxic Vasodilation in Humans: Evidence for Nitric Oxide-Dependent and S-Nitrosothiol Mediated Signal Transduction. *J. Cereb. Blood Flow Metab.* **2023**, *43*, 1519–1531. [CrossRef] [PubMed]
86. Lavi, S.; Gaitini, D.; Milloul, V.; Jacob, G. Impaired Cerebral CO2 Vasoreactivity: Association with Endothelial Dysfunction. *Am. J. Physiol. Heart Circ. Physiol.* **2006**, *291*, H1856–H1861. [CrossRef] [PubMed]
87. Fathi, A.R.; Yang, C.; Bakhtian, K.D.; Qi, M.; Lonser, R.R.; Pluta, R.M. Carbon Dioxide Influence on Nitric Oxide Production in Endothelial Cells and Astrocytes: Cellular Mechanisms. *Brain Res.* **2011**, *1386*, 50–57. [CrossRef] [PubMed]
88. Garry, P.S.; Ezra, M.; Rowland, M.J.; Westbrook, J.; Pattinson, K.T.S. The Role of the Nitric Oxide Pathway in Brain Injury and Its Treatment--from Bench to Bedside. *Exp. Neurol.* **2015**, *263*, 235–243. [CrossRef] [PubMed]
89. Patel, J.K.; Schoenfeld, E.; Hou, W.; Singer, A.; Rakowski, E.; Ahmad, S.; Patel, R.; Parikh, P.B.; Smaldone, G. Inhaled Nitric Oxide in Adults with In-Hospital Cardiac Arrest: A Feasibility Study. *Nitric Oxide* **2021**, *115*, 30–33. [CrossRef] [PubMed]
90. Lenz, I.J.; Plesnila, N.; Terpolilli, N.A. Role of Endothelial Nitric Oxide Synthase for Early Brain Injury after Subarachnoid Hemorrhage in Mice. *J. Cereb. Blood Flow Metab.* **2021**, *41*, 1669–1681. [CrossRef] [PubMed]
91. Qu, W.; Cheng, Y.; Peng, W.; Wu, Y.; Rui, T.; Luo, C.; Zhang, J. Targeting INOS Alleviates Early Brain Injury After Experimental Subarachnoid Hemorrhage via Promoting Ferroptosis of M1 Microglia and Reducing Neuroinflammation. *Mol. Neurobiol.* **2022**, *59*, 3124–3139. [CrossRef] [PubMed]
92. Li, H.; Wu, W.; Liu, M.; Zhang, X.; Zhang, Q.R.; Ni, L.; Hang, C.H. Increased Cerebrospinal Fluid Concentrations of Asymmetric Dimethylarginine Correlate with Adverse Clinical Outcome in Subarachnoid Hemorrhage Patients. *J. Clin. Neurosci.* **2014**, *21*, 1404–1408. [CrossRef]
93. Ng, W.H.; Moochhala, S.; Yeo, T.T.; Ong, P.L.; Ng, P.Y. Nitric Oxide and Subarachnoid Hemorrhage: Elevated Level in Cerebrospinal Fluid and Their Implications. *Neurosurgery* **2001**, *49*, 622–627. [CrossRef]
94. Fung, C.; Z'Graggen, W.J.; Jakob, S.M.; Gralla, J.; Haenggi, M.; Rothen, H.U.; Mordasini, P.; Lensch, M.; Söll, N.; Terpolilli, N.; et al. Inhaled Nitric Oxide Treatment for Aneurysmal SAH Patients With Delayed Cerebral Ischemia. *Front. Neurol.* **2022**, *13*, 817072. [CrossRef] [PubMed]
95. Kozlov, A.V.; Bahrami, S.; Redl, H.; Szabo, C. Alterations in Nitric Oxide Homeostasis during Traumatic Brain Injury. *Biochim. Biophys. Acta Mol. Basis Dis.* **2017**, *1863*, 2627–2632. [CrossRef] [PubMed]

96. Angelis, D.; Savani, R.; Chalak, L. Nitric Oxide and the Brain. Part 2: Effects Following Neonatal Brain Injury-Friend or Foe? *Pediatr. Res.* **2021**, *89*, 746–752. [CrossRef] [PubMed]
97. Lauer, T.; Preik, M.; Rassaf, T.; Strauer, B.E.; Deussen, A.; Feelisch, M.; Kelm, M. Plasma Nitrite Rather than Nitrate Reflects Regional Endothelial Nitric Oxide Synthase Activity but Lacks Intrinsic Vasodilator Action. *Proc. Natl. Acad. Sci. USA* **2001**, *98*, 12814–12819. [CrossRef] [PubMed]
98. Ignarro, L.J.; Gruetter, C.S. Requirement of Thiols for Activation of Coronary Arterial Guanylate Cyclase by Glyceryl Trinitrate and Sodium Nitrite: Possible Involvement of S-Nitrosothiols. *Biochim. Biophys. Acta* **1980**, *631*, 221–231. [CrossRef] [PubMed]
99. Ignarro, L.J.; Byrns, R.E.; Buga, G.M.; Wood, K.S. Endothelium-Derived Relaxing Factor from Pulmonary Artery and Vein Possesses Pharmacologic and Chemical Properties Identical to Those of Nitric Oxide Radical. *Circ. Res.* **1987**, *61*, 866–879. [CrossRef]
100. Gladwin, M.T.; Shelhamer, J.H.; Schechter, A.N.; Pease-Fye, M.E.; Waclawiw, M.A.; Panza, J.A.; Ognibene, F.P.; Cannon, R.O. Role of Circulating Nitrite and S-Nitrosohemoglobin in the Regulation of Regional Blood Flow in Humans. *Proc. Natl. Acad. Sci. USA* **2000**, *97*, 11482–11487. [CrossRef] [PubMed]
101. Furchgott, R.; Bhadrakom, S. Reactions of Strips of Rabbit Aorta to Epinephrine, Isopropylarterenol, Sodium Nitrite and Other Drugs. *J. Pharmacol. Exp. Ther.* **1953**, *2*, 129–143.
102. Brücken, A.; Derwall, M.; Bleilevens, C.; Stoppe, C.; Götzenich, A.; Gaisa, N.T.; Weis, J.; Nolte, K.W.; Rossaint, R.; Ichinose, F.; et al. Brief Inhalation of Nitric Oxide Increases Resuscitation Success and Improves 7-Day-Survival after Cardiac Arrest in Rats: A Randomized Controlled Animal Study. *Crit. Care* **2015**, *19*, 408. [CrossRef]
103. Wu, M.; Pritchard, K.A.; Kaminski, P.M.; Fayngersh, R.P.; Hintze, T.H.; Wolin, M.S. Involvement of Nitric Oxide and Nitrosothiols in Relaxation of Pulmonary Arteries to Peroxynitrite. *Am. J. Physiol.* **1994**, *266*, H2108–H2113. [CrossRef]
104. Liu, S.; Beckman, J.S.; Ku, D.D. Peroxynitrite, a Product of Superoxide and Nitric Oxide, Produces Coronary Vasorelaxation in Dogs. *J. Pharmacol. Exp. Ther.* **1994**, *268*, 1114–1121.
105. Wei, E.P.; Kontos, H.A.; Beckman, J.S.; Faraci, F.M. Antioxidants Inhibit ATP-Sensitive Potassium Channels in Cerebral Arterioles. *Stroke* **1998**, *29*, 817–823. [CrossRef]
106. Nossaman, B.D.; Kadowitz, P.J. Potential Benefits of Peroxynitrite. *Open Pharmacol. J.* **2008**, *2*, 31–53. [CrossRef] [PubMed]
107. Daneva, Z.; Marziano, C.; Ottolini, M.; Chen, Y.L.; Baker, T.M.; Kuppusamy, M.; Zhang, A.; Ta, H.Q.; Reagan, C.E.; Mihalek, A.D.; et al. Caveolar Peroxynitrite Formation Impairs Endothelial TRPV4 Channels and Elevates Pulmonary Arterial Pressure in Pulmonary Hypertension. *Proc. Natl. Acad. Sci. USA* **2021**, *118*, e2023130118. [CrossRef] [PubMed]
108. Ottolini, M.; Hong, K.; Cope, E.L.; Daneva, Z.; Delalio, L.J.; Sokolowski, J.D.; Marziano, C.; Nguyen, N.Y.; Altschmied, J.; Haendeler, J.; et al. Local Peroxynitrite Impairs Endothelial Transient Receptor Potential Vanilloid 4 Channels and Elevates Blood Pressure in Obesity. *Circulation* **2020**, *141*, 1318–1333. [CrossRef] [PubMed]
109. Ronson, R.S.; Nakamura, M.; Vinten-Johansen, J. The Cardiovascular Effects and Implications of Peroxynitrite. *Cardiovasc. Res.* **1999**, *44*, 47–59. [CrossRef] [PubMed]
110. Andrews, K.L.; Irvine, J.C.; Tare, M.; Apostolopoulos, J.; Favaloro, J.L.; Triggle, C.R.; Kemp-Harper, B.K. A Role for Nitroxyl (HNO) as an Endothelium-Derived Relaxing and Hyperpolarizing Factor in Resistance Arteries. *Br. J. Pharmacol.* **2009**, *157*, 540–550. [CrossRef] [PubMed]
111. Andrews, K.L.; Lumsden, N.G.; Farry, J.; Jefferis, A.M.; Kemp-Harper, B.K.; Chin-Dusting, J.P.F. Nitroxyl: A Vasodilator of Human Vessels That Is Not Susceptible to Tolerance. *Clin. Sci.* **2015**, *129*, 179–187. [CrossRef]
112. Paolocci, N.; Jackson, M.I.; Lopez, B.E.; Miranda, K.; Tocchetti, C.G.; Wink, D.A.; Hobbs, A.J.; Fukuto, J.M. The Pharmacology of Nitroxyl (HNO) and Its Therapeutic Potential: Not Just the Janus Face of NO. *Pharmacol. Ther.* **2007**, *113*, 442–458. [CrossRef]
113. Favaloro, J.L.; Kemp-Harper, B.K. The Nitroxyl Anion (HNO) Is a Potent Dilator of Rat Coronary Vasculature. *Cardiovasc. Res.* **2007**, *73*, 587–596. [CrossRef]
114. Kemp-Harper, B.K.; Horowitz, J.D.; Ritchie, R.H. Therapeutic Potential of Nitroxyl (HNO) Donors in the Management of Acute Decompensated Heart Failure. *Drugs* **2016**, *76*, 1337–1348. [CrossRef]
115. Zhu, G.; Groneberg, D.; Sikka, G.; Hori, D.; Ranek, M.J.; Nakamura, T.; Takimoto, E.; Paolocci, N.; Berkowitz, D.E.; Friebe, A.; et al. Soluble Guanylate Cyclase Is Required for Systemic Vasodilation But Not Positive Inotropy Induced by Nitroxyl in the Mouse. *Hypertension* **2014**, *65*, 385–392. [CrossRef]
116. Eberhardt, M.; Dux, M.; Namer, B.; Miljkovic, J.; Cordasic, N.; Will, C.; Kichko, T.I.; De La Roche, J.; Fischer, M.; Suárez, S.A.; et al. H_2S and NO Cooperatively Regulate Vascular Tone by Activating a Neuroendocrine HNO–TRPA1–CGRP Signalling Pathway. *Nat. Commun.* **2014**, *5*, 4381. [CrossRef]
117. Senoner, T.; Dichtl, W. Oxidative Stress in Cardiovascular Diseases: Still a Therapeutic Target? *Nutrients* **2019**, *11*, 90. [CrossRef]
118. Gryglewski, R.J.; Palmer, R.M.J.; Moncada, S. Superoxide Anion Is Involved in the Breakdown of Endothelium-Derived Vascular Relaxing Factor. *Nature* **1986**, *320*, 454–456. [CrossRef]
119. Zhang, M.S.; Liang, J.H.; Yang, M.J.; Ren, Y.R.; Cheng, D.H.; Wu, Q.H.; He, Y.; Yin, J. Low Serum Superoxide Dismutase Is Associated With a High Risk of Cognitive Impairment After Mild Acute Ischemic Stroke. *Front. Aging Neurosci.* **2022**, *14*, 834114. [CrossRef] [PubMed]
120. Gómez-Marcos, M.A.; Blázquez-Medela, A.M.; Gamella-Pozuelo, L.; Recio-Rodriguez, J.I.; García-Ortiz, L.; Martínez-Salgado, C. Serum Superoxide Dismutase Is Associated with Vascular Structure and Function in Hypertensive and Diabetic Patients. *Oxid. Med. Cell. Longev.* **2016**, *2016*, 9124676. [CrossRef] [PubMed]

121. Fesharaki-Zadeh, A. Oxidative Stress in Traumatic Brain Injury. *Int. J. Mol. Sci.* **2022**, *23*, 13000. [CrossRef] [PubMed]
122. Younus, H. Therapeutic Potentials of Superoxide Dismutase. *Int. J. Health Sci.* **2018**, *12*, 88–93.
123. McGirt, M.J.; Parra, A.; Sheng, H.; Higuchi, Y.; Oury, T.D.; Laskowitz, D.T.; Pearlstein, R.D.; Warner, D.S. Attenuation of Cerebral Vasospasm after Subarachnoid Hemorrhage in Mice Overexpressing Extracellular Superoxide Dismutase. *Stroke* **2002**, *33*, 2317–2323. [CrossRef] [PubMed]
124. Hazell, A.S.; Faim, S.; Wertheimer, G.; Silva, V.R.; Marques, C.S. The Impact of Oxidative Stress in Thiamine Deficiency: A Multifactorial Targeting Issue. *Neurochem. Int.* **2013**, *62*, 796–802. [CrossRef] [PubMed]
125. Bozic, I.; Lavrnja, I. Thiamine and Benfotiamine: Focus on Their Therapeutic Potential. *Heliyon* **2023**, *9*, e21839. [CrossRef] [PubMed]
126. Burk, R.F.; Hill, K.E. Glutathione Peroxidases. In *Comprehensive Toxicology*, 2nd ed.; Volume 4: Biotransformation; Elsevier Science: Amsterdam, The Netherlands, 2010; pp. 229–242. [CrossRef]
127. Angstwurm, M.W.A.; Engelmann, L.; Zimmermann, T.; Lehmann, C.; Spes, C.H.; Abel, P.; Strauß, R.; Meier-Hellmann, A.; Insel, R.; Radke, J.; et al. Selenium in Intensive Care (SIC): Results of a Prospective Randomized, Placebo-Controlled, Multiple-Center Study in Patients with Severe Systemic Inflammatory Response Syndrome, Sepsis, and Septic Shock. *Crit. Care Med.* **2007**, *35*, 118–126. [CrossRef] [PubMed]
128. Jaff, S.; Zeraattalab-Motlagh, S.; Amiri Khosroshahi, R.; Gubari, M.; Mohammadi, H.; Djafarian, K. The Effect of Selenium Therapy in Critically Ill Patients: An Umbrella Review of Systematic Reviews and Meta-Analysis of Randomized Controlled Trials. *Eur. J. Med. Res.* **2023**, *28*, 104. [CrossRef] [PubMed]
129. Aoyama, K. Glutathione in the Brain. *Int. J. Mol. Sci.* **2021**, *22*, 5010. [CrossRef] [PubMed]
130. Matuz-Mares, D.; Riveros-Rosas, H.; Vázquez-Meza, H.; Vilchis-Landeros, M.M. Glutathione Participation in the Prevention of Cardiovascular Diseases. *Antioxidants* **2021**, *10*, 1220. [CrossRef] [PubMed]
131. Schmitt, B.; Vicenzi, M.; Garrel, C.; Denis, F.M. Effects of N-Acetylcysteine, Oral Glutathione (GSH) and a Novel Sublingual Form of GSH on Oxidative Stress Markers: A Comparative Crossover Study. *Redox Biol.* **2015**, *6*, 198–205. [CrossRef] [PubMed]
132. Uemura, T.; Watanabe, K.; Ko, K.; Higashi, K.; Kogure, N.; Kitajima, M.; Takayama, H.; Takao, K.; Sugita, Y.; Sakamoto, A.; et al. Protective Effects of Brain Infarction by N-Acetylcysteine Derivatives. *Stroke* **2018**, *49*, 1727–1733. [CrossRef]
133. Sabetghadam, M.; Mazdeh, M.; Abolfathi, P.; Mohammadi, Y.; Mehrpooya, M. Evidence for a Beneficial Effect of Oral N-Acetylcysteine on Functional Outcomes and Inflammatory Biomarkers in Patients with Acute Ischemic Stroke. *Neuropsychiatr. Dis. Treat.* **2020**, *16*, 1265–1278. [CrossRef]
134. Olesen, H.Ø.; Pors, S.E.; Jensen, L.B.; Grønning, A.P.; Lemser, C.E.; Nguyen Heimbürger, M.T.H.; Mamsen, L.S.; Getreu, N.; Christensen, S.T.; Andersen, C.Y.; et al. N-Acetylcysteine Protects Ovarian Follicles from Ischemia-Reperfusion Injury in Xenotransplanted Human Ovarian Tissue. *Hum. Reprod.* **2021**, *36*, 429–443. [CrossRef]
135. Cayuela, N.C.; Koike, M.K.; Jacysyn, J.d.F.; Rasslan, R.; Cerqueira, A.R.A.; Costa, S.K.P.; Diniz-Júnior, J.A.P.; Utiyama, E.M.; de Souza Montero, E.F. N-Acetylcysteine Reduced Ischemia and Reperfusion Damage Associated with Steatohepatitis in Mice. *Int. J. Mol. Sci.* **2020**, *21*, 4106. [CrossRef]
136. Raghu, G.; Berk, M.; Campochiaro, P.A.; Jaeschke, H.; Marenzi, G.; Richeldi, L.; Wen, F.-Q.; Nicoletti, F.; Calverley, P.M.A. The Multifaceted Therapeutic Role of N-Acetylcysteine (NAC) in Disorders Characterized by Oxidative Stress. *Curr. Neuropharmacol.* **2021**, *19*, 1202–1224. [CrossRef]
137. Ballaz, S.J.; Rebec, G.V. Neurobiology of Vitamin C: Expanding the Focus from Antioxidant to Endogenous Neuromodulator. *Pharmacol. Res.* **2019**, *146*, 104321. [CrossRef]
138. Harrison, F.E.; May, J.M. Vitamin C Function in the Brain: Vital Role of the Ascorbate Transporter SVCT2. *Free Radic. Biol. Med.* **2009**, *46*, 719–730. [CrossRef]
139. Rice, M.E. Ascorbate Regulation and Its Neuroprotective Role in the Brain. *Trends Neurosci.* **2000**, *23*, 209–216. [CrossRef]
140. Grossmann, M.; Dobrev, D.; Himmel, H.M.; Ravens, U.; Kirch, W. Ascorbic Acid–Induced Modulation of Venous Tone in Humans. *Hypertension* **2001**, *37*, 949–954. [CrossRef] [PubMed]
141. May, J.M. How Does Ascorbic Acid Prevent Endothelial Dysfunction? *Free Radic. Biol. Med.* **2000**, *28*, 1421–1429. [CrossRef] [PubMed]
142. Barak, O.F.; Caljkusic, K.; Hoiland, R.L.; Ainslie, P.N.; Thom, S.R.; Yang, M.; Jovanov, P.; Dujic, Z. Differential Influence of Vitamin C on the Peripheral and Cerebral Circulation after Diving and Exposure to Hyperoxia. *Am. J. Physiol. Regul. Integr. Comp. Physiol.* **2018**, *315*, R759–R767. [CrossRef] [PubMed]
143. Salvagno, M.; Taccone, F.S.; Bogossian, E.G. Tissue Hyperoxia Is Not a Risk Factor for Cerebral Vasospasm Following Subarachnoid Hemorrhage. *J. Neurol. Sci.* **2023**, *445*, 120535. [CrossRef] [PubMed]
144. Kawakami, M.; Kodama, N.; Toda, N. Suppression of the Cerebral Vasospastic Actions of Oxyhemoglobin by Ascorbic Acid. *Neurosurgery* **1991**, *28*, 33. [CrossRef] [PubMed]
145. Abdullah, M.; Jamil, R.T.; Attia, F.N. Vitamin C (Ascorbic Acid). In *Encyclopedia of Toxicology*, 3rd ed.; Elsevier: Amsterdam, The Netherlands, 2023; pp. 962–963. [CrossRef]
146. Engin, K.N. Alpha-Tocopherol: Looking beyond an Antioxidant. *Mol. Vis.* **2009**, *15*, 855–860.
147. La Torre, M.E.; Villano, I.; Monda, M.; Messina, A.; Cibelli, G.; Valenzano, A.; Pisanelli, D.; Panaro, M.A.; Tartaglia, N.; Ambrosi, A.; et al. Role of Vitamin E and the Orexin System in Neuroprotection. *Brain Sci.* **2021**, *11*, 1098. [CrossRef]

148. Motoyama, T.; Kawano, H.; Kugiyama, K.; Hirashima, O.; Ohgushi, M.; Tsunoda, R.; Moriyama, Y.; Miyao, Y.; Yoshimura, M.; Ogawa, H.; et al. Vitamin E Administration Improves Impairment of Endothelium-Dependent Vasodilation in Patients with Coronary Spastic Angina. *J. Am. Coll. Cardiol.* **1998**, *32*, 1672–1679. [CrossRef]
149. Rasool, A.H.G.; Rahman, A.R.A.; Yuen, K.H.; Wong, A.R. Arterial Compliance and Vitamin E Blood Levels with a Self Emulsifying Preparation of Tocotrienol Rich Vitamin E. *Arch. Pharm. Res.* **2008**, *31*, 1212–1217. [CrossRef]
150. Heitzer, T.; Ylä Herttuala, S.; Wild, E.; Luoma, J.; Drexler, H. Effect of Vitamin E on Endothelial Vasodilator Function in Patients with Hypercholesterolemia, Chronic Smoking or Both. *J. Am. Coll. Cardiol.* **1999**, *33*, 499–505. [CrossRef]
151. Cheng, P.; Wang, L.; Ning, S.; Liu, Z.; Lin, H.; Chen, S.; Zhu, J. Vitamin E Intake and Risk of Stroke: A Meta-Analysis. *Br. J. Nutr.* **2018**, *120*, 1181–1188. [CrossRef] [PubMed]
152. Loh, H.C.; Lim, R.; Lee, K.W.; Ooi, C.Y.; Chuan, D.R.; Looi, I.; Kah Hay, Y.; Abdul Karim Khan, N. Effects of Vitamin E on Stroke: A Systematic Review with Meta-Analysis and Trial Sequential Analysis. *Stroke Vasc. Neurol.* **2021**, *6*, 109–120. [CrossRef] [PubMed]
153. Pfister, H.W.; Ködel, U.; Dirnagl, U.; Haberl, R.L.; Ruckdeschel, G.; Einhäupl, K.M. Effect of Catalase on Regional Cerebral Blood Flow and Brain Edema during the Early Phase of Experimental Pneumococcal Meningitis. *J. Infect. Dis.* **1992**, *166*, 1442–1445. [CrossRef]
154. Iida, Y.; Katusic, Z.S.; Wei, E.P. Mechanisms of Cerebral Arterial Relaxations to Hydrogen Peroxide. *Stroke* **2000**, *31*, 2224–2230. [CrossRef] [PubMed]
155. Bondonno, N.P.; Bondonno, C.P.; Blekkenhorst, L.C.; Considine, M.J.; Maghzal, G.; Stocker, R.; Woodman, R.J.; Ward, N.C.; Hodgson, J.M.; Croft, K.D. Flavonoid-Rich Apple Improves Endothelial Function in Individuals at Risk for Cardiovascular Disease: A Randomized Controlled Clinical Trial. *Mol. Nutr. Food Res.* **2018**, *62*, 1700674. [CrossRef]
156. Vauzour, D.; Vafeiadou, K.; Rodriguez-Mateos, A.; Rendeiro, C.; Spencer, J.P.E. The Neuroprotective Potential of Flavonoids: A Multiplicity of Effects. *Genes Nutr.* **2008**, *3*, 115–126. [CrossRef]
157. Gül, Ş.; Aydoğmuş, E.; Bahadir, B.; Büyükuysal, Ç.; Güven, B. Neuroprotective Effects of Quercetin on Cerebral Vasospasm Following Experimental Subarachnoid Haemorrhage in Rats. *Turk. J. Med. Sci.* **2020**, *50*, 1106–1110. [CrossRef]
158. Zhang, L.; Ma, J.; Yang, F.; Li, S.; Ma, W.; Chang, X.; Yang, L. Neuroprotective Effects of Quercetin on Ischemic Stroke: A Literature Review. *Front. Pharmacol.* **2022**, *13*, 854249. [CrossRef]
159. Lee, J.M.; Jeong, S.W.; Kim, M.Y.; Park, J.B.; Kim, M.S. The Effect of Vitamin D Supplementation in Patients with Acute Traumatic Brain Injury. *World Neurosurg.* **2019**, *126*, e1421–e1426. [CrossRef] [PubMed]
160. Wei, S.; Yuan, X.; Li, D.; Fan, F.; Guo, X.; Xu, Y.; Guan, S. Vitamin D Level Is Associated with Rupture of Intracranial Aneurysm in Patients with Subarachnoid Hemorrhage. *Front. Neurol.* **2022**, *13*, 890950. [CrossRef]
161. Della Nera, G.; Sabatino, L.; Gaggini, M.; Gorini, F.; Vassalle, C. Vitamin D Determinants, Status, and Antioxidant/Anti-Inflammatory-Related Effects in Cardiovascular Risk and Disease: Not the Last Word in the Controversy. *Antioxidants* **2023**, *12*, 948. [CrossRef] [PubMed]
162. Tagliaferri, S.; Porri, D.; De Giuseppe, R.; Manuelli, M.; Alessio, F.; Cena, H. The Controversial Role of Vitamin D as an Antioxidant: Results from Randomised Controlled Trials. *Nutr. Res. Rev.* **2019**, *32*, 99–105. [CrossRef]
163. Dao, D.Q.; Ngo, T.C.; Thong, N.M.; Nam, P.C. Is Vitamin A an Antioxidant or a Pro-Oxidant? *J. Phys. Chem. B* **2017**, *121*, 9348–9357. [CrossRef]
164. Hummel, R.; Ulbrich, S.; Appel, D.; Li, S.; Hirnet, T.; Zander, S.; Bobkiewicz, W.; Gölz, C.; Schäfer, M.K.E. Administration of All-Trans Retinoic Acid after Experimental Traumatic Brain Injury Is Brain Protective. *Br. J. Pharmacol.* **2020**, *177*, 5208–5223. [CrossRef] [PubMed]
165. Bonney, S.; Harrison-Uy, S.; Mishra, S.; MacPherson, A.M.; Choe, Y.; Li, D.; Jaminet, S.C.; Fruttiger, M.; Pleasure, S.J.; Siegenthaler, J.A. Diverse Functions of Retinoic Acid in Brain Vascular Development. *J. Neurosci.* **2016**, *36*, 7786–7801. [CrossRef]
166. Sautin, Y.Y.; Johnson, R.J. Uric Acid: The Oxidant–Antioxidant Paradox. *Nucleosides Nucleotides Nucleic Acids* **2008**, *27*, 608–619. [CrossRef]
167. Halvorson, B.; Frisbee, J.; Halvorson, B.; Frisbee, J. Cerebral Vascular Tone Regulation: Integration and Impact of Disease. In *Basic and Clinical Understanding of Microcirculation*; IntechOpen: London, UK, 2020. [CrossRef]
168. Hsieh, H.J.; Liu, C.A.; Huang, B.; Tseng, A.H.; Wang, D.L. Shear-Induced Endothelial Mechanotransduction: The Interplay between Reactive Oxygen Species (ROS) and Nitric Oxide (NO) and the Pathophysiological Implications. *J. Biomed. Sci.* **2014**, *21*, 3. [CrossRef]
169. Demchenko, I.T.; Boso, A.E.; O'Neill, T.J.; Bennett, P.B.; Piantadosi, C.A. Nitric Oxide and Cerebral Blood Flow Responses to Hyperbaric Oxygen. *J. Appl. Physiol.* **2000**, *88*, 1381–1389. [CrossRef]
170. Zhilyaev, S.Y.; Moskvin, A.N.; Platonova, T.F.; Gutsaeva, D.R.; Churilina, I.V.; Demchenko, I.T. Hyperoxic Vasoconstriction in the Brain Is Mediated by Inactivation of Nitric Oxide by Superoxide Anions. *Neurosci. Behav. Physiol.* **2003**, *33*, 783–787. [CrossRef]
171. Jelinek, M.; Jurajda, M.; Duris, K. Oxidative Stress in the Brain: Basic Concepts and Treatment Strategies in Stroke. *Antioxidants* **2021**, *10*, 1886. [CrossRef] [PubMed]
172. Nguyen, A.; Patel, A.B.; Kioutchoukova, I.P.; Diaz, M.J.; Valenti, D.; Nguyen, A.; Patel, A.B.; Kioutchoukova, I.P.; Diaz, M.J.; Lucke-Wold, B. Mechanisms of Mitochondrial Oxidative Stress in Brain Injury: From Pathophysiology to Therapeutics. *Oxygen* **2023**, *3*, 163–178. [CrossRef]
173. Chen, X.; Guo, C.; Kong, J. Oxidative Stress in Neurodegenerative Diseases. *Neural Regen. Res.* **2012**, *7*, 376–385. [CrossRef] [PubMed]

174. Villalba, N.; Sonkusare, S.K.; Longden, T.A.; Tran, T.L.; Sackheim, A.M.; Nelson, M.T.; Wellman, G.C.; Freeman, K. Traumatic Brain Injury Disrupts Cerebrovascular Tone Through Endothelial Inducible Nitric Oxide Synthase Expression and Nitric Oxide Gain of Function. *J. Am. Heart Assoc. Cardiovasc. Cerebrovasc. Dis.* **2014**, *3*, e001474. [CrossRef] [PubMed]
175. Szarka, N.; Pabbidi, M.R.; Amrein, K.; Czeiter, E.; Berta, G.; Pohoczky, K.; Helyes, Z.; Ungvari, Z.; Koller, A.; Buki, A.; et al. Traumatic Brain Injury Impairs Myogenic Constriction of Cerebral Arteries: Role of Mitochondria-Derived H2O2 and TRPV4-Dependent Activation of BKca Channels. *J. Neurotrauma* **2018**, *35*, 930–939. [CrossRef] [PubMed]
176. Spranger, M.; Krempien, S.; Schwab, S.; Donneberg, S.; Hacke, W. Superoxide Dismutase Activity in Serum of Patients With Acute Cerebral Ischemic Injury. *Stroke* **1997**, *28*, 2425–2428. [CrossRef] [PubMed]
177. Wang, K.; Yin, L.; Song, Y.; Zhang, M.; Lu, Y.; Wang, S. The Use of Hydrocortisone, Ascorbic Acid and Thiamine in Patients with Sepsis and Septic Shock—A Systematic Review. *J. Pharm. Pract.* **2023**, *36*, 933–940. [CrossRef] [PubMed]
178. Lamontagne, F.; Masse, M.-H.; Menard, J.; Sprague, S.; Pinto, R.; Heyland, D.K.; Cook, D.J.; Battista, M.-C.; Day, A.G.; Guyatt, G.H.; et al. Intravenous Vitamin C in Adults with Sepsis in the Intensive Care Unit. *N. Engl. J. Med.* **2022**, *386*, 2387–2398. [CrossRef] [PubMed]
179. Bowton, D.L.; Bertels, N.H.; Prough, D.S.; Stump, D.A. Cerebral Blood Flow Is Reduced in Patients with Sepsis Syndrome. *Crit. Care Med.* **1989**, *17*, 399–403. [CrossRef]
180. Margaritelis, N.V.; Paschalis, V.; Theodorou, A.A.; Vassiliou, V.; Kyparos, A.; Nikolaidis, M.G. Rapid Decreases of Key Antioxidant Molecules in Critically Ill Patients: A Personalized Approach. *Clin. Nutr.* **2020**, *39*, 1146–1154. [CrossRef] [PubMed]

Disclaimer/Publisher's Note: The statements, opinions and data contained in all publications are solely those of the individual author(s) and contributor(s) and not of MDPI and/or the editor(s). MDPI and/or the editor(s) disclaim responsibility for any injury to people or property resulting from any ideas, methods, instructions or products referred to in the content.

International Journal of
Molecular Sciences

MDPI

Article

The Effect of Targeted Hyperoxemia on Brain Immunohistochemistry after Long-Term, Resuscitated Porcine Acute Subdural Hematoma and Hemorrhagic Shock

Franziska Münz [1,2,*], Thomas Datzmann [1], Andrea Hoffmann [1], Michael Gröger [1], René Mathieu [3], Simon Mayer [3], Fabian Zink [1], Holger Gässler [4], Eva-Maria Wolfschmitt [1], Melanie Hogg [1], Enrico Calzia [1], Pierre Asfar [5], Peter Radermacher [1], Thomas Kapapa [6,†] and Tamara Merz [1,2,*,†]

1 Institute for Anesthesiological Pathophysiology and Process Engineering, Ulm University, 89081 Ulm, Germany; peter.radermacher@uni-ulm.de (P.R.)
2 Department of Anesthesiology and Intensive Care Medicine, University Hospital Ulm, 89081 Ulm, Germany
3 Department of Neurosurgery, German Federal Armed Forces Hospital Ulm, 89081 Ulm, Germany
4 Department of Anesthesiology, Intensive Care Medicine, Emergency Medicine and Pain Therapy, German Armed Forces Hospital Ulm, 89081 Ulm, Germany
5 Department of Intensive Care and Hyperbaric Medicine, University Hospital Angers, 49045 Angers, France
6 Department of Neurosurgery, University Hospital Ulm, 89081 Ulm, Germany
* Correspondence: franziska.muenz@uni-ulm.de (F.M.); tamara.merz@uni-ulm.de (T.M.)
† These authors contributed equally to this work.

Abstract: Epidemiological data suggest that moderate hyperoxemia may be associated with an improved outcome after traumatic brain injury. In a prospective, randomized investigation of long-term, resuscitated acute subdural hematoma plus hemorrhagic shock (ASDH + HS) in 14 adult, human-sized pigs, targeted hyperoxemia ($200 < P_aO_2 < 250$ mmHg vs. normoxemia $80 < P_aO_2 < 120$ mmHg) coincided with improved neurological function. Since brain perfusion, oxygenation and metabolism did not differ, this post hoc study analyzed the available material for the effects of targeted hyperoxemia on cerebral tissue markers of oxidative/nitrosative stress (nitrotyrosine expression), blood–brain barrier integrity (extravascular albumin accumulation) and fluid homeostasis (oxytocin, its receptor and the H_2S-producing enzymes cystathionine-β-synthase and cystathionine-γ-lyase). After 2 h of ASDH + HS (0.1 mL/kgBW autologous blood injected into the subdural space and passive removal of 30% of the blood volume), animals were resuscitated for up to 53 h by re-transfusion of shed blood, noradrenaline infusion to maintain cerebral perfusion pressure at baseline levels and hyper-/normoxemia during the first 24 h. Immediate postmortem, bi-hemispheric (i.e., blood-injected and contra-lateral) prefrontal cortex specimens from the base of the sulci underwent immunohistochemistry (% positive tissue staining) analysis of oxidative/nitrosative stress, blood–brain barrier integrity and fluid homeostasis. None of these tissue markers explained any differences in hyperoxemia-related neurological function. Likewise, hyperoxemia exerted no deleterious effects.

Keywords: traumatic brain injury; blood–brain barrier; oxidative/nitrosative stress; cystathionine-β-synthase; cystathionine-γ-lyase; oxytocin; oxytocin receptor

1. Introduction

The post-traumatic mortality and morbidity are contingent upon the presence or absence of traumatic brain injury (TBI) and/or hemorrhagic shock (HS) [1]. Throughout HS treatment, supplementary O_2 is often administered to enhance the amount of physically dissolved O_2, aiming to expedite the restoration of tissue O_2 levels during impairment of O_2 transport caused by blood loss [2].

Hyperoxemia, however, may exert potentially adverse effects, including elevated generation of reactive oxygen species (ROS), in particular during ischemia/reperfusion sequences, e.g., restoration of blood flow during resuscitation from HS [2]. Nonetheless, after TBI, epidemiological data showed that the presence of moderate hyperoxemia ($150 < P_aO_2 < 200$ mmHg during the initial 24 h of intensive care unit (ICU) stay) coincided with improved functional outcomes and survival [3]. In contrast, more recent data from the Center–TBI cohort found that long-term morbidity and mortality were aggravated with every 10 mmHg increase in supranormal arterial O_2 partial pressure (P_aO_2) [4]. Finally, in a long-term, resuscitated porcine model of acute subdural hematoma (ASDH) and HS in adult and cardiovascular healthy animals, hyperoxemia targeting P_aO_2 of 200–250 mmHg was associated with improved neurological function when compared to standard treatment (P_aO_2 80–120 mmHg) [5]. In these experiments, neither parameters of cerebral tissue perfusion (intracranial and cerebral perfusion pressure) and oxygenation (brain tissue O_2 partial pressure) nor metabolism (tissue microdialysis for glucose, lactate, pyruvate, and glutamate) showed any differences between the two experimental groups. Hence, the mechanisms allowing us to explain any effects of this targeted hyperoxemia on neurological function remain largely underexplored.

In a long-term, resuscitated porcine model, we had previously shown that ASDH alone, i.e., without additional HS, was associated both with markedly higher extravascular albumin accumulation as a marker of blood–brain barrier dysfunction, as well as nitrotyrosine formation as a marker of oxidative and nitrosative stress in the blood-injected brain hemisphere when compared to the contralateral regions, which had only undergone neurosurgical instrumentation [6]. Hippocampal nitrotyrosine staining was also significantly increased in hyperoxia-exposed rats after controlled cortical impact-induced TBI [7]. However, delayed analysis of neuronal survival in that study did not show any significant difference between the hyperoxic and normoxic groups. In mice that had undergone combined TBI and HS, hyperoxia was also associated with signs of aggravated tissue oxidative stress, as demonstrated by increased ascorbate depletion, but, in contrast, hippocampal neuron survival improved [8].

Both oxytocin (OT) as well as its receptor (OT-R) and the hydrogen sulfide (H_2S) system are believed to be of pivotal importance in the stress response to physical and psychological trauma, but also in fluid homeostasis, e.g., blood loss. In fact, in hemorrhaged rats, OT formation was significantly decreased both in the hypothalamus and in the neurohypophysis [9]. Moreover, tissue OT was shown to be significantly decreased in the ipsilateral striatum in a mouse model of intracerebral hemorrhage, whereas the OT-R expression showed the opposite response, i.e., a significant increase [10]. Our immunohistochemical characterization of the H_2S and OT systems in brain specimen from swine that had undergone ASDH alone without HS showed expression of the OT-R on both sides, i.e., in the brain hemisphere affected by the acute subdural hematoma (ipsilateral) as well as in the control (contralateral) hemisphere. OT, however, was only expressed on the ipsilateral side. Similarly, cystathionine-β-synthase (CBS), one of the two major H_2S-producing enzymes, was also predominantly detected on the ipsilateral side. In contrast, the staining for cystathionine-γ-lyase (CSE), the other of the two major H_2S-producing enzymes, was primarily present in the contralateral hemisphere, i.e., that without subdural blood injection [11]. Finally, after murine TBI, the expression of CBS was significantly decreased in the ipsilateral hemisphere, but reached basal level after 7 days [12]. It is noteworthy that the aforementioned rodent studies were conducted without hemodynamic support to maintain cerebral perfusion pressure (CPP), which is crucial for the outcome of TBI patients. Moreover, animals breathed pure O_2 rather than an inspiratory O_2 concentration titrated to achieve pre-defined P_aO_2 targets; in other words, they were exposed to potentially excessive hyperoxia.

Hence, the effect of targeted hyperoxemia after combined ASDH-induced TBI and HS on brain immunohistochemistry is still unknown. Therefore, this post hoc study of brain tissue specimens available as part of the above-mentioned interventional study [5] investigated the effect of targeted hyperoxemia on cerebral tissue markers of oxidative/nitrosative stress, blood–brain barrier integrity and fluid homeostasis.

2. Results

Figures 1 and 2 show representative images (left side) and the quantitative analysis (right panels) of the cerebral tissue detection of albumin (Figure 1) as, when occurring outside of the vasculature, a marker of blood–brain barrier integrity in both gray (upper graphs) and white matter (lower graphs) as well as for nitrotyrosine (Figure 2) as a marker of oxidative and nitrosative stress. Neither nitrotyrosine expression nor extravascular albumin accumulation showed any significant intergroup difference, regardless of the presence/absence of ASDH or of hyperoxemia. While a substantial amount of albumin was detected in the gray matter and a noteworthy portion of tissue in the white matter, indicating compromised blood–brain barrier function, nearly no nitrotyrosine was present in the gray matter, and very little in the white matter.

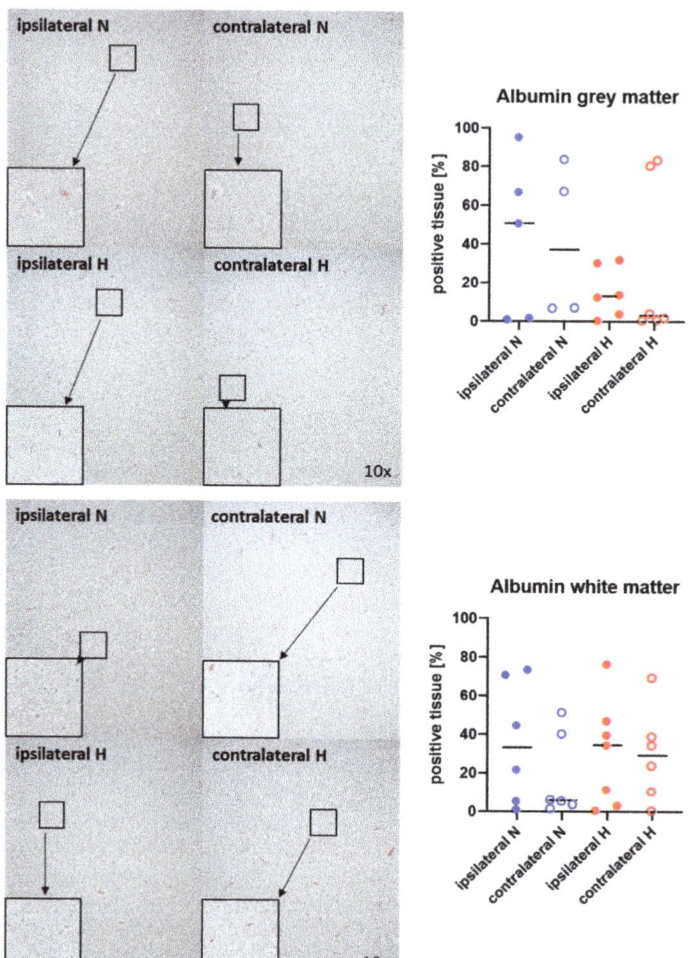

Figure 1. Albumin in the gray matter (**upper panel**; n = 4–6) and white matter (**lower panel**; n = 6–7) of the prefrontal cortex. Representative images (**left panel**), 30× magnified images originating from the black box in the 10× magnified image and quantification of immunohistochemical staining as positive tissue [pink, %] (**right graph**). N: Normoxemia (blue symbols); H: Hyperoxemia (red symbols); ipsilateral: blood-injected hemisphere (solid circles); contralateral: instrumented-only hemisphere (open circles).

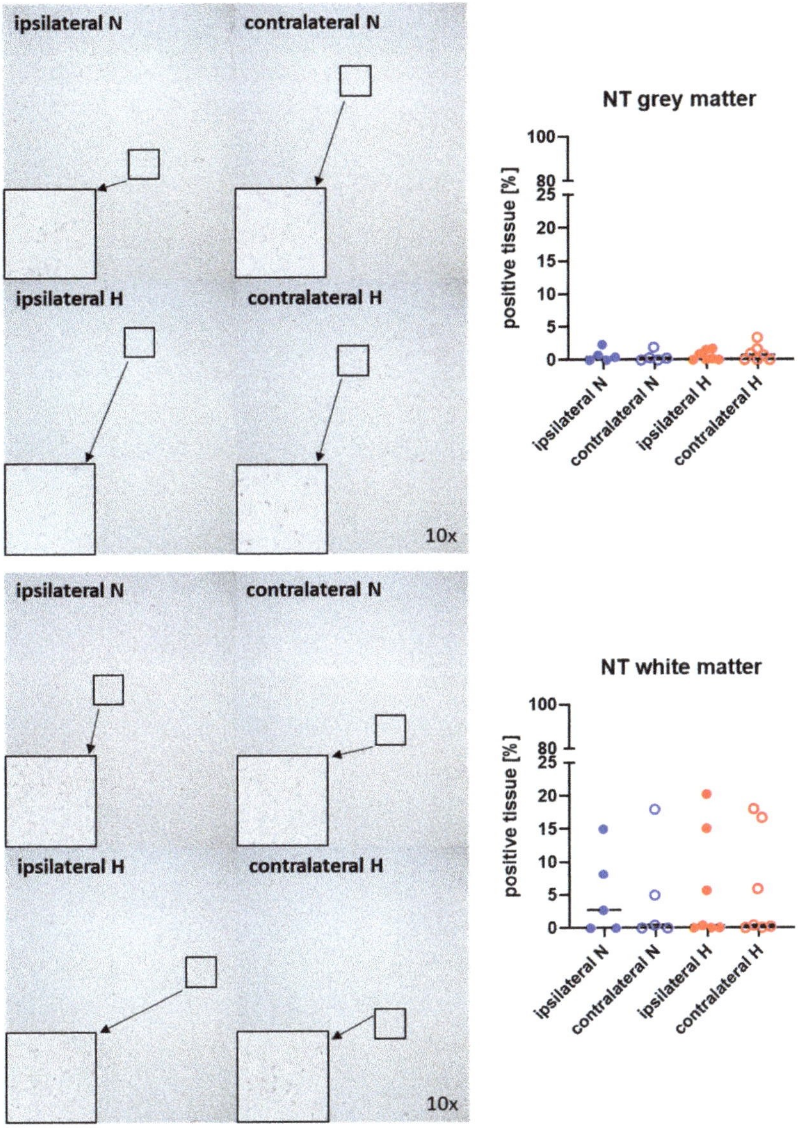

Figure 2. Nitrotyrosine (NT) in the gray matter (**upper panel**; n = 5–7) and white matter (**lower panel**; n = 5–7) of the prefrontal cortex. Representative images (**left panel**), 30× magnified images originating from the black box in the 10× magnified image and quantification of immunohistochemical staining as positive tissue [pink, %] (**right graph**). N: Normoxemia (blue symbols); H: Hyperoxemia (red symbols); ipsilateral: blood-injected hemisphere (solid circles); contralateral: instrumented-only hemisphere (open circles).

Figures 3 and 4 show representative images (left panels) and the quantitative analysis (right panels) of the cerebral tissue staining for oxytocin (Figure 3) and oxytocin receptor (Figure 4) in both gray (top graphs) and white matter (bottom graphs). Neither oxytocin nor the expression of oxytocin receptor exhibited any significant intergroup variance, irrespective of the presence or absence of ASDH or hyperoxemia.

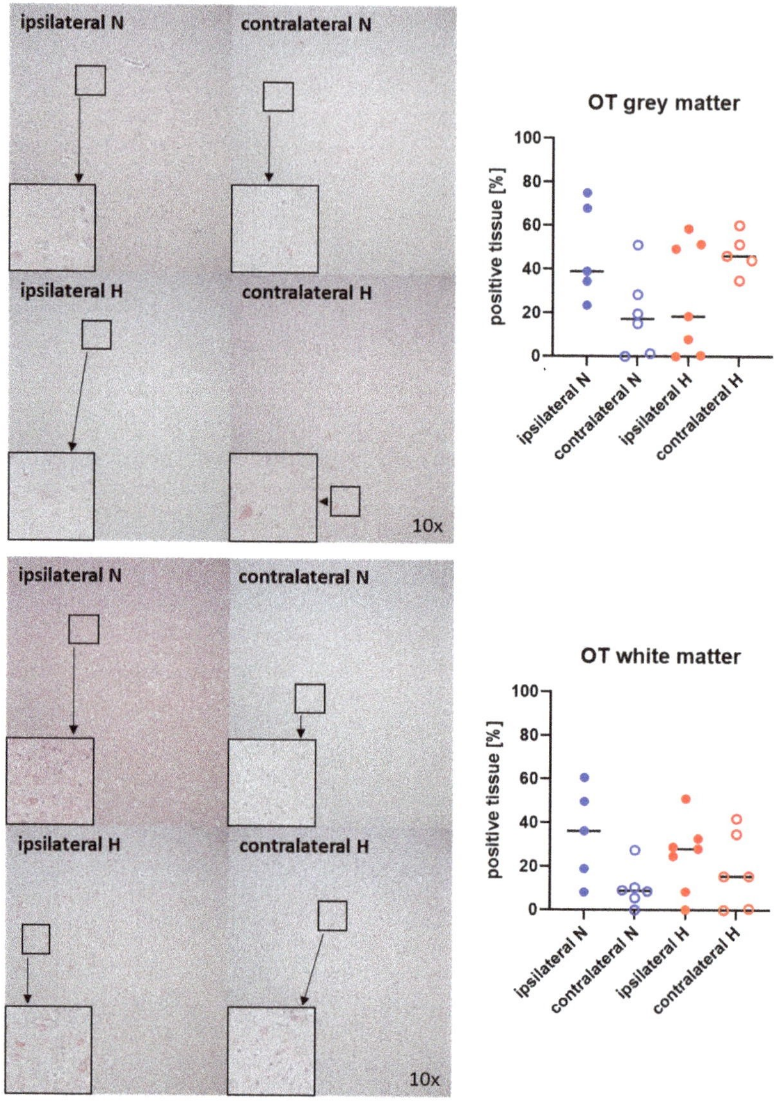

Figure 3. Oxytocin (OT) in the gray matter (**upper panel**; n = 5–7) and white matter (**lower panel**; n = 5–7) of the prefrontal cortex. Representative images (**left panel**), 30× magnified images originating from the black box in the 10× magnified image and quantification of immunohistochemical staining as positive tissue [pink, %] (**right graph**). N: Normoxemia (blue symbols); H: Hyperoxemia (red symbols); ipsilateral: blood-injected hemisphere (solid circles); contralateral: instrumented-only hemisphere (open circles).

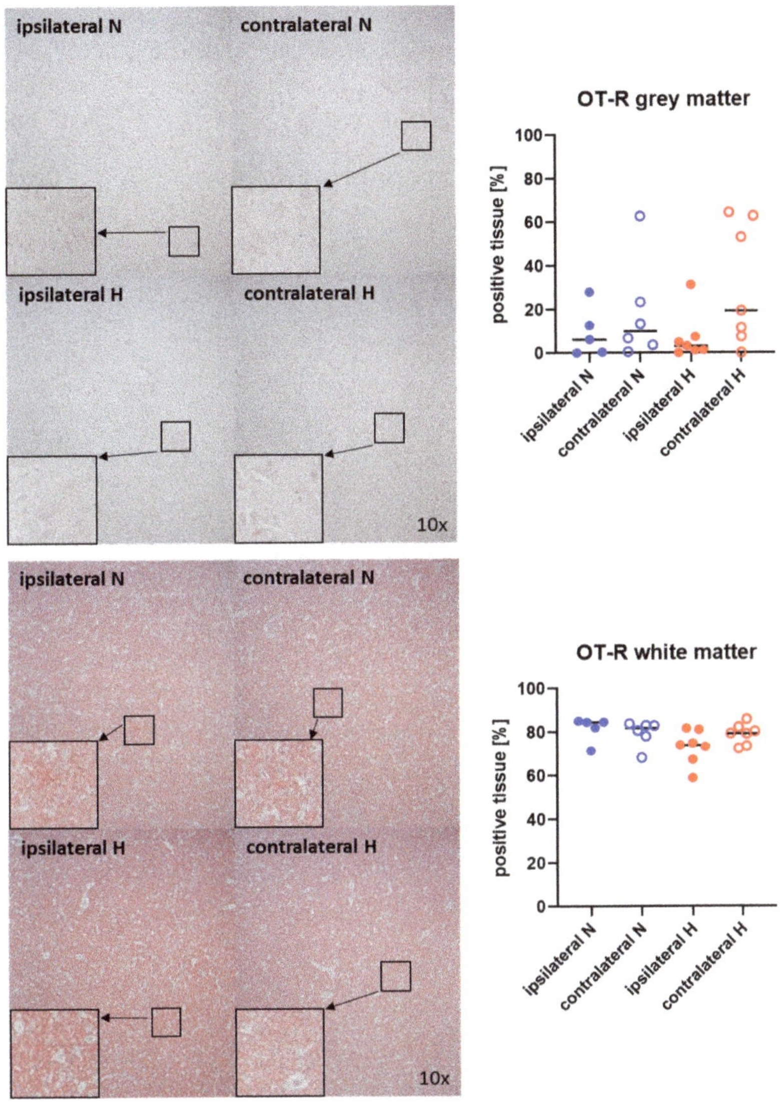

Figure 4. Oxytocin receptor (OT-R) in the gray matter (**upper panel**; n = 5–7) and white matter (**lower panel**; n = 5–7) of the prefrontal cortex. Representative images (**left panel**), 30× magnified images originating from the black box in the 10× magnified image and quantification of immunohistochemical staining as positive tissue [pink, %] (**right graph**). N: Normoxemia (blue symbols); H: Hyperoxemia (red symbols); ipsilateral: blood-injected hemisphere (solid circles); contralateral: instrumented-only hemisphere (open circles).

Representative images (left panels) and the quantitative analysis (right panels) of the cerebral tissue staining for the H_2S-producing enzymes CBS and CSE are presented in Figures 5 and 6 (gray matter: upper graphs; white matter: lower graphs). Neither CBS (Figure 5) nor CSE (Figure 6) showed any significant intergroup differences.

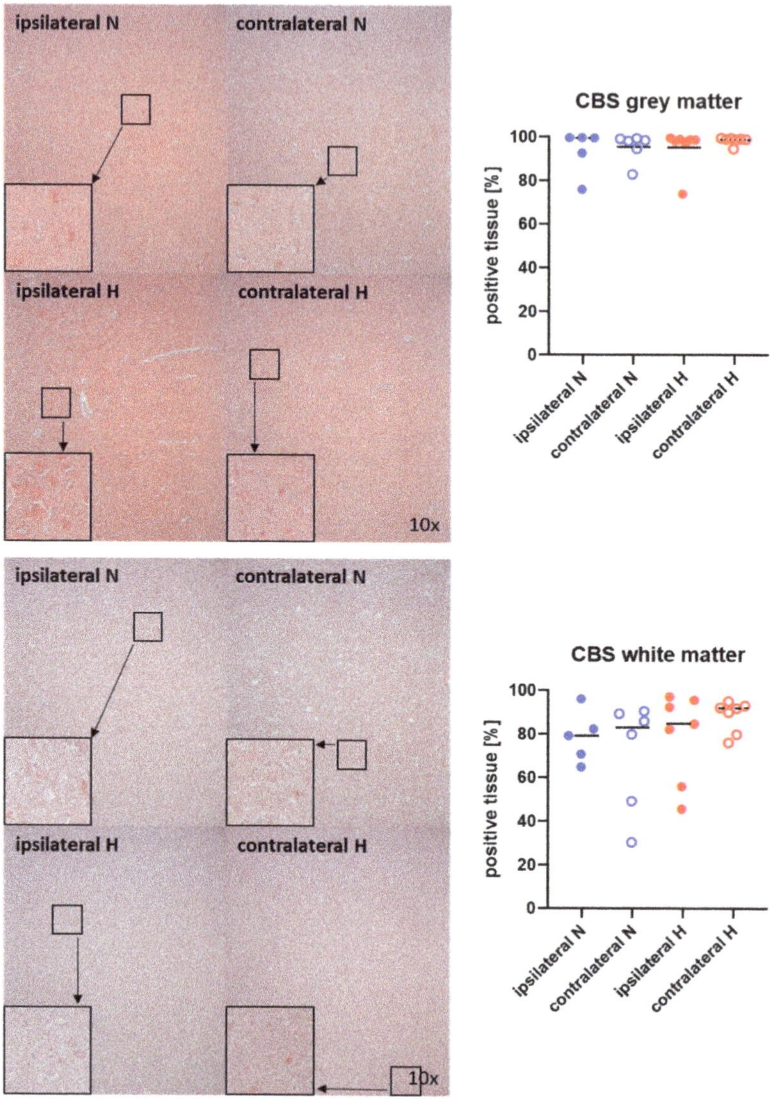

Figure 5. H_2S-producing enzyme cystathionine-β-synthase (CBS) in the gray matter (**upper panel**; n = 5–7) and white matter (**lower panel**; n = 5–7) of the prefrontal cortex. Representative images (**left panel**), 30× magnified images originating from the black box in the 10× magnified image and quantification of immunohistochemical staining as positive tissue [pink, %] (**right graph**). N: Normoxemia (blue symbols); H: Hyperoxemia (red symbols); ipsilateral: blood-injected hemisphere (solid circles); contralateral: instrumented-only hemisphere (open circles).

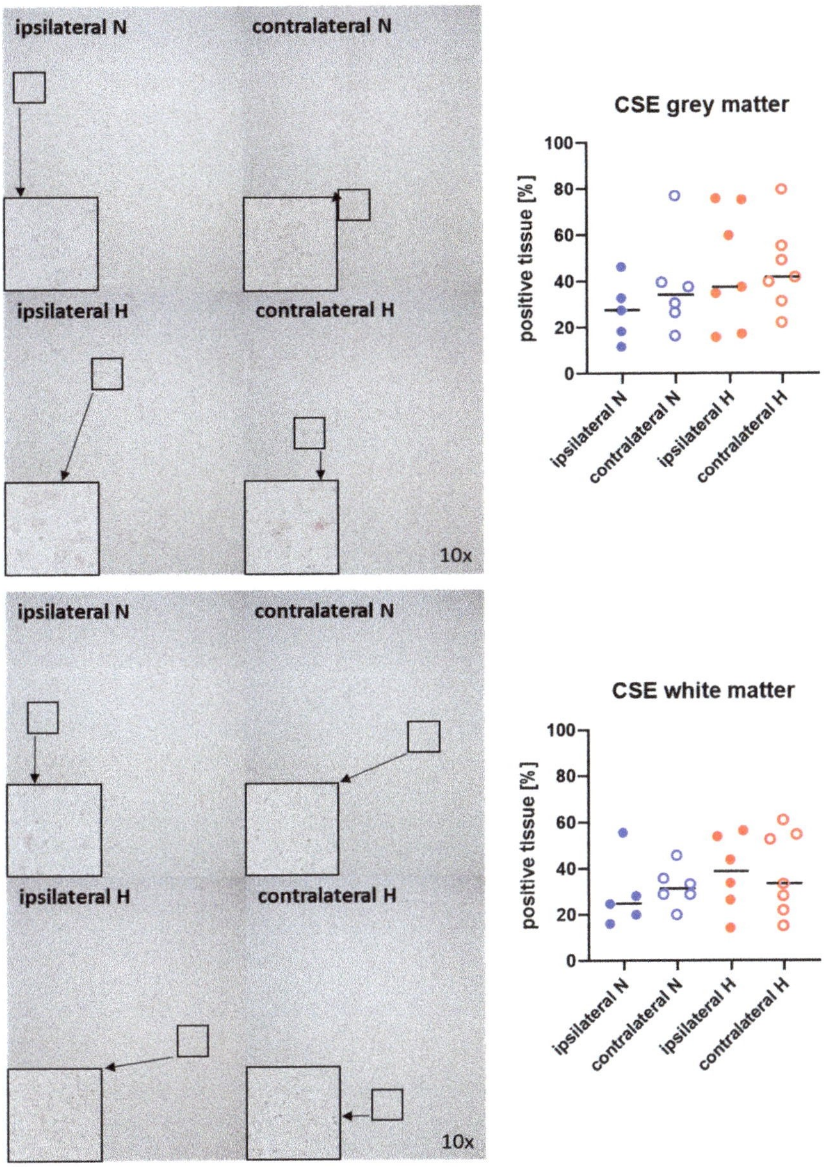

Figure 6. H_2S-producing enzyme cystathionine-γ-lyase (CSE) in the gray matter (**upper panel**; n = 5–7) and white matter (**lower panel**; n = 5–7) of the prefrontal cortex. Representative images (**left panel**), 30× magnified images originating from the black box in the 10× magnified image and quantification of immunohistochemical staining as positive tissue [pink, %] (**right graph**). N: Normoxemia (blue symbols); H: Hyperoxemia (red symbols); ipsilateral: blood-injected hemisphere (solid circles); contralateral: instrumented-only hemisphere (open circles).

3. Discussion

The aim of this investigation was to assess the protein levels of extravascular albumin, nitrotyrosine, CBS, CSE, OT, and OT-R in the prefrontal cortex following ASDH and HS, and subsequent resuscitation with targeted hyperoxemia vs. standard treatment. The main findings of the present study were (i) no significant differences in expression of any of these parameters, (ii) without major effect at all of hyperoxemia.

In our study, the presence of albumin extravasation served as an indication of the destruction of the blood–brain barrier, which is consistent with findings from a previous study conducted on gerbils, wherein immunohistochemical analysis demonstrated increased permeability of the blood–brain barrier to serum albumin after infarction in the hippocampus [13]. In comparison to our prior investigations in swine, the following disparities were observed: following HS alone without simultaneous ASDH or any other direct acute brain injury, no alterations in the levels of extravascular albumin had been noted [14], whereas following ASDH alone, i.e., direct acute brain injury, but without concomitant circulatory depression, a significant increase in extravascular albumin was detected in the ipsilateral, i.e., blood-injected brain hemisphere [6]. In the present study, the concurrent occurrence of ASDH and HS induced an extravasation of albumin. Overall, these findings suggest that only the combined presence of acute brain injury and circulatory (in other words, simultaneous regional (cerebral) and systemic (circulatory shock)) challenge is mandatory to produce disruption of the blood–brain barrier in the contralateral hemisphere, i.e., that without blood injection, ultimately resulting in albumin extravasation.

The present study revealed only a little nitrotyrosine expression, regardless of the blood-injected vs. instrumented-only hemisphere. In comparison, in the previously mentioned study focusing on HS alone, no expression of nitrotyrosine was detected [14]. Conversely, following ASDH alone, a significantly higher level of nitrotyrosine could be observed in the ipsilateral hemisphere [6]. This might suggest that ASDH alone per se may induce ipsilateral oxidative stress. It should be noted, however, that in that study, the volume of blood injected into the subdural was markedly higher, i.e., 20 mL corresponding to approximately 12.5% of the brain volume, than in the present study, i.e., 0.1 mL/kgBW $\approx$ 7–8 mL in animals with slightly higher body weight (median 75 [5] vs. 65 [6] kg). This approach was chosen to keep the volume of blood injected into the subdural below 10% of the intracranial volume and, therefore, to avoid major intracranial hypertension with a subsequent fall of CPP during the HS phase with potentially irreversible brain injury.

Targeted hyperoxemia neither influenced the levels of nitrotyrosine (a marker of oxidative and nitrosative stress) in the ipsilateral nor in the contralateral hemisphere. In both experimental animals and patients, the available data on the impact of hyperoxemia on oxidative stress following TBI is inconclusive, with reports of exacerbated [7], unchanged [15,16], or even diminished [17] markers of radical damage. Even prolonged hyperoxemia, comparable to our investigation, for up to 14 days did not impact serum markers related to oxidative stress, inflammation, or neurological injury [16]. Moreover, it is worth noting that most of the aforementioned studies focused on short-term (up to 4 h) pure O_2 ventilation, resulting in P_aO_2 levels between 300 and 450 mmHg, rather than moderate hyperoxemia within a well-defined target range, as in our experiment. Thus, the results from that study align with our own findings, indicating that moderate hyperoxia within the chosen limits may be safe with respect to serum or cerebral tissue markers of oxidative stress.

Targeted hyperoxemia suppressed the elevation of oxytocin in the ipsilateral brain hemisphere. Moreover, there was reduced expression of oxytocin receptor in the same hemisphere. To date, to the best of our knowledge there are no available data in the literature regarding the impact of hyperoxemia on the cerebral protein levels of oxytocin and oxytocin receptor. In contrast to our findings, divergent expression of oxytocin/oxytocin receptor following intracerebral hemorrhage in a mouse model has been described previously [10]. In rats undergoing subarachnoid hemorrhage by blood injection into the great cistern, oxytocin release sharply increased in the hypothamalic supraoptic nucleus, while no effect was observed in the paraventricular nucleus [18]. It should be underscored, however, that any direct comparison between these rodents and our porcine models is difficult: in addition to the fundamental difference of the rodent, lissencephalic macroscopic brain anatomy when compared to the gyrencephalic porcine brain, in the aforementioned studies animals did not receive any ICU care after blood injection, i.e., no mechanical ventilation (e.g., to control for effects of anesthesia on respiratory drive and, thus, on arterial PCO_2-related changes in intracranial pressure (ICP)) and/or circulatory support to maintain CPP. Moreover, the breathing gas consisted of pure O_2 during the instrumentation and blood injection and room air during the observation periods, respectively. Hence, possible effects of excess systemic hyperoxemia and/or later hypoxemia would have remained undetectable. Regardless of the differences in the experimental design, the elevation of OT expression in the damaged brain areas may represent a physiological response of the body utilizing the protective effects of oxytocin [19].

While the OT/OT-R system exhibits interaction with the H_2S system, it is noteworthy that targeted hyperoxemia, as previously delineated, exerts an influence on the expression of OT and its receptor, yet fails to impact the expression of CBS and CSE within the gray and white matter. While the existing data on CBS expression are currently inconclusive, in the ipsilateral hemisphere, reports indicate both increased expression in swine receiving ICU care [11] and decreased expression in mice without ICU care [12]. There is, to the best of our knowledge, no available data regarding the expression of CSE. However, our study noted consistent expression of CBS and CSE in both hemispheres. This disparity may also be attributed to the substantial difference in the injected blood volume inducing ASDH between our present study (0.1 mL/kgBW) and the previous one by Denoix et al. (20 mL). As mentioned above, this approach had been guided by the reasoning that, in prior investigations of porcine ASDH, injection of a blood volume maximally approaching 10% of the intracranial volume represents the threshold for supratentorial volume tolerance [20,21]. In addition, this approach aimed to prevent pronounced intracranial hypertension and a subsequent fall of CPP during the HS phase in order to avoid potentially irreversible brain damage resulting from low CPP. Finally, as outlined above, a major divergence from Zhang et al. [12] pertains to the utilization of swine in contrast to mice.

The pig serves as a highly relevant translational model due to its structural similarity to the human brain. The presence of gyri and sulci (gyrencephalic brain), a proportional white matter to gray matter ratio and the existence of a tentorium cerebelli distinguish it from the rodent brain and reflect human pathophysiology [19,22]. A critical consideration in translational TBI research pertains to the surface anatomy of the brain: the lissencephalic nature of the rodent brain renders it unsuitable for extrapolation to humans with gyrencephalic brains. The morphology of the gyrencephalic pig brain allows for both gray and white matter responses to injury, closely mirroring human physiology [22]. In lissencephalic brains, "maximum mechanical stress" is experienced proximate to the surface and evenly distributed. Conversely, in gyrencephalic brains, maximum stress is redirected from the surface towards the depths at the base of the sulci, which is reminiscent of conditions in humans [23]. This suggests that the pathophysiology of traumatic injuries in lissencephalic rodents might significantly differ from that in gyrencephalic brains in more developed species like pigs, which share anatomical and morphological features not only in the presence of gyri and sulci but also in the distribution of white matter. Furthermore, an additional limitation of rodent models lies in their failure to replicate the ICU interventions akin to those received by TBI patients, notably the targeted surveillance and adjustment of the CPP.

Limitations of the Study

Clearly, the results of our study are constrained by the relatively short 55 h timeframe for injury and resuscitation, a limitation imposed by practicability and staff availability for continuous ICU care, which is in sharp contrast to the medical reality, as TBI patients typically remain in the intensive care unit for significantly longer periods. Nevertheless, a recent study emphasized that our swine model incorporating ICU care is of a considerably longer duration when compared to other pig trials [22].

Moreover, it could be argued that the prefrontal cortex is not the appropriate region because the hypothalamus would be more sensitive. However, this region was selected to maintain comparability with our prior study using swine with identical genetic background and of comparable age and body weight, which had focused on the consequences of ASDH alone [6]. Indeed, this approach enabled the detection of specific differences in the consequences of ASDH alone vs. combined ASDH and HS. In both studies, the decision to focus on the prefrontal cortex was driven by its role in coordinating a multitude of complex cognitive processes and regulating behavior. In humans, injuries to this brain region can result in impaired cognitive control, social behavior, and emotional regulation [24]. We reasoned that this selection would be of particular relevance, aiming to identify a correlate elucidating any impact on neurological function (Modified Glasgow Coma Scale) subsequent to targeted hyperoxemia therapy.

4. Materials and Methods

4.1. Animals

Ethical approval was granted by the Federal Authorities (Tuebingen, Germany) for Animal Research (#1316) and the Animal Care Committee of the University of Ulm. All experiments were conducted in compliance with the European Union Directive 2010/63/EU on the protection of animals used for scientific purposes. Fourteen adult pigs (body weight: 75 kg (73; 76), age: 16 months (15; 18), comprising four females and ten castrated males) were investigated. The pigs belonged to the Bretoncelles–Meishan–Willebrand strain, which is characterized by a diminished activity of the von Willebrand factor, thereby emulating the human coagulation system [6], in contrast to the hypercoagulatory state observed in domestic swine strains [25].

4.2. Experimental Protocol

This study is a post hoc analysis of brain sections from a model of combined ASDH and HS in adult pigs in good cardiovascular health [5]. Induction of anesthesia and surgical instrumentation, as well as the experimental protocol of induction of ASDH, HS and resuscitation, has been described in detail previously [5,6] and is graphically illustrated once again in the Supplementary Material (Figure S1). The volume of blood used to induce ASDH was selected based on the following insights: Firstly, previous studies on porcine ASDH have demonstrated that injecting a blood volume of maximally 10% of the intracranial volume represents the threshold for supra-tentorial volume tolerance [20,21]. Secondly, preliminary work from our own research group on pigs, which only received an ASDH without hemorrhagic shock but with an absolute injected blood volume of 20 mL [6], showed a marked increase in ICP within the first 30 min, in individual animals even reaching values of 80–100 mmHg [6]. Moreover, in that study, even at 2 h after ASDH induction, ICP values were still more than twice as high at the baseline levels, while only a moderate increase was observed in the present experiment. Based on the aforementioned findings, in this experiment, induction of ASDH was performed by injection of 0.1 mL/kgBW of autologous blood through the subdural catheter [5]. Therefore, the cranial vault was exposed, and a craniotomy was executed by perforating openings over the left and right parietal cortices, accompanied by a modest incision of the dura. Adhering to the principles of the 3Rs, the manipulation extended to the contralateral hemisphere to obviate the necessity for supplementary sham experiments. Microdialysis catheters for the determination of glutamate, glucose, pyruvate and lactate, as well as multimodal brain monitoring probes for ICP, brain tissue partial O_2 pressure ($P_{bt}O_2$) and temperature measurements were introduced bilaterally into the cerebral parenchyma [5,6]. HS was initiated by passive withdrawal of blood targeting 30% of the calculated blood volume. The deceleration of blood extraction was implemented, as required, to uphold CPP, i.e., the difference between mean arterial pressure (MAP) and ICP $\geq$ 50 mmHg. Subsequent to 2 h of concurrent ASDH and HS, resuscitation was initiated. This encompassed the re-transfusion of shed blood within 30 min, fluid resuscitation and the continuous intravenous administration of noradrenaline, titrated to sustain MAP at pre-shock levels and CPP > 60 mmHg [5]. Albeit already presented in Datzmann et al. [5], the data are shown in the supplementary material upon the reviewer's request (Table S1). During the first 24 h of resuscitation, the animals were randomly assigned to the control group receiving normoxemia (P_aO_2 80–120 mmHg) or to the intervention group obtaining targeted hyperoxemia (P_aO_2 200–250 mmHg). To this end, blood gas analyses were conducted hourly during the initial 24 h, and subsequently every 2 h. Any deviations from the target P_aO_2 were promptly addressed by adjusting the inspiratory oxygen fraction (F_iO_2). After a maximum of 53 h of intensive care treatment or premature cessation of the experiment in accordance with pre-defined termination criteria (i.e., CPP < 60 mmHg despite receiving the maximum vasopressor dose, acute anuric kidney failure and overall survival [5]; at the reviewer's request, the survival analysis is graphically represented in the Supplementary Material (Figure S2)), pigs were euthanized by intravenous injection of KCl after further deepening of anesthesia. Immediately postmortem, the brain was removed for further tissue analysis.

4.3. Immunohistochemistry

Immunohistochemistry was employed to assess cerebral expression levels of extravascular albumin, serving as an indicator of blood–brain barrier integrity, nitrotyrosine as a marker of oxidative and nitrosative stress within the tissue, OT and its receptor, along with the principal H_2S-producing enzymes CBS and CSE. Immunohistochemistry was selected for several reasons: (i) it is well documented in the literature that densitometric analysis of colorimetric immunohistochemical staining is comparably reliable to Western blotting for quantifying protein levels [26], (ii) significant correlations were observed between densitometric values and those derived from Western blotting analysis [27], and (iii) unlike Western blotting, immunohistochemical evaluation of tissue permits the identification of spatial distribution and protein expression in distinct cell types within the tissue specimen. All brain specimens underwent uniform fixation in a 4% formalin solution for 6 days. Subsequently, each brain was dissected into consecutive coronal sections with a thickness of 4 mm, spanning from the frontal to occipital regions. In instances where the macroscopic section exceeded the dimensions of the embedding cassette (26 × 3 × 4 mm), it was laid flat and further dissected into a maximum of five pieces. This dissection process was conducted in such a way as to facilitate subsequent reconstruction of the complete section. For the purposes of this investigation, the macroscopic section, encompassing the prefrontal cortex, was specifically chosen for detailed analysis. The prefrontal cortex was selected (i) because of its sufficient distance from the ASDH, which primarily affected the parietal cortex, thereby ensuring its macro- and microscopic structure remains intact, (ii) the prefrontal cortex is of great significance in swine, as it is in other mammals, playing a variety of roles in cognitive processing, behavior, and adaptation to the environment, and (iii) to allow for comparison with our previous work in swine that had undergone ASDH alone without HS [6]. The tissue was subsequently dehydrated and encased in paraffin blocks. Sections with a thickness of 3–5 µm underwent de-paraffinization using xylene, followed by rehydration through a graded series of ethanol and deionized water.

Immunohistochemistry was conducted in accordance with the previously outlined methodology [11]. In brief, following de-paraffinization, heat-induced antigen retrieval was performed in citrate solution (pH 6). Subsequently, blocking was achieved using normal goat serum (10%) before incubation with the following primary antibodies: anti-pig Albumin (Abcam, abab79960, RRID:AB_1658916, Cambridge, UK) as a marker of blood–brain barrier dysfunction, H_2S-producing enzymes anti-CBS (Protein Tech, Planegg-Martinsried, Germany 14787-1-AP, RRID: AB_2070970) and anti-CSE (Protein Tech, Planegg-Martinsried, Germany 12217-1-AP, RRID:AB_2087497), anti-OT (Merck SA, an affiliate of Merck KGaA, Darmstadt, Germany, AB911, RRID:AB_2157629), anti-OT-R (Protein Tech, 2304523045-1-AP, RRID:AB_2827435) and anti-Nitrotyrosine (Merck SA, an affiliate of Merck KGaA, Darmstadt, Germany, ab5411, RRID:AB_177459) as a marker of nitrosative and oxidative stress.

All primary antibodies were adjusted to their optimal dilution based on the manufacturer's recommendations (Table 1). Negative controls were concurrently conducted [11] by incubating with the diluent instead of the primary antibody to monitor the specificity of the secondary system. Alternatively, when possible, pre-incubation of the primary antibody with the corresponding immunogen peptide was performed. In such cases, brain tissue was incubated with the pre-absorbed primary antibody rather than the regular primary antibody [11]. The primary antibodies were detected utilizing the Dako REAL detection system, which employed alkaline phosphatase-conjugated secondary antibodies (anti-mouse; anti-rabbit). Visualization was achieved using a Fast Red-type chromogen. For each animal, one slide per hemisphere was observed with a Zeiss Axio Imager A1 microscope equipped with a 10× objective. Quantification was performed on 800,000-μm² sections using the Zen Image Analysis Software (Version 3.0, Zeiss, Oberkochen, Germany). The results are reported as the percentage of the positive stained area as a fraction of the total area.

Table 1. Primary antibodies.

Primary Antibody (Source, Catalog No., RRID)	Host Species	Immunogen Sequence	Concentration Used for IHC
anti-Albumin (Abcam, ab79960, AB_1658916)	Rabbit Polyclonal	Pig Albumin purified from pig plasma	1:2000
anti-CBS (Protein Tech, 14787-1-AP, AB_2070970)	Rabbit Polyclonal	CBS fusion protein Ag6437	1:200
anti-CSE (Protein Tech, 12217-1-AP, AB_2087497)	Rabbit Polyclonal	Gamma cystathionse fusion protein Ag2872	1:200
anti-Nitrotyrosine (Merck Millipore, ab5411, AB_177459)	Rabbit Polyclonal	Nitrated KLH	1:200
anti-OT (Millipore, Ab911, AB_2157629)	Rabbit Polyclonal	CYIQNCPLG (Synthetic oxytocin (Sigma) conjugated to thyroglobulin)	1:500
anti-OT-R (Protein Tech, 123045-1-AP, AB_2827425)	Rabbit Polyclonal	Oxytocin Receptor fusion protein Ag19074	1:100

4.4. Statistical Analysis

Statistical analysis was conducted using GraphPad Prism Version 8. Inter-group differences were examined utilizing the Kruskal–Wallis test. The data are presented as individual representation with a corresponding median.

5. Conclusions

In this post hoc analysis of material from a long-term, resuscitated porcine model with ASDH and HS, the expression levels of cerebral tissue markers associated with oxidative and nitrosative stress, indicators of blood–brain barrier integrity, as well as regulators of fluid homeostasis, did not provide an explanatory framework for the observed variations in neurological function related to targeted hyperoxemia. However, it is noteworthy that targeted hyperoxemia during resuscitation from combined ASDH and HS did not exhibit any apparent adverse effects.

Supplementary Materials: The following supporting information can be downloaded at https://www.mdpi.com/article/10.3390/ijms25126574/s1.

Author Contributions: Conceptualization, P.A., P.R., T.K. and T.M.; Data curation, P.R., T.K. and T.M.; Formal analysis, F.M.; Funding acquisition, F.M., P.R. and T.M.; Investigation, F.M., A.H., P.R., T.K. and T.M.; Methodology, F.M., T.D., A.H., R.M., S.M., H.G., E.C., P.R., T.K. and T.M.; Project administration, E.C., P.R. and T.M.; Resources, P.R. and T.M.; Software, F.M. and T.M.; Supervision, P.R. and T.M.; Validation, P.R., T.K. and T.M.; Visualization, F.M.; Writing—original draft, F.M. and P.R.; Writing—review and editing, T.D., A.H., M.G., R.M., S.M., F.Z., H.G., E.-M.W., M.H., E.C., T.K. and T.M. All authors have read and agreed to the published version of the manuscript.

Funding: This study was funded by grants to P.R. and T.M. (Collaborative Research Center 1149, project number 251293561; Research Group 5417, project number 465409392) by the Deutsche Forschungsgemeinschaft (DFG). F.M. received funding by means of a "GEROK Rotation" (rotation as clinician scientist) by the Collaborative Research Center 1149, DFG. The funders had no role in the design of this study, data collection, interpretation, or the decision to submit the results.

Institutional Review Board Statement: Ethical approval was granted by the Animal Care Committee of the University Ulm and the Federal Authorities (Tuebingen, Germany) for Animal Research (Regierungspräsidium Tübingen; Reg.-Nr. 1316, approval 6 December 2016).

Informed Consent Statement: Not applicable.

Data Availability Statement: The data presented in this study are available on request from the corresponding author.

Acknowledgments: We thank Stefanie Kranz, Sandra Kress, Rosemarie Mayer, Carolin Renner, Bettina Stahl, Tanja Schulz, and Andrea Seifritz for their excellent technical assistance.

Conflicts of Interest: The authors declare no conflicts of interest.

References

1. Cannon, J.W. Hemorrhagic Shock. *N. Engl. J. Med.* **2018**, *378*, 370–379. [CrossRef] [PubMed]
2. Demiselle, J.; Calzia, E.; Hartmann, C.; Messerer, D.A.C.; Asfar, P.; Radermacher, P.; Datzmann, T. Target arterial PO_2 according to the underlying pathology: A mini-review of the available data in mechanically ventilated patients. *Ann. Intensive Care* **2021**, *11*, 88. [CrossRef] [PubMed]
3. Alali, A.S.; Temkin, N.; Vavilala, M.S.; Lele, A.V.; Barber, J.; Dikmen, S.; Chesnut, R.M. Matching early arterial oxygenation to long-term outcome in severe traumatic brain injury: Target values. *J. Neurosurg.* **2019**, *132*, 537–544. [CrossRef] [PubMed]
4. Rezoagli, E.; Petrosino, M.; Rebora, P.; Menon, D.K.; Mondello, S.; Cooper, D.J.; Maas, A.I.R.; Wiegers, E.J.A.; Galimberti, S.; Citerio, G.; et al. High arterial oxygen levels and supplemental oxygen administration in traumatic brain injury: Insights from CENTER-TBI and OzENTER-TBI. *Intensive Care Med.* **2022**, *48*, 1709–1725. [CrossRef] [PubMed]
5. Datzmann, T.; Münz, F.; Hoffmann, A.; Moehrke, E.; Binzenhöfer, M.; Gröger, M.; Kapapa, T.; Mathieu, R.; Mayer, S.; Zink, F.; et al. An exploratory study investigating the effect of targeted hyperoxemia in a randomized controlled trial in a long-term resuscitated model of combined acute subdural hematoma and hemorrhagic shock in cardiovascular healthy pigs. *Front. Immunol.* **2023**, *14*, 1123196. [CrossRef]
6. Datzmann, T.; Kapapa, T.; Scheuerle, A.; McCook, O.; Merz, T.; Unmuth, S.; Hoffmann, A.; Mathieu, R.; Mayer, S.; Mauer, U.M.; et al. In-depth characterization of a long-term, resuscitated model of acute subdural hematoma-induced brain injury. *J. Neurosurg.* **2021**, *134*, 223–234. [CrossRef] [PubMed]
7. Ahn, E.S.; Robertson, C.L.; Vereczki, V.; Hoffman, G.E.; Fiskum, G. Normoxic ventilatory resuscitation following controlled cortical impact reduces peroxynitrite-mediated protein nitration in the hippocampus. *J. Neurosurg.* **2008**, *108*, 124–131. [CrossRef] [PubMed]
8. Blasiole, B.; Bayr, H.; Vagni, V.A.; Janesko-Feldman, K.; Cheikhi, A.; Wisniewski, S.R.; Long, J.B.; Atkins, J.; Kagan, V.; Kochanek, P.M. Effect of hyperoxia on resuscitation of experimental combined traumatic brain injury and hemorrhagic shock in mice. *Anesthesiology* **2013**, *118*, 649–663. [CrossRef] [PubMed]
9. Ciosek, J.; Cisowska, A.; Dabrowski, R. Galanin affects vasopressin and oxytocin release from the hypothalamo-neurohypophysial system in haemorrahaged rats. *J. Physiol. Pharmacol.* **2003**, *54*, 233–246. [PubMed]
10. Yang, M.; Deng, S.; Jiang, J.; Tian, M.; Xiao, L.; Gong, Y. Oxytocin Improves Intracerebral Hemorrhage Outcomes by Suppressing Neuronal Pyroptosis and Mitochondrial Fission. *Stroke* **2023**, *54*, 1888–1900. [CrossRef] [PubMed]
11. Denoix, N.; Merz, T.; Unmuth, S.; Hoffmann, A.; Nespoli, E.; Scheuerle, A.; Huber-Lang, M.; Gündel, H.; Waller, C.; Radermacher, P.; et al. Cerebral Immunohistochemical Characterization of the H_2S and the Oxytocin Systems in a Porcine Model of Acute Subdural Hematoma. *Front. Neurol.* **2020**, *11*, 649. [CrossRef] [PubMed]
12. Zhang, M.; Shan, H.; Wang, Y.; Wang, T.; Liu, W.; Wang, L.; Zhang, L.; Chang, P.; Dong, W.; Chen, X.; et al. The expression changes of cystathionine-β-synthase in brain cortex after traumatic brain injury. *J. Mol. Neurosci.* **2013**, *51*, 57–67. [CrossRef] [PubMed]
13. Kitagawa, K.; Matsumoto, M.; Ohtsuki, T.; Tagaya, M.; Okabe, T.; Hata, R.; Ueda, H.; Handa, N.; Sobue, K.; Kamada, T. The characteristics of blood-brain barrier in three different conditions—Infarction, selective neuronal death and selective loss of presynaptic terminals--following cerebral ischemia. *Acta Neuropathol.* **1992**, *84*, 378–386. [CrossRef] [PubMed]
14. Denoix, N.; McCook, O.; Scheuerle, A.; Kapapa, T.; Hoffmann, A.; Gündel, H.; Waller, C.; Szabo, C.; Radermacher, P.; Merz, T. Brain Histology and Immunohistochemistry after Resuscitation from Hemorrhagic Shock in Swine with Pre-Existing Atherosclerosis and Sodium Thiosulfate ($Na_2S_2O_3$) Treatment. *Front. Med.* **2022**, *9*, 925433. [CrossRef] [PubMed]
15. Puccio, A.M.; Hoffman, L.A.; Bayir, H.; Zullo, T.G.; Fischer, M.; Darby, J.; Alexander, S.; Dixon, C.E.; Okonkwo, D.O.; Kochanek, P.M. Effect of short periods of normobaric hyperoxia on local brain tissue oxygenation and cerebrospinal fluid oxidative stress markers in severe traumatic brain injury. *J. Neurotrauma* **2009**, *26*, 1241–1249. [CrossRef] [PubMed]

16. Lång, M.; Skrifvars, M.B.; Siironen, J.; Tanskanen, P.; Ala-Peijari, M.; Koivisto, T.; Djafarzadeh, S.; Bendel, S. A pilot study of hyperoxemia on neurological injury, inflammation and oxidative stress. *Acta Anaesthesiol. Scand.* **2018**, *62*, 801–810. [CrossRef] [PubMed]
17. Vidal-Jorge, M.; Sánchez-Guerrero, A.; Mur-Bonet, G.; Castro, L.; Rădoi, A.; Riveiro, M.; Fernández-Prado, N.; Baena, J.; Poca, M.A.; Sahuquillo, J. Does Normobaric Hyperoxia Cause Oxidative Stress in the Injured Brain? A Microdialysis Study Using 8-Iso-Prostaglandin F2α as a Biomarker. *J. Neurotrauma* **2017**, *34*, 2731–2742. [CrossRef] [PubMed]
18. Kleindienst, A.; Hildebrandt, G.; Kroemer, S.A.; Franke, G.; Gaab, M.R.; Landgraf, R. Hypothalamic neuropeptide release after experimental subarachnoid hemorrhage: In vivo microdialysis study. *Acta Neurol. Scand.* **2004**, *109*, 361–368. [CrossRef] [PubMed]
19. McCook, O.; Scheuerle, A.; Denoix, N.; Kapapa, T.; Radermacher, P.; Merz, T. Localization of the hydrogen sulfide and oxytocin systems at the depth of the sulci in a porcine model of acute subdural hematoma. *Neural Regen. Res.* **2021**, *16*, 2376–2382. [CrossRef]
20. Zwetnow, N.N.; Orlin, J.R.; Wu, W.H.; Tajsic, N. Studies on supratentorial subdural bleeding using a porcine model. *Acta Neurochir.* **1993**, *121*, 58–67. [CrossRef]
21. Timaru-Kast, R.; Meissner, A.; Heimann, A.; Hoelper, B.; Kempski, O.; Alessandri, B. Acute subdural hematoma in pigs: Role of volume on multiparametric neuromonitoring and histology. *J. Neurotrauma* **2008**, *25*, 1107–1119. [CrossRef] [PubMed]
22. O'Donnell, J.C.; Browne, K.D.; Kvint, S.; Makaron, L.; Grovola, M.R.; Karandikar, S.; Kilbaugh, T.J.; Cullen, D.K.; Petrov, D. Multimodal Neuromonitoring and Neurocritical Care in Swine to Enhance Translational Relevance in Brain Trauma Research. *Biomedicines* **2023**, *11*, 1336. [CrossRef] [PubMed]
23. Cloots, R.J.; Gervaise, H.M.; van Dommelen, J.A.; Geers, M.G. Biomechanics of traumatic brain injury: Influences of the morphologic heterogeneities of the cerebral cortex. *Ann. Biomed. Eng.* **2008**, *36*, 1203–1215. [CrossRef] [PubMed]
24. Arnould, A.; Rochat, L.; Azouvi, P.; Van der Linden, M. A multidimensional approach to apathy after traumatic brain injury. *Neuropsychol. Rev.* **2013**, *23*, 210–233. [CrossRef] [PubMed]
25. Read, M.S.; Potter, J.Y.; Brinkhous, K.M. Venom coagglutinin for detection of von Willebrand factor activity in animal plasmas. *J. Lab. Clin. Med.* **1983**, *101*, 74–82. [PubMed]
26. Hinson, J.A.; Michael, S.L.; Ault, S.G.; Pumford, N.R. Western blot analysis for nitrotyrosine protein adducts in livers of saline-treated and acetaminophen-treated mice. *Toxicol. Sci.* **2000**, *53*, 467–473. [CrossRef] [PubMed]
27. Merz, T.; Lukaschewski, B.; Wigger, D.; Rupprecht, A.; Wepler, M.; Gröger, M.; Hartmann, C.; Whiteman, M.; Szabo, C.; Wang, R.; et al. Interaction of the hydrogen sulfide system with the oxytocin system in the injured mouse heart. *Intensive Care Med. Exp.* **2018**, *6*, 41. [CrossRef] [PubMed]

Disclaimer/Publisher's Note: The statements, opinions and data contained in all publications are solely those of the individual author(s) and contributor(s) and not of MDPI and/or the editor(s). MDPI and/or the editor(s) disclaim responsibility for any injury to people or property resulting from any ideas, methods, instructions or products referred to in the content.

International Journal of
Molecular Sciences

MDPI

Article

Exposure to Non-Steady-State Oxygen Is Reflected in Changes to Arterial Blood Gas Values, Prefrontal Cortical Activity, and Systemic Cytokine Levels

Elizabeth G. Damato [1], Joseph S. Piktel [2], Seunghee P. Margevicius [3], Seth J. Fillioe [4,†], Lily K. Norton [5,†], Alireza Abdollahifar [1], Kingman P. Strohl [1], David S. Burch [6] and Michael J. Decker [1,*]

1 Department of Physiology & Biophysics, Center for Aerospace Physiology, School of Medicine, Case Western Reserve University, Cleveland, OH 44106, USA; egd@case.edu (E.G.D.)
2 Department of Emergency Medicine, MetroHealth Medical Center, School of Medicine, Case Western Reserve University, Cleveland, OH 44106, USA
3 Department of Population and Quantitative Health Sciences, School of Medicine, Case Western Reserve University, Cleveland, OH 44106, USA
4 Cuyahoga Community College, Cleveland, OH 44122, USA
5 Jacobs School of Medicine and Biomedical Sciences, University at Buffalo, Buffalo, NY 14203, USA
6 711th Human Performance Wing, Biomedical Impact of Flight Branch, Air Force Research Laboratory, United States Air Force, Wright-Patterson Air Force Base, Dayton, OH 45433, USA
* Correspondence: mjd6@case.edu
† Formerly of the Department of Physiology & Biophysics, School of Medicine, Case Western Reserve University, Cleveland, OH 44106, USA.

Abstract: Onboard oxygen-generating systems (OBOGSs) provide increased inspired oxygen (F_iO_2) to mitigate the risk of neurologic injury in high altitude aviators. OBOGSs can deliver highly variable oxygen concentrations oscillating around a predetermined F_iO_2 set point, even when the aircraft cabin altitude is relatively stable. Steady-state exposure to 100% F_iO_2 evokes neurovascular vasoconstriction, diminished cerebral perfusion, and altered electroencephalographic activity. Whether non-steady-state F_iO_2 exposure leads to similar outcomes is unknown. This study characterized the physiologic responses to steady-state and non-steady-state F_iO_2 during normobaric and hypobaric environmental pressures emulating cockpit pressures within tactical aircraft. The participants received an indwelling radial arterial catheter while exposed to steady-state or non-steady-state F_iO_2 levels oscillating ± 15% of prescribed set points in a hypobaric chamber. Steady-state exposure to 21% F_iO_2 during normobaria produced arterial blood gas values within the anticipated ranges. Exposure to non-steady-state F_iO_2 led to P_aO_2 levels higher upon cessation of non-steady-state F_iO_2 than when measured during steady-state exposure. This pattern was consistent across all F_iO_2 ranges, at each barometric condition. Prefrontal cortical activation during cognitive testing was lower following exposure to non-steady-state F_iO_2 >50% and <100% during both normobaria and hypobaria of 494 mmHg. The serum analyte levels (IL-6, IP-10, MCP-1, MDC, IL-15, and VEGF-D) increased 48 h following the exposures. We found non-steady-state F_iO_2 levels >50% reduced prefrontal cortical brain activation during the cognitive challenge, consistent with an evoked pattern of neurovascular constriction and dilation.

Keywords: hypobaric; oxygen; arterial; brain; neurovascular; spectroscopy

1. Introduction

Hypobaric hypoxia and decompression injury are among the risks awaiting tactical aviators within their austere, high-altitude environment. The life-support equipment providing a continuous fraction of inspired oxygen (F_iO_2), typically between 35 and 100%, is an intended neuroprotection against those hazards. Exposure to enhanced oxygen concentrations also conveys a risk. Prolonged exposure is pathologic to multiple organ systems [1,2] while short term exposure reduces cerebral perfusion and alters cortical electroencephalographic activity [3].

The original technology to provide the increased F_iO_2 levels necessary for survival within high altitude environments was first implemented during World War I. Those systems used liquid oxygen, a relatively simple approach [4,5]. As the liquid oxygen transitioned into a gaseous state, it flowed into the aircrew's breathing system. There, it was diluted with air to deliver a specific level of F_iO_2 to the aviator, with that level determined by cockpit ambient pressure [6]. Further dilution of the F_iO_2 could occur within the gas regulators, such as that found within diluter demand masks. The success of liquid-oxygen systems led to their further development and, beginning in the early 1940s, the installation of a small refillable liquid oxygen container within almost every tactical aircraft. The simplicity of the liquid-oxygen systems contributes to their continued use.

Onboard oxygen-generation systems (OBOGs) began replacing liquid-oxygen-based life-support systems during the 1970s [7]. Their operation is dependent upon a stream of ambient air being forced through a molecular sieve. Only oxygen molecules pass through the sieve and into a series of small storage tanks [8]. Upon release from the storage tanks, dilution occurs in diluter-demand regulators. The criteria of both minimum and maximum F_iO_2 delivery are determined according to the aircraft cockpit pressure. The OBOGs typically incorporate "safety pressure", which is a continuous positive pressure within the pilot's mask of 1.25–4 cm of water (cmH_2O). Systems without safety pressure, or when safety pressure is turned off, will provide 0–0.5 cmH_2O pressure within the mask. In contrast with liquid-oxygen systems that deliver a relatively constant F_iO_2 concentration into the life support system, the F_iO_2 delivery from the OBOGs system follows a sinusoidal pattern [6].

Oxygen-induced reductions in cerebral perfusion, and subsequently, oxygen delivery to the brain, was first characterized in healthy humans with indwelling arterial and venous catheters by Lambertsen et al., in 1953 [9]. Those findings have since been replicated using noninvasive techniques [10,11], with more recent studies revealing that reductions in cerebral perfusion begin during exposure to an F_iO_2 of 60% [12]. Inspired oxygen levels > 60% not only influence neurovascular tone; systemic sequelae can range from decreased cardiac output [13] and the onset of lung alveolar collapse and atelectasis [14], to tonic-clonic seizure activity when hyperoxia occurs during hyperbaric conditions [15].

In contrast with well characterized neuro- and physiological outcomes of exposure to steady-state F_iO_2, fewer studies have focused upon the outcomes of exposure to non-steady-state F_iO_2. Those findings, often derived from cell [16], rodent, or swine models [17] reveal inflammation of the pulmonary epithelium. Those observations concur with studies by Formenti et al. [18,19] revealing that non-steady-state F_iO_2 levels, induced by altering the ventilatory inspiratory and expiratory ratios, lead to non-steady-state arterial blood oxygen (P_aO_2) levels [17]. While those studies affirm that exposure to non-steady-state F_iO_2 induces non-steady-state P_aO_2 levels, there is an absence of peer-reviewed publications assessing the impact of non-steady-state F_iO_2 and P_aO_2 upon functional activity within the human cerebral cortex. Our objective for this study was to address that void.

To inform our understanding of the central nervous system's functional response to non-steady-state F_iO_2, we measured prefrontal cortical activity during a cognitive task immediately following exposure to non-steady F_iO_2 and again 120 s later following exposure to steady-state F_iO_2. This enabled us to test the following hypotheses: (1) Following exposure to non-steady-state F_iO_2, arterial blood oxygen (P_aO_2) levels will reflect the F_iO_2 at the time which the sample was obtained; (2) The prefrontal cortex will achieve a different level of activation during a cognitive task following exposure to non-steady-state F_iO_2 when compared to exposure to steady-state F_iO_2; and (3) Exposure to increased F_iO_2 levels, both steady and non-steady-state, will be followed by increased levels of systemic proinflammatory serum analytes.

2. Results

Thirty-seven candidates received a verbal description of the study protocol and provided written informed consent to participate. Of those 37, seven withdrew prior to participating due to scheduling conflicts or concerns regarding COVID-19. Of the remaining 30 people who began the study, six were excluded from continuing the protocol following a vasovagal response during arterial catheter placement. The remaining 24 participants completed all phases of the protocol. Their basic demographics are presented in Table 1; there were no differences between male and female study participant's age or BMI.

Table 1. Study participant demographics.

Sex	Race	Age (Years) M ± SD (Range)	BMI (kg/m^2) M ± SD (Range)
Males n = 17	Asian = 2 Black = 5 White = 10	31.12 ± 11.03 (21–57)	28.80 ± 5.52 (22.12–45.84)
Females n = 7	Asian = 2 Black = 0 White = 5	29.57 ± 6.29 (24–42)	28.89 ± 5.77 (21.07–39.30)
p-value	0.2020 [a]	0.8731 [b]	0.9241 [b]

No age or BMI differences were found between males and females. [a] p-value from Fisher's exact test. [b] p-values from Wilcoxon rank sum test.

2.1. Non-Steady-State/Steady-State F_iO_2 Exposure

Continuous tracing from an oxygen sensor attached to the study participant's facemask validated that the F_iO_2 delivered to the participant matched the intended output from the air/oxygen blender. The signal hysteresis depicted in Figure 1, especially at the top of each square wave, represents nitrogen washout from the lungs, which can take several minutes [20]. The hysteresis/nitrogen washout reveals the heterogeneity in lung ventilation and confirms that a steady-state, homogenous level of oxygen within the lungs was not achieved during the 60 s cycle time of each F_iO_2 oscillation.

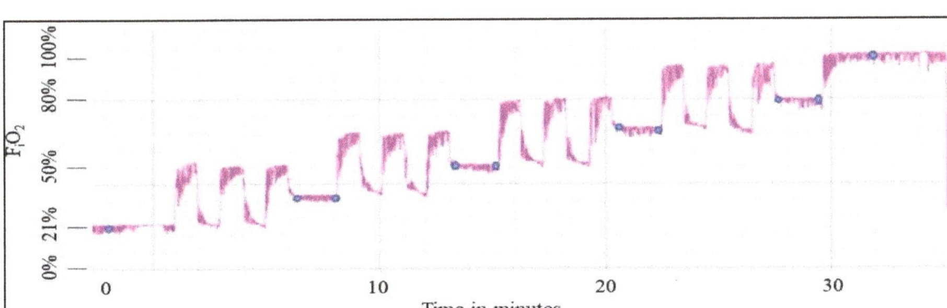

Figure 1. Output from mask oxygen sensor.

This graph displays the output from the mask oxygen sensor from one study participant. The x-axis is time in minutes with each block representing two minutes. The y-axis is oxygen concentration measured within the mask, with each block representing 8.0 percent. The blue circles represent the time points of each arterial blood sample. The series of three pegboard tests (not indicated on this figure) were initiated after each collection of each arterial blood sample.

2.2. Arterial Blood Gas Results

Table 2 illustrates that during normobaric ambient pressure (749 mmHg), the P_aO_2 levels measured during exposure to steady-state 21% F_iO_2 were 95.63 ± 13.21 mmHg (mean ± 1 SD), while exposure to steady-state 100% F_iO_2 produced P_aO_2 levels of 541.83 ± 47.62 mmHg. Those values were within the anticipated range for healthy people [21]. Table 2 also presents the P_aO_2 levels measured during exposure to steady-state 21% and 100% F_iO_2 at the simulated altitudes of 8000 ft (565 mmHg) and 15,000 ft (494 mmHg). Those P_aO_2 levels were also within the anticipated ranges [22]. The accompanying values of P_aCO_2, pH, HCO_3, S_aO_2, glucose, and hematocrit are provided in Supplementary Tables S1–S6.

The values of P_aO_2 measured at the conclusion of each non-steady-state F_iO_2 sequence were significantly greater than the P_aO_2 values measured 120 s later during exposure to steady-state F_iO_2. This pattern was consistent during all non-steady-state F_iO_2 sequences administered at 749 mmHg (normobaric conditions), 565 mmHg (8000 ft), and 494 mmHg (15,000 ft). However, the magnitude of difference between the P_aO_2 values observed immediately post non-steady-state F_iO_2 with those observed following 120 s of steady-state F_iO_2 increased as ambient environmental pressure decreased. Whereas the mean percent change was 12.81% during normobaric conditions at 749 mmHg, that mean percent change increased to 15.37% for P_aO_2 values measured at 565 mmHg and 17.55% for P_aO_2 values measured at 494 mmHg.

Table 2. Arterial blood P_aO_2 comparisons.

	F_iO_2 Range during Non-Steady-State/Steady-State Hyperoxia Exposure	N †	P_aO_2 Measured upon Reaching Predetermined F_iO_2 Level Following Non-Steady-State/Steady-State Hyperoxia Exposure (Mean ± SD) Range	P_aO_2 Measured after Maintaining Predetermined F_iO_2 Level for 120 s (Mean ± SD) Range	*p*-Value	Adj. *p*-Value
749 mmHg	21% steady state	24		95.63 ± 13.21 (68–122)	n/a	
(% Change) 17.73%	35% ± 15%	24	216.67 ± 29.53 (115–264)	178.25 ± 26.73 (90–210)	<0.0001	<0.0001
13.75%	50% ± 15%	24	296.92 ± 37.53 (166–356)	255.50 ± 34.59 (121–288)	<0.0001	<0.0001
9.73%	65% ± 15%	24	382.50 ± 42.99 (227–431)	345.29 ± 44.56 (171–396)	<0.0001	<0.0001
10.01%	80% ± 15%	24	470.96 ± 55.59 (318–548)	423.83 ± 49.81 (225–471)	<0.0001 *	<0.0001
	100% steady state	24		541.83 ± 47.62 (385–613)	n/a	
565 mmHg	21% steady state	24		66.71 ± 6.10 (51–83)	n/a	
21.02%	35% ± 15%	24	154.21 ± 19.72 (105–195)	121.79 ± 17.99 (78–163)	<0.0001	<0.0001
18.79%	50% ± 15%	24	218.25 ± 25.10 (134–264)	177.25 ± 27.34 (77–208)	<0.0001	<0.0001
11.68%	65% ± 15%	23	274.35 ± 22.37 (218–301)	242.30 ± 27.11 (161–273)	<0.0001	<0.0001
9.97%	80% ± 15%	23	336.52 ± 41.60 (174–391)	302.96 ± 40.47 (141–342)	<0.0001	<0.0001

Table 2. *Cont.*

	F_iO_2 Range during Non-Steady-State/Steady-State Hyperoxia Exposure	N †	P_aO_2 Measured upon Reaching Predetermined F_iO_2 Level Following Non-Steady-State/Steady-State Hyperoxia Exposure (Mean ± SD) Range	P_aO_2 Measured after Maintaining Predetermined F_iO_2 Level for 120 s (Mean ± SD) Range	*p*-Value	Adj. *p*-Value
	100% steady state	23		379.29 ± 46.56 (189–420)	n/a	
494 mmHg	21% steady state	23		47.17 ± 5.51 (36–58)	n/a	
27.26%	35% ± 15%	23	107.65 ± 16.38 (77–136)	78.30 ± 10.61 (53–93)	<0.0001	<0.0001
18.09%	50% ± 15%	23	153.83 ± 20.75 (93–186)	126.00 ± 17.22 (79–152)	<0.0001	<0.0001
13.64%	65% ± 15%	23	199.26 ± 25.32 (111–229)	172.09 ± 23.19 (94–197)	<0.0001	<0.0001
11.21%	80% ± 15%	23	242.39 ± 21.26 (184–267)	215.22± 28.16 (112–237)	<0.0001	<0.0001
	100% steady state	23		273.22 ± 29.27 (184–306)	n/a	

Comparisons of arterial blood P_aO_2 sampled immediately following 5 min of exposure to oscillatory F_iO_2 were made with those sampled immediately following 120 s of exposure to steady-state F_iO_2. Comparisons were performed using paired *t*-tests unless otherwise indicated. * *p*-values from Wilcoxon signed rank test; adj. *p*-values from false discovery rate (FDR). † Sample size for ABG measurements decreased as a result of one participant whose arterial line catheter became non-functional during the latter part of the experimental protocol.

2.3. fNIRS Results

Table 3 reports comparisons of fNIRS contrasts performed during the grooved pegboard task immediately following exposure to oscillatory F_iO_2 with those performed during a grooved pegboard task following 120 s of exposure to steady-state F_iO_2. We found exposure to non-steady-state cyclic F_iO_2 > 50% and < 100% led to reduced prefrontal cortical activation levels immediately following 5 min of exposure to oscillatory F_iO_2 at both normobaric pressure and during exposure to a reduced barometric pressure of 494 mmHg. These results are graphically illustrated in Figure 2.

Table 3. Prefrontal cortical activation levels.

	F_iO_2 Range during Non-Steady-State/Steady-State Hyperoxia Exposure	N †	Activation Level during Pegboard Task #1 (Mean ± SD) Range	Activation Level during Pegboard Task #3 (Mean ± SD) Range	*p*-Value	Adj. *p*-Value
749 mmHg	21% steady state	23	0.992 ± 0.918 (−0.873–2.525)	1.02 ±1.051 (−1.009–2.676)	0.4625	0.6508
	35% ± 15%	24	0.779 ± 1.029 (−0.692–2.81)	0.726 ± 0.955 (−1.153–2.576)	0.5872	0.6508
	50% ± 15%	24	0.662 ± 1.061 (−0.999–2.954)	0.731 ± 0.822 (−0.562–2.317)	0.5438	0.6508
	65% ± 15%	24	0.632 ± 0.932 (−1.36–2.692)	0.92 ± 0.871 (−0.356–2.892)	0.0146	0.0876
	80% ± 15%	24	0.609 ± 0.815 (−0.778–2.176)	0.856 ± 0.885 (−1.071–2.649)	0.0321	0.0963
	100% steady state	23	0.431 ± 0.969 (−1.293–2.782)	0.467 ± 0.931 (−1.243–2.988)	0.6508	0.6508

Table 3. *Cont.*

	F_iO_2 Range during Non-Steady-State/Steady-State Hyperoxia Exposure	N †	Activation Level during Pegboard Task #1 (Mean ± SD) Range	Activation Level during Pegboard Task #3 (Mean ± SD) Range	*p*-Value	Adj. *p*-Value
565 mmHg	21% steady state	22	0.476 ± 0.987 (−1.154–2.601)	0.741 ± 1.081 (−0.723–3.614)	0.0466	0.2190
	35% ± 15%	22	0.756 ± 0.673 (−0.17–2.324)	0.794 ± 0.845 (−0.673–2.449)	0.7181	0.8554
	50% ± 15%	24	0.501 ± 1.048 (−1.548–2.951)	0.695 ± 0.965 (−1.375–2.322)	0.0730	0.2190
	65% ± 15%	22	0.662 ± 1.056 (−1.177–4.221)	0.687 ± 0.945 (−0.819–3.677)	0.8554	0.8554
	80% ± 15%	23	0.555 ± 1.055 (−1.817–2.549)	0.592 ± 1.031 (−1.769–2.381)	0.4351	0.6527
	100% steady state	23	0.791 ± 0.885 (−1.223–2.455)	0.887 ± 0.916 (−1.675–2.36)	0.1820	0.3640
494 mmHg	21% steady state	22	0.434 ± 1.006 (−1.577–2.639)	0.874 ± 0.764 (−0.631–2.035)	0.0340	0.0680
	35% ± 15%	23	0.997 ± 1.076 (−1.041–3.164)	0.943 ± 1.061 (−0.749–3.776)	0.6663	0.6663
	50% ± 15%	21	0.666 ± 0.791 (−0.526–2.466)	0.879 ± 1.071 (−0.674–3.611)	0.0335	0.0680
	65% ± 15%	22	0.798 ± 0.948 (−0.558–2.968)	0.872 ± 0.949 (−0.942–2.829)	0.5564	0.6663
	80% ± 15%	22	0.605 ± 0.949 (−0.715–2.583)	0.726 ± 0.915 (−0.47–3.205)	0.0271 *	0.0680
	100% steady state	22	0.762 ± 1.075 (−1.455–2.721)	0.61 ± 0.992 (−1.361–2.439)	0.1838 *	0.2757

fNIRS contrasts performed during the grooved pegboard task immediately following exposure to oscillatory F_iO_2 were compared with those performed during a grooved pegboard task following 120 s of exposure to steady-state F_iO_2. Comparisons were performed using paired *t*-tests unless otherwise indicated. † Sample size variation is due to artifact rejection which deleted some sequences of fNIRS data. * *p*-values from Wilcoxon signed rank test.

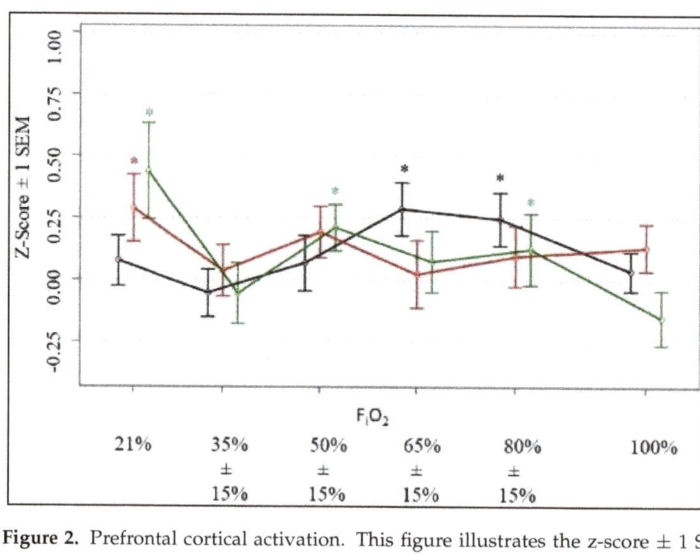

Figure 2. Prefrontal cortical activation. This figure illustrates the z-score ± 1 SEM of prefrontal cortical activation levels as measured by fNIRS between Task #1 and Task #3 at each barometric pressure. The black line represents data generated at 749 mmHg, red is 565 mmHg and green is 494 mmHg. The values for z-scores are staggered on the *x*-axis only for the purpose of visualization. * Represents significant differences between Task #1 and Task #3 as reported in Table 3.

2.3.1. Pressure of 749mmHg (Normobaria)

No differences in levels of prefrontal cortical activation occurred at normobaric pressure between Task #1 and Task #3 during exposure to a steady-state F_iO_2 of 21%. The prefrontal cortical activation levels also did not differ between pegboard Task #1 and Task #3 during exposure to a non-steady-state F_iO_2 of 35% ± 15% and F_iO_2 of 50% ± 15%. However, significant differences in prefrontal cortical activation did emerge between Task #1 and Task #3 during exposure to a non-steady-state F_iO_2 of 65% ± 15% as well as F_iO_2 of 80% ± 15%. At those oxygen concentrations, prefrontal cortical activation levels were significantly lower immediately after exposure to non-steady-state F_iO_2 (Task #1) than during steady-state F_iO_2 (Task #3). Those differences resolved upon exposure to a steady-state F_iO_2 of 100%.

2.3.2. Pressure of 565 mmHg (8000 ft)

Prefrontal cortical activation levels only differed between Task #1 and Task #3 at 565 mmHg following exposure to a steady-state F_iO_2 of 21%. Exposure to increased oxygen concentrations > 21%, presented as either non-steady-state or steady-state, did not elicit differences in prefrontal cortex activation levels between pegboard Task #1 and Task #3.

2.3.3. Pressure of 494 mmHg (15,000 ft)

Prefrontal cortical activation levels at 494 mmHg differed between Task #1 and Task #3 during exposure to a steady-state F_iO_2 of 21%. Prefrontal cortical activation levels also differed between Task #1 and Task #3 while the participant was exposed to non-steady-state F_iO_2 levels of 50% ± 15% and F_iO_2 levels of 80% ± 15%. Those differences resolved upon exposure to steady-state F_iO_2 of 100%.

2.4. Blood Serum Results

The levels of 37 serum analytes were measured in blood samples obtained at each of the two data collection time points. Of those 37 analytes, the serum levels of six analytes differed significantly between the values obtained prior to exposure to increased F_iO_2 and hypobaria with those values measured 48 h after completion of all exposures. Serum levels for those six analytes and the outcomes of the statistical comparisons are provided in Table 4. This table reveals that IL-6, measured by the proinflammatory plate, was increased. The chemokine plate showed increases in IP-10, MCP-1, and MDC. The cytokine plate revealed increased levels of IL-15 while the angiogenesis plate demonstrated that VEGF-D was also increased post exposure.

Table 4. Serum analytes.

Analyte	N [†]	Baseline M ± S.D (Range)	Post-Hypobaria and Hyperoxia Exposure M ± S.D (Range)	*p*-Value [a]	Adj. *p*-Value
Proinflammatory Plate (pg/mL)					
IL-6	23	1.367 ± 3.201 (0.010–15.898)	1.973 ± 3.790 (0.305–17.981)	0.014 *	0.0268
Chemokine Plate (pg/mL)					
IP-10	23	146.535 ± 76.353 (34.809–394.060)	245.677 ± 183.548 (91.328–770.989)	<0.0001 *	0.0004
MCP-1	23	84.383 ± 43.204 (15.264–152.951)	119.536 ± 60.249 (46.300–303.390)	0.023	0.0268
MDC	23	*495.726 ± 204.249* (160.135–1066.029)	592.515 ± 207.538 (324.178–1015.837)	0.004	0.0140

Table 4. *Cont.*

Analyte	N †	Baseline M ± S.D (Range)	Post-Hypobaria and Hyperoxia Exposure M ± S.D (Range)	*p*-Value [a]	Adj. *p*-Value
			Cytokine (pg/mL)		
IL-15	23	1.464 ± 0.613 (0.678–2.832)	1.671 ± 0.558 (0.817–2.628)	0.023	0.0268
			Angiogenesis (pg/mL)		
VEGF-D	23	1423.960 ± 343.450 (853.415–2225.042)	1529.171 ± 417.718 (824.415–2636.861)	0.023	0.0268

Six serum analyte levels changed significantly from baseline when compared to serum analyte levels measured following exposure to hypobaria and hyperoxia. † N = 23, due to one missing post-exposure venous blood sample; * *p*-values from Wilcoxon signed rank test; [a] *p*-values from paired *t*-tests; adj. *p*-values from false discovery rate (FDR).

3. Discussion

Our objective was to characterize physiologic responses to exposure to both non-steady-state and steady-state F_iO_2 during normobaric and hypobaric environmental pressures. The primary outcomes included serial measurements of arterial blood gases (ABG) and prefrontal cortical activity during cognitive challenge. The secondary outcomes included measures of general blood chemistry and the quantification of selected serum analytes within the circulatory system both before and after exposure.

The results indicate that steady-state exposure to 21% F_iO_2 during normobaric environmental pressures produced ABG values within the anticipated ranges (control condition). Exposure to non-steady-state F_iO_2 levels led to transient elevations of P_aO_2 values that were higher upon cessation of non-steady-state F_iO_2 than when measured 120 s later during steady-state exposure to the same F_iO_2 level (Table 2). This pattern of increased P_aO_2 levels following exposure to non-steady-state F_iO_2 was consistent across all F_iO_2 ranges, and present at each of the three barometric pressure conditions.

When exposed to both steady-state and non-steady-state F_iO_2 levels < 50%, prefrontal cortical activation measured during pegboard Task #1 was not different from levels measured 120 s later during pegboard Task #3. In contrast, exposure to non-steady-state cyclic F_iO_2 > 50% and <100% led to reduced prefrontal cortical activation levels during Task #1 when compared with levels measured 120 s later during Task #3. These differences emerged at both normobaric pressure and during exposure to a reduced barometric pressure of 494 mmHg, which simulated an altitude of 15,000 feet.

In addition to acute transient changes in the ABG values and levels of prefrontal cortical activation, we also observed that six serum analyte levels were increased 48 h following exposure to increased F_iO_2 and hypobaria. Those included IL-6, IP-10, MCP-1, MDC, and IL-15. The vascular endothelial growth factor, VEGF-D, was also increased.

Arterial blood gas values of P_aO_2, measured within two to three breaths following cessation of non-steady-state F_iO_2, suggest that the oxygen content within each inspired breath was rapidly conveyed into the circulatory system. During exposure to non-steady-state F_iO_2 levels of 65% ± 15% F_iO_2, an atmospheric pressure of 749 mmHg, a P_aCO_2 of 41.9 mmHg with presumed partial pressure of water vapor in the airway of 47 mmHg, and a respiratory quotient (R.Q.) of 0.8, the alveolar pressure of oxygen (PAO_2) was predicted to be 403.9 mmHg. When accounting for the alveolar–arterial (Aa) gradient, which reduces the partial pressure of oxygen by 5–10 mmHg, the anticipated P_aO_2 within those participants should have been between 389.9 and 393.9 mmHg. Table 2 reveals that following the non-steady-state F_iO_2 sequence of 65% ± 15%, the actual P_aO_2 values were 382.5 ± 42.9 mmHg (mean ± 1 SD), which closely approximates to the expected value.

In a recently reported study [23], human participants were exposed to 60 s oscillations of 80% F_iO_2 and 20% nitrogen (N_2) and between 70% F_iO_2 and 30% N_2 in a hypobaric chamber at 8000 feet in two exposure cycles of 45 min alternating with a 45 min break. Measurements were taken at ground level before, between, and after the oscillatory exposures and comparisons were made between baseline and hyperoxic oscillatory exposures while remaining at 8000 ft. No differences were found in arterial P_aO_2 across the measurement time points but statistically significant reductions in P_aCO_2 were noted between and following the oscillatory exposures. Conversely, our study compared P_aO_2 and P_aCO_2 levels following 120 s exposures of steady-state F_iO_2 of 65% and 80% to P_aO_2 and P_aCO_2 levels obtained following three 60 s oscillations $\pm$ 15% of those respective steady-state values at 8000 feet. Key differences between the two experimental designs prevent meaningful comparisons of our study with the Kelley et al. publication. Additional barriers to comparing the two studies include the lack of explanation for the very low P_aCO_2 levels at baseline and the omission of pH, bicarbonate, and other ABG components that would allow interpretation. Ambiguity as to whether baseline blood gas measurements used for statistical comparisons were obtained at sea level or at 8000 feet prior to oscillatory exposure also limit inter-study comparisons.

If significant mixing occurred between the newly inspired oxygen content contained within each inspiration with the pre-existing oxygen content within the residual lung volume, the P_aO_2 value measured following each non-steady-state F_iO_2 sequence would have been much higher. During the non-steady-state F_iO_2 sequence of 65% $\pm$ 15%, the alveolar air equation estimates that an F_iO_2 of 80%, which was the peak F_iO_2 prior to the drop to 65% F_iO_2, would produce P_aO_2 values of 499–504 mmHg [24]. If "mixing" occurred between an existing residual lung volume of gas containing 80% F_iO_2 with an incoming gas containing an F_iO_2 of 65%, the predicted P_aO_2 would have been ~440.5 mmHg. However, actual P_aO_2 levels were not in that range; they were instead 382.5 $\pm$ 42.9 mmHg. This suggests that during the two to three breaths occurring during the transition from 80% F_iO_2 to 65% F_iO_2, the newly inspired oxygen content was immediately transferred from the alveoli into the circulatory system. This would be consistent with observations by Formenti and Farmery [19], who revealed breath-by-breath oscillations in P_aO_2 do occur, and those oscillations correspond with the inspiratory and expiratory phases of the respiratory cycle. Their studies suggest that the actual oxygen content within each inspired breath is rapidly transferred across the alveolar epithelium and into the systemic circulation.

Exposure to non-steady-state F_iO_2 sequences evoked a systematic and reproducible outcome on P_aO_2 levels, regardless of ambient environmental pressures. In contrast, non-steady-state F_iO_2 influences upon prefrontal cortical activation were less systematic and were constrained to F_iO_2 exposures >50% but <100%. The potential mechanisms influencing these changes in prefrontal cortical activation levels have been informed by studies characterizing the relationship between increased F_iO_2 with cerebral perfusion. Those studies [3,12], conducted under normobaric conditions, revealed that cerebral perfusion is unaffected by F_iO_2 levels $\geq$ 21% but $\leq$50%. Beginning with F_iO_2 levels of 60%, cerebral perfusion begins to decline and continues to fall with each incremental increase in F_iO_2. Upon reaching an F_iO_2 of 80%, cerebral perfusion is reduced by ~25% of baseline values (mean $\pm$ 1 SD), dropping from 46.16 $\pm$ 10.11 milliliters per minute per 100 g of tissue (mL/min/100 g) to 34.58 $\pm$ 8.59 mL/min/100 g. During exposure to 100% F_iO_2, cerebral perfusion is 32.46 $\pm$ 7.24 mL/min/100 g, a five percent reduction from levels observed during exposure to 80% F_iO_2. Collectively, these findings suggest that exposure to F_iO_2 levels of ~60% evokes onset of neurovascular constriction. Increasing F_iO_2 beyond 60% prompts further neurovascular constriction, which becomes maximal during exposure to F_iO_2 levels between 80% and 100%.

Our collective observations from this and prior studies suggest that (1) P_aO_2 levels are increased following exposure to non-steady-state F_iO_2 compared to when measured following the subsequent 120 s of steady-state F_iO_2 (Table 2), and (2) F_iO_2 levels $\geq$ 60% reduce cerebral perfusion via neurovascular constriction [12], and finally, (3) lowering the F_iO_2 from 100% to 21% leads to neurovascular dilation with the restoration of cerebral perfusion to baseline levels [12]. Those findings lead us to suspect that exposure to non-steady-state, cyclic F_iO_2 levels within the range of 65% $\pm$ 15% induces non-steady-state, cyclic neurovascular constriction and dilation. During exposure to 80% F_iO_2, the peak level delivered during the non-steady-state F_iO_2 sequence of 65% ± 15%, maximal neurovascular constriction with a concomitant reduction in cerebral perfusion would have existed. We believe the reduced levels of prefrontal cortical activity observed during pegboard Task #1 reflected the reduced cerebral perfusion occurring at the peak F_iO_2 during non-steady-state exposures.

Due to the inherent circulatory delay between the lungs and brain [25,26], the change in F_iO_2 from 80% to 65% followed by neurovascular dilation with increased cerebral perfusion, would not have occurred until after completion of pegboard Task #1. Beginning with pegboard Task #3, which commenced following 120 s of steady-state F_iO_2, neurovascular dilation with increased cerebral perfusion would have achieved a constant level. The relative increase in cerebral perfusion at F_iO_2 of 65% versus that following exposure to an F_iO_2 of 80% would have led to increased oxygen delivery. We believe that during pegboard Task #3, the increase in cerebral perfusion and oxygen delivery could have accounted for the increased prefrontal cortical activation levels that we observed. While that hypothesis is biologically plausible, confirming or refuting it would have required additional studies and experimental techniques on cortical connectivity that were beyond the intent and scope of this study.

In addition to the changes in P_aO_2 and levels of prefrontal cortical activation that emerged during exposure to non-steady-state F_iO_2, we also observed increased levels of six blood serum analytes 48 h later, following the conclusion of the experimental protocol. Comparison of our serum analyte levels to previously published reports is limited by different analysis techniques (enzyme-linked immunosorbent assay (ELISA)) vs. the more sensitive multi-array technology we used) and the scarcity of studies documenting inter-subject variation and temporal changes in baseline levels within non-clinical populations. Two studies conducted in healthy individuals concluded that significant variability exists in the baseline levels between healthy individuals, and most cytokines remain stable across serial measurements [27,28]. The baseline and post-exposure serum analyte levels we report appear to reside within published normative reference range measurements [27,29–32]. However, comparisons are limited between ELISA-derived values and those obtained from ultrasensitive assay methods that are essential for characterizing cytokine levels [28]. More importantly, the increase in the serum analyte levels in our study concurs with prior observations that exposure either to steady state or non-steady-state F_iO_2 levels $\geq$ 50% elicits the onset of proinflammatory biochemical cascades within the pulmonary epithelium and other cell types [17]. In addition, the placement of the radial artery catheter could also have initiated the release of several of the proinflammatory serum analytes presented in Table 4. Although baseline levels of MCP-1 have been reported to vary across time in healthy individuals [27], MCP-1 influences the movement of monocytes out of the bloodstream, across the endothelium and into the tissues to engage in immunologic surveillance and inflammatory responses [33] and could explain the increase we observed. Determining the specific mechanisms underlying increased analyte levels is beyond the scope of this project but may represent an adaptive or maladaptive physiological stress response.

Strengths and Limitations

The intent of this study was to characterize the physiologic responses of healthy individuals to exposure to both steady-state and non-steady F_iO_2 levels above 21%. Specific F_iO_2 levels were delivered in a non-steady-state, square wave cycle which ranged ±15% around a pre-specified level or "dose" of oxygen. That experimental design was intended to model oxygen delivery provided by aviation life support systems that employ onboard oxygen-generating systems, some of which can potentially deliver oxygen concentrations of ±15% around a pre-defined level. Study participants were exposed to those non-steady F_iO_2 levels within a hypobaric chamber that provided three different barometric pressures: 749 mmHg, which was the normobaric pressure of the study location, 565 mmHg paralleling an altitude of 8000 feet, and 494 mmHg, which was equivalent to an altitude of

15,000 feet. Each pressure was chosen as representative of cockpit pressures encountered by tactical aviators. The simultaneous and conscious manipulation of the key experimental variables of F_iO_2 and environmental pressure could induce inherent confounds to the data analyses and interpretation, and thereby, present a study weakness. In contrast, our a priori intent was to recreate an exposure matrix of non-steady-state F_iO_2 levels delivered within a normobaric and hypobaric environment, thereby emulating the life support system and ambient cockpit pressures that many tactical aviators routinely experience.

Statistical analyses revealed that P_aO_2 levels differed immediately following exposure to non-steady-state F_iO_2 compared to P_aO_2 levels 120 s later during steady-state exposure to steady-state F_iO_2. Levels of prefrontal cortical activity, which were measured at the same time as the ABG samples were taken, also differed but only during F_iO_2 exposures $\geq$ 60%. In addition, six of thirty-seven blood serum analytes differed between baseline and the study endpoint. However, our experimental design, which included placement of an arterial line catheter, precludes a defensible discussion of how hyperoxia/hypobaria may have contributed to the changes in the serum analytes that we observed.

It remains unclear why non-steady-state F_iO_2 levels > 50% but <100% led to changes in prefrontal cortical activation between Task #1 and Task #3 only at normobaric pressure (749 mmHg) and again at a barometric pressure of 494 mmHg, equivalent to 15,000 feet. Figure 2 suggests that at an atmospheric pressure of 565 mmHg simulating an altitude of 8000 feet, the pegboard Task #1 to Task #3 patterns of prefrontal cortical activation were similar to those seen during at an atmospheric pressure of 494 mmHg, equivalent to 15,000 feet. The difference was that the individual range of the prefrontal cortical activation levels at 565 mmHg between pegboard Task #1 and Task #3 was much greater than that observed at either 749 mmHg or 494 mmHg (Table 3). As the participants in our study had never before been inside a hypobaric chamber, their novel experience with depressurization may have led to a temporary state of heightened arousal that subsequently masked statistically changes in the prefrontal cortical activation between pegboard Task #1 and Task #3. Acclimatization to the experience of hypobaria at 565 mmHg could have reduced the likelihood of anxiety during the transition to the lower barometric pressure of 494 mmHg, enabling changes in the prefrontal cortical activation between pegboard Task #1 and Task #3 to be observed during that phase of the study. However, this is only speculation, and no defensible reason exists to exclude those persons who experienced the wider range of variability of prefrontal cortical activation during pegboard testing at 565 mmHg. While a sham condition may have reduced any confounding effect of participant anxiety, the invasiveness of arterial line placement and continued data collection during the decreasing but ever-present exposure risks of the pandemic, precluded this option.

To inform our decision as to whether Type I error was necessary, we identified recent studies of a similar sample size, N = 20 [34] and a larger N = 51 [35], using similar technologies to those employed in this study. Neither study applied Bonferroni corrections. Nonetheless, we felt that controlling for Type I error could enhance the rigor of our analyses and the defensibility of findings. As the application of Bonferroni corrections in a study such as this could obscure pertinent findings [36], we chose to present all significant findings and annotate those that remained significant following false discovery rate (FDR) correction. We consider this level of transparency to be a strength rather than a limitation of this study.

We do not believe that this study's limitations impact the significance of our findings that exposure to non-steady F_iO_2 levels are followed by changes in arterial blood oxygen content, changes in prefrontal cortical activation levels, and enhanced systemic levels of proinflammatory serum analytes. Although neurovascular tone was not directly measured in this study, our findings pose the hypothesis that neurovascular constriction and dilation may potentially exist during exposure to non-steady-state F_iO_2 levels $\geq$ 60%. If it does indeed occur, executive functioning, cognitive performance, and visuomotor speed and accuracy could be impacted. Addressing that relevant question will require additional studies employing experimental protocols, cognitive assessments, and other physiologic measurement techniques beyond those employed in this study.

4. Materials and Methods

The objective of this study was to define the neurophysiologic and systemic responses to non-steady-state levels of inspired oxygen concentrations at barometric pressures of 749 mmHg (normobaric pressure at the study site), 565 mmHg (equivalent to an altitude of 2438 m or 8000 feet), and 494 mmHg (equivalent to an altitude of 4572 m or 15,000 feet). Measurements of ABG levels and prefrontal cortical brain activity were obtained from healthy volunteers during exposure to non-steady-state and steady-state F_iO_2.

The study protocol was approved by the Institutional Review Board of University Hospitals, STUDY20191540 and the United States Air Force Human Research Protection Office (HRPO), Protocol Number: FWR20200056X. Candidate study participants were required to be non-smokers between the ages of 18 and 61 years, and without exposure to a high-altitude environment >8000 ft. within the previous two weeks. Exclusion criteria included a medically conferred diagnosis of pulmonary and/or cardiac disease, a current or previous neurologic issue (e.g., epilepsy or seizure disorder), known history of sickle cell disease or sickle cell trait, elevated risk for bleeding or a bleeding disorder, recent (within the past 5 years) history of inner ear problems, a positive urine pregnancy test or currently attempting pregnancy, or a history of claustrophobia. Upon verifying the absence of exclusion criteria, all candidate participants were provided with, and then signed, an informed consent document.

To establish an appropriate sample size, we first conducted a series of preliminary studies in which patterns of prefrontal cortical activity were assessed with functional near infrared spectroscopy during a task-on and task-off cognitive challenge. During that testing, participants were exposed to both non-steady-state and steady-state F_iO_2 conditions, as described below.

Outcomes from those studies revealed that an N = 24 would provide sufficient data to achieve a minimum statistical power of 0.80 at a two-tailed significance of <0.05 to detect differences in prefrontal cortical activity during pegboard testing between exposures to non-steady-state and steady-state F_iO_2.

A detailed explanation of the experimental protocol and study methods follows (see Figure 3).

4.1. Health Screening and Protocol Familiarization

Upon arrival for the day of experimental exposure, participants were queried about current medications followed by measurements of height and weight, body temperature, vital signs, and self-reported outcome of their most recent coronavirus disease (COVID-19) test. Those assessments were followed by a focused neurological and physical examination performed by a licensed clinician.

Participants were next instructed on procedures that would occur during the experimental exposures. This included a practice session on the grooved pegboard test (Model 32025 Lafayette Instrument, Lafayette, IN, USA) which was employed to activate the prefrontal cortex using a task-on/task-off paradigm [37] executed in sequence three times. The pegboard contains 25 holes with randomly positioned slots in which metal pegs can be placed. The pegs have a key shape along one side and must be rotated to match the hole before they can be inserted. During the 20-s "task-on" phase, participants were instructed to pick up the pegs, one at a time, and place them into the board. When cued by the researcher for the 20-s "task-off" phase, participants were instructed to stop placing pegs, not move their hands or speak, and try to clear their minds. Participants were coached to not achieve a personal best during any of the tests. Rather, the goal was to complete the task as consistently as possible.

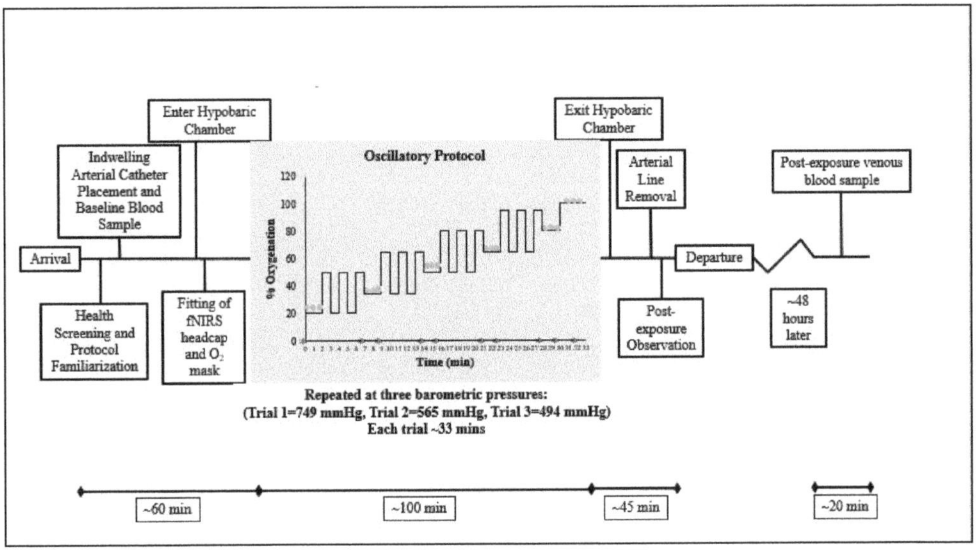

Figure 3. Study data collection overview. This figure illustrates the study protocol at each barometric pressure. The portion of the study in which the participant was exposed to steady-state and non-steady-state inspired oxygen is within the gray shaded box. Each exposure to non-steady-state oxygen appears as a series of cyclic square waves. Green circles represent the time points of each pegboard test. Red asterisks represent the time points of each arterial blood sample.

4.2. Indwelling Radial Arterial Catheter Placement

With the study participant seated comfortably, an Allen's test was performed to ensure adequate collateral perfusion throughout both the right and left hands [38]. A small heating pad was then placed into the participant's non-dominant hand to promote vasodilation of the target artery and the wrist was prepped and draped to provide a sterile field. A 1.0 milliliter (mL) subdermal injection of 1% lidocaine was injected into ventral aspect of the wrist to provide local anesthesia. Using ultrasound guidance, a 20 gauge angiocatheter was inserted through the anesthetized area into the radial artery and advanced until a flash of blood was observed in the catheter. The catheter endcap was removed, the catheter's internal stylet withdrawn, and the catheter secured in place with gauze, tape, and a sterile transparent film dressing. One end of a 6-inch extension tubing was attached to the hub of the arterial catheter, with a three-way stopcock attached to the other end. A 500 mL warmed bag of normal saline was placed into a pressure cuff, and the output of the bag attached to the three-way stopcock via a 60-inch intravenous tubing gravity set.

Baseline Blood Sample Collection for Serum Analyte Analyses

Following placement of the arterial catheter, a single 8 mL arterial blood sample was obtained via the three-way stopcock, using a 10 mL syringe. Blood was then injected into an 8.5 mL BD Vacutainer® tiger top serum separator tube (Benton, Dickinson & Company, Franklin Lakes, NJ, USA) and the tube was centrifuged at 3000 rpm for 8–10 min. The separated serum was pipetted into 1.5 mL Eppendorf tubes, which were immediately placed into dry ice for transport to −80 °C storage.

4.3. Hypobaric Chamber

Following placement of the indwelling arterial catheter, the study participant entered the human hypobaric chamber (Silvan Industries, Marinette, WI, USA). The chamber was 16 ft. long by 7 ft. wide by 7.5 ft. tall, and able to accommodate 4–6 persons. Although structurally capable of depressurizing to an atmospheric pressure of 8.17 mmHg, equivalent to an altitude of 30,480 m (100,000 feet), it was programmed to never exceed a barometric pressure below 226 mmHg, which is equivalent to an altitude of 9144 m (30,000 feet).

4.4. Functional Near Infrared Spectroscopy (fNIRS)

Once seated inside the chamber, an fNIRS microfiber headcap was placed securely across the participant's scalp and connected to the NIRScout system (NIRx Medical Technologies, LLC, Glen Head, NY, USA). The fNIRS system was used to detect, measure, and quantify changes in the brain's functional response to stimuli by measuring changes in oxygenated and deoxygenated hemoglobin in cortical areas [39]. Based upon the brain's functional response or lack of response to stimuli, neuronal activity within discrete regions can increase, decrease, or remain the same. The subsequent level of activity modifies the volume of blood delivered to those brain regions, leading to a brief change in the concentration of oxygenated and deoxygenated hemoglobin [40]. Patterns of prefrontal cortical brain activation patterns were measured with fNIRS throughout pegboard task-on/task-off sequences.

The fNIRS headcap was equipped with 32 optodes consisting of 16 light emitting diodes (sources) and 16 receivers (detectors). Optode locations concurred with the bilateral prefrontal cortices. A dark cloth hood was then placed over the headcap to minimize ambient light intrusion to the optodes while also reducing risk of optode movement. Signal quality of optodes was confirmed using internal calibration sequences of the system's software (nirsLAB 2017.6, NIRx Medical Technologies, LLC, Glen Head, NY, USA). If poor signal quality was detected, the hood was removed and the offending optode adjusted. Signal quality was again assessed, and those steps repeated until desired results were attained. One final measurement of signal quality was conducted after placement of the oxygen delivery mask on the participant, as described below. Continuous fNIRS data collection began at the onset of the study protocol and was recorded throughout the course of the study, which was approximately 120 mins' duration.

fNIRS Analysis

Acquisition data files were downloaded from the fNIRS system computer and imported into Homer3 open-source software in MATLAB R2022a (The Mathworks, Inc., Natick, MA, USA) for analysis [41]. Preprocessing of data included selecting, from the entire data stream, only those sections occurring within the pegboard "task-on" and corresponding "task-off" periods with 2-s of data on either side. This condensed the data file into 128 discrete conditions of 20 s duration per condition of task-on or task-off. The condensed dataset was uploaded to the Homer3 GUI where a software pipeline converted raw data to "beta values" for each of the 128, 20-s discrete data conditions. Each data channel was assessed for signal strength and flagged for additional review if the signal strength or the moving average of standard deviations exceeded pre-determined threshold levels. In those cases, we employed recursive principle component analyses as defined by Yücel [42]. In addition, each channel was assessed for motion artifact. If the artifact involved multiple channels and exceeded pre-established thresholds, the entire 20-s data condition was rejected and excluded from further analyses. A high-pass and low-pass band filter was applied over the remaining data set. The optical density signals were then converted to oxyhemoglobin and deoxyhemoglobin concentrations followed by block averaging of each of the 128, 20-s data conditions. General Linear Model (GLM) analysis was then used to estimate the hemodynamic response function (HRF) [43]. Values for both oxyhemoglobin and deoxyhemoglobin were derived and exported to Statistical Analysis Software (SAS) version 9.4 (SAS Institute, Inc., Cary, NC, USA) for further statistical analysis.

Upon completion of signal processing, we then determined patterns of prefrontal cortical brain activity during pegboard testing, first immediately upon cessation of non-steady-state F_iO_2, and then following 120 s of exposure to steady-state F_iO_2. This was accomplished by comparing levels of prefrontal cortical activity during the first 20-s pegboard "task-on" time period with the following 20-s "task-off" time period. We defined the difference between levels of prefrontal cortical activity between those two conditions as "brain activation." We then compared levels of prefrontal cortical activation between pegboard Task #1, which occurred immediately after cessation of non-steady-state F_iO_2, with pegboard Task #3 which occurred following 120 s of steady-state F_iO_2 exposure.

4.5. Delivery of Non-Steady-State F_iO_2

Following placement of the fNIRS headcap and system calibration, a gel foam-sealed facemask (Hans Rudolph Inc., Shawnee, KS, USA) was strapped securely over the participant's nose and mouth. A 2-way non-rebreather T-shape valve (Hans Rudolph, Series 2700) was inserted into the single large bore opening on the front of the mask. The left side of the connector was attached to an inspiratory circuit while the right side of the connector was attached to the expiratory circuit. A one-way valve within the inspiratory circuit adjacent to the facemask, coupled with constant flow of gas through both the inspiratory and expiratory circuits, insured that the participant did not rebreathe previously exhaled gas.

Delivery of precise oxygen concentrations was achieved by attaching the inspiratory side of the circuit to a PM5200M Air/Oxygen Blender (Precision Medical Inc., Northampton, PA, USA). The blender was connected to compressed air (21% oxygen and 79% nitrogen) and oxygen (100%) supply lines and used to titrate specific oxygen concentrations delivered to the study participant. A BIOPAC MP160 data acquisition and analysis system (BIOPAC Systems, Inc. Goleta, CA, USA) with the BIOPAC oxygen (O_2) 100C Module and a carbon dioxide (CO_2) 100C Module was attached to the participant's face mask to provide a continuous measure of actual mask levels of F_iO_2, CO_2, and respiratory rate. An additional O_2 100C Module was connected to the analyzer to monitor ambient O_2 levels within the hypobaric chamber.

As illustrated in Figure 1, the participant was exposed to steady-state 21% F_iO_2 for three minutes duration. A baseline ABG sample was then obtained from the indwelling arterial catheter using a syringe treated with dry lithium heparin. That initial ABG sample, as well as all subsequent ABG samples, were immediately passed from inside the hypobaric chamber to the outside via a small, sealed steel tube passage. Once received by a research team member outside the hypobaric chamber, the blood sample was immediately injected (within 1–2 min) into an iSTAT blood analyzer (Abbott Point of Care, Princeton, NJ, USA) equipped with a CG8+ cartridge for analysis of sodium (Na^+), potassium (K^+), ionized calcium (iCa^{+2}), Glucose, Hematocrit, Hemoglobin, pH, partial pressure of carbon dioxide ($PaCO_2$), partial pressure of oxygen (P_aO_2), total carbon dioxide content (TCO_2), bicarbonate (HCO_3^-), base excess (BE), and oxygen saturation (SaO_2).

4.6. Non-Steady-State/Steady-State F_iO_2 Exposures and Arterial Blood Gas Sampling

Following collection of the initial arterial blood sample, the participant executed the pegboard task for 20 s, and then rested quietly for 20 s before completing two additional pegboard task-on/task-off sequences. Following the third task, the first sequence of non-steady-state F_iO_2 exposure was initiated by a rapid increase from 21% to 50%, where it was maintained for 60 s, followed by a return to 21% F_iO_2 that was maintained for 60 s. That non-steady-state cycle was repeated a second and third time. Following the third non-steady-state cycle, the F_iO_2 was reduced to 35% (the midpoint between 21% and 50%) and participants completed the three task-on and task-off grooved pegboard sequences. Figure 1 illustrates that following the third oscillation of each F_iO_2, a 0.5 mL arterial blood sample was obtained from the arterial catheter line, followed by a 0.5 mL flush of normal saline. The F_iO_2 was then maintained at a steady-state level for 120 s, during which time the participant again completed the three task-on and task-off grooved pegboard sequences. At the completion of the pegboard tasks, a second (companion) 0.5 mL arterial blood sample was obtained, followed by a 0.5 mL heparinized saline (100 u/mL) flush to maintain catheter line patency. This pattern of non-steady-state F_iO_2 oscillations, ABG sampling, and pegboard task-on/task-off sequences was repeated at F_iO_2 levels of 50% ± 15%, 65% ± 15%, and 80% ± 15%, as illustrated in Figure 1. Following the final non-steady-state F_iO_2 exposure, the F_iO_2 was increased to 100% and maintained for 120 s, at which point participants completed a final series of three pegboard task-on/task-off sequences, followed by collection of a single 0.5 mL arterial blood sample.

After completing the initial 33 min exposure protocol conducted at 749 mmHg (Trial 1), the hypobaric chamber was depressurized to a barometric pressure of 565 mmHg, paralleling an altitude of 8000 ft. The same protocol of exposure to F_iO_2 oscillations, arterial blood sampling, and pegboard task-on/task-off sequences was again delivered over the next 33 min (Trial 2). The hypobaric chamber was then depressurized to a barometric pressure of 494 mmHg, paralleling an altitude of 15,000 ft and same exposure protocol repeated for the third and final time (Trial 3).

Following completion of Trial 3, the chamber was slowly repressurized over a 10–15 min period. Upon reaching 749 mmHg, the participant was escorted from the chamber, seated in a chair, and the arterial line removed. The participant was monitored for 30–60 min to insure absence of any potential adverse effects resulting from hypobaric conditions or arterial line placement, and then released.

4.7. Post-Exposure Study Visit

Within 48 h following the experimental exposure, a member of the investigative team met with the participant to assess the site of the arterial catheterization and to obtain a post-exposure blood sample for proinflammatory serum analyte analysis. At that time, a tourniquet was applied approximately 2–3 inches above the right or left antecubital vein. A 23-gauge butterfly needle with tubing was used to puncture the vein. An 8.5 mL BD Vacutainer® serum separation tube was attached to the butterfly tubing, followed by collection of ~8 mL of venous blood. The venous sample was processed in the same manner as the prior arterial sample, with serum stored at −80 °C until analyses.

4.8. Serum Analyte Analyses

Blood serum samples were collected prior to exposure to non-steady-state F_iO_2 and hypobaria and again 48 h after experimental exposure. These serum samples were analyzed using multi-array technology (QuickPlex 120; MesoScale Diagnostics, Rockville, MD, USA) coupled with the V-PLEX neuroinflammation panel (Catalog No. K15210D). To establish measurement reproducibility, each sample was divided between two adjacent wells of each 96-well plate. The neuroinflammation panel included the proinflammatory plate measuring interleukin 1 beta (IL-1β), interleukin 2 (IL-2), interleukin 4 (IL-4), interleukin 6 (IL-6), interleukin 8 (IL-8), interleukin 10 (IL-10), interleukin 13 (IL-13), tumor necrosis factor alpha (TNF-α), and interferon-gamma (IFN-γ). The chemokine plate measured monocyte chemoattractant protein-1 (MCP-1), monocyte chemoattractant protein-4 (MCP-4), eotaxin, macrophage inflammatory protein-1 alpha (MIP-1α), eotaxin-3, thymus activation regulated chemokine (TARC), macrophage inflammatory protein-1 beta (MIP-1β), macrophage-derived chemokine (MDC), and interferon gamma inducible protein-10 (IP-10). The cytokine plate measured interleukin 1 alpha (IL-1α), interleukin 5 (IL-5), interleukin 7 (IL-7), interleukin 12 (IL-12), interleukin 15 (IL-15), interleukin 16 (IL-16), interleukin 17A (IL-17A), tumor necrosis factor beta (TNF-β), and vascular endothelial growth factor A (VEGF-A). The angiogenesis plate measured basic fibroblastic growth factor (bFGF), vascular endothelial growth factor C (VEGF-C), vascular endothelial growth factor D (VEGF-D), vascular endothelial growth factor receptor 1 (Flt-1), placental growth factor (PlGF), and tyrosine kinase 2 (Tie-2). The vascular injury plate measured serum amyloid A (SAA), C-reactive protein (CRP), intercellular adhesion molecule-1 (ICAM-1), and vascular cell adhesion molecule-1 (VCAM-1).

4.9. Statistical Approach

Comparisons of participants' race, age, sex, and BMI were tested using Fisher's Exact test and Wilcoxon rank sum test. fNIRS-derived measures of cortical activation levels within each brain region during pegboard Task #1 and pegboard Task #3 were explored using paired t-tests or Wilcoxon signed rank tests. ABG values obtained following exposures to non-steady-state F_iO_2 and again after steady-state F_iO_2 was sustained for 120 s were summarized as mean, standard deviation (SD), and range (minimum, maximum) and then compared using paired t-tests or Wilcoxon signed rank tests. Serum analytes measured at baseline and again at 48 h following the experimental exposures to hypobaria and to non-steady-state and steady-state FiO2 were evaluated using the same approach. The false discovery rate (FDR) method was applied to control Type I error from multiple comparison testing. All tests were two-sided and adjusted p-values from the FDR less than 0.05 were considered to be statistically significant. Data were analyzed using SAS version 9.4 (SAS Institute, Inc., Cary, NC, USA) and Statistical Package for Social Sciences (SPSS) version 28 (IBM Corp; Armonk, NY, USA).

Supplementary Materials: The following supporting information can be downloaded at: https://www.mdpi.com/article/10.3390/ijms25063279/s1.

Author Contributions: M.J.D., E.G.D., J.S.P., L.K.N., D.S.B. and K.P.S. contributed to the study design; M.J.D., E.G.D., J.S.P., S.J.F., L.K.N. and A.A. collected data; M.J.D., E.G.D., S.P.M., S.J.F. and L.K.N. analyzed the data; M.J.D., S.P.M. and E.G.D. developed and performed statistical analyses; M.J.D., E.G.D., S.P.M., K.P.S. and D.S.B. interpreted the data; M.J.D., E.G.D. and S.P.M. prepared the initial draft; K.P.S. wrote sections of the manuscript. All authors contributed to manuscript revision, proofreading, and approval of the submitted version. All authors have read and agreed to the published version of the manuscript.

Funding: This project was supported through FA8650-19-C-6103, Department of Defense—Air Force Research Laboratory 711th Human Performance Wing, Airman Systems Directorate, Airman Biosciences Division, Biomedical Impact of Flight Branch, Wright-Patterson Air Force Base, OH, 45433, USA.

Institutional Review Board Statement: The study was conducted in accordance with the Declaration of Helsinki and approved by the Institutional Review Board University Hospitals of Cleveland, Ohio, STUDY20191540 on 17 January 2020 and the United States Air Force Human Research Protection Office (HRPO), Protocol Number: FWR20200056X on 14 February 2020 for studies involving humans.

Informed Consent Statement: Informed consent was obtained from all subjects involved in the study.

Data Availability Statement: Data are subject to third party restrictions. The data are not openly available due to privacy or ethical restrictions. Data supporting the findings of this study may be available from the United States Air Force upon reasonable request submitted to the corresponding author.

Acknowledgments: Appreciation is extended to Jessica Beebe and Naji Saker for assistance with generating preliminary data for sample size estimation and to Noel Samsum and Ian Vannix for their assistance with data management.

Conflicts of Interest: The authors declare no conflicts of interest.

References

1. Asfar, P.; Singer, M.; Radermacher, P. Understanding the benefits and harms of oxygen therapy. *Intensive Care Med.* **2015**, *41*, 1118–1121. [CrossRef] [PubMed]
2. Brugniaux, J.V.; Coombs, G.B.; Barak, O.F.; Dujic, Z.; Sekhon, M.S.; Ainslie, P.N. Highs and lows of hyperoxia: Physiological, performance, and clinical aspects. *Am. J. Physiol. Regul. Integr. Comp. Physiol.* **2018**, *315*, R1–R27. [CrossRef] [PubMed]
3. Damato, E.G.; Flak, T.A.; Mayes, R.S.; Strohl, K.P.; Ziganti, A.M.; Abdollahifar, A.; Flask, C.A.; LaManna, J.C.; Decker, M.J. Neurovascular and cortical responses to hyperoxia: Enhanced cognition and electroencephalographic activity despite reduced perfusion. *J. Physiol.* **2020**, *598*, 3941–3956. [CrossRef] [PubMed]
4. Griffiths, E.A. The production of liquid oxygen for use on aircraft. *Trans. Faraday Soc.* **1922**, *18*, 224–239. [CrossRef]
5. Grayson-Smith, H.; Findlay, J.C. Liquid oxygen in aircraft. *Chem. Rev.* **1946**, *39*, 397–402. [CrossRef]
6. Elliott, L.C.J.J.; Schmitt, M.D.R. Unexplained Physiological Episodes: A Pilot's Perspective. *Air Space Power J.* **2019**, *33*, 15–32.
7. Manatt, S.A. Onboard oxygen generation systems. *Aviat. Space Environ. Med.* **1981**, *52*, 645–653.
8. Bhat, A.A.; Mang, H.; Rajkumar, S.; Kotresh, T.; Singh, U. On-board oxygen generation using high performance molecular sieve. *Def. Life Sci. J.* **2017**, *2*, 380–384. [CrossRef]

9. Lambertsen, C.J.; Dough, R.H.; Cooper, D.Y.; Emmel, G.L.; Loeschcke, H.H.; Schmidt, C.F. Oxygen toxicity; effects in man of oxygen inhalation at 1 and 3.5 atmospheres upon blood gas transport, cerebral circulation and cerebral metabolism. *J. Appl. Physiol.* **1953**, *5*, 471–486. [CrossRef]
10. Floyd, T.F.; Clark, J.M.; Gelfand, R.; Detre, J.A.; Ratcliffe, S.; Guvakov, D.; Lambertsen, C.J.; Eckenhoff, R.G. Independent cerebral vasoconstrictive effects of hyperoxia and accompanying arterial hypocapnia at 1 ATA. *J. Appl. Physiol.* **2003**, *95*, 2453–2461. [CrossRef]
11. Mattos, J.D.; Campos, M.O.; Rocha, M.P.; Mansur, D.E.; Rocha, H.N.M.; Garcia, V.P.; Rocha, N.G.; Silveira Alvares, T.; Secher, N.H.; Claudio Lucas da Nobrega, A.; et al. Differential Vasomotor Responses to Isocapnic Hyperoxia: Cerebral vs. Peripheral Circulation. *Am. J. Physiol. Regul. Integr. Comp. Physiol.* **2019**, *318*, R182–R187. [CrossRef] [PubMed]
12. Damato, E.G.; Fillioe, S.J.; Vannix, I.S.; Norton, L.K.; Margevicius, S.P.; Beebe, J.L.; Decker, M.J. Characterizing the Dose Response of Hyperoxia with Brain Perfusion. *Aerosp. Med. Hum. Perform.* **2022**, *93*, 493–498. [CrossRef] [PubMed]
13. Lodato, R.F. Decreased O2 consumption and cardiac output during normobaric hyperoxia in conscious dogs. *J. Appl. Physiol.* **1989**, *67*, 1551–1559. [CrossRef] [PubMed]
14. Dussault, C.; Gontier, E.; Verret, C.; Soret, M.; Boussuges, A.; Hedenstierna, G.; Montmerle-Borgdorff, S. Hyperoxia and hypergravity are independent risk factors of atelectasis in healthy sitting humans: A pulmonary ultrasound and SPECT/CT study. *J. Appl. Physiol.* **2016**, *121*, 66–77. [CrossRef] [PubMed]
15. Ciarlone, G.E.; Hinojo, C.M.; Stavitzski, N.M.; Dean, J.B. CNS function and dysfunction during exposure to hyperbaric oxygen in operational and clinical settings. *Redox Biol.* **2019**, *27*, 101159. [CrossRef] [PubMed]
16. Tiboldi, A.; Hunyadi-Gulyas, E.; Wohlrab, P.; Schmid, J.A.; Markstaller, K.; Klein, K.U.; Tretter, V. Effects of Hyperoxia and Hyperoxic Oscillations on the Proteome of Murine Lung Microvascular Endothelium. *Antioxidants* **2022**, *11*, 2349. [CrossRef] [PubMed]
17. Boehme, S.; Hartmann, E.K.; Tripp, T.; Thal, S.C.; David, M.; Abraham, D.; Baumgardner, J.E.; Markstaller, K.; Klein, K.U. PO_2 oscillations induce lung injury and inflammation. *Crit. Care* **2019**, *23*, 102. [CrossRef]
18. Formenti, F.; Bommakanti, N.; Chen, R.; Cronin, J.N.; McPeak, H.; Holopherne-Doran, D.; Hedenstierna, G.; Hahn, C.E.W.; Larsson, A.; Farmery, A.D. Respiratory oscillations in alveolar oxygen tension measured in arterial blood. *Sci. Rep.* **2017**, *7*, 7499. [CrossRef]
19. Formenti, F.; Farmery, A.D. Intravascular oxygen sensors with novel applications for bedside respiratory monitoring. *Anaesthesia* **2017**, *72* (Suppl. 1), 95–104. [CrossRef]
20. Culver, B.H. Chapter 9—Pulmonary Function Testing. In *Clinical Respiratory Medicine*, 4th ed.; Spiro, S.G., Silvestri, G.A., Agustí, A., Eds.; W.B. Saunders: Philadelphia, PA, USA, 2012; pp. 133–142.
21. Crapo, R.O.; Jensen, R.L.; Hegewald, M.; Tashkin, D.P. Arterial blood gas reference values for sea level and an altitude of 1,400 meters. *Am. J. Respir. Crit. Care Med.* **1999**, *160*, 1525–1531. [CrossRef]
22. Gonzalez-Garcia, M.; Maldonado, D.; Barrero, M.; Casas, A.; Perez-Padilla, R.; Torres-Duque, C.A. Arterial blood gases and ventilation at rest by age and sex in an adult Andean population resident at high altitude. *Eur. J. Appl. Physiol.* **2020**, *120*, 2729–2736. [CrossRef]
23. Kelley, E.F.; Carlson, A.R.; Wentz, R.J.; Ziegler, B.L.; Johnson, B.D. Influence of rapidly oscillating inspired O_2 and N_2 concentrations on pulmonary vascular function and lung fluid balance in healthy adults. *Front. Physiol.* **2022**, *13*, 1018057. [CrossRef]
24. Rahn, H. A concept of mean alveolar air and the ventilation-blood flow relationships during pulmonary gas exchange. *Am. J. Physiol.* **1949**, *158*, 21–30. [CrossRef]
25. Oldendorf, W.H.; Kitano, M. Radioisotope measurement of brain blood turnover time as a clinical index of brain circulation. *J. Nucl. Med.* **1967**, *8*, 570–587. [PubMed]
26. Mapleson, W.W. Circulation-time models of the uptake of inhaled anaesthetics and data for quantifying them. *Br. J. Anaesth.* **1973**, *45*, 319–334. [CrossRef] [PubMed]
27. Biancotto, A.; Wank, A.; Perl, S.; Cook, W.; Olnes, M.J.; Dagur, P.K.; Fuchs, J.C.; Langweiler, M.; Wang, E.; McCoy, J.P. Baseline Levels and Temporal Stability of 27 Multiplexed Serum Cytokine Concentrations in Healthy Subjects. *PLoS ONE* **2013**, *8*, e76091. [CrossRef] [PubMed]
28. Wu, D.; Dinh, T.L.; Bausk, B.P.; Walt, D.R. Long-Term Measurements of Human Inflammatory Cytokines Reveal Complex Baseline Variations between Individuals. *Am. J. Pathol.* **2017**, *187*, 2620–2626. [CrossRef] [PubMed]
29. Glasgow, C.G.; Avila, N.A.; Lin, J.P.; Stylianou, M.P.; Moss, J. Serum vascular endothelial growth factor-D levels in patients with lymphangioleiomyomatosis reflect lymphatic involvement. *Chest* **2009**, *135*, 1293–1300. [CrossRef] [PubMed]
30. Lev, S.; Gottesman, T.; Sahaf Levin, G.; Lederfein, D.; Berkov, E.; Diker, D.; Zaidman, A.; Nutman, A.; Ilan Ber, T.; Angel, A.; et al. Observational cohort study of IP-10's potential as a biomarker to aid in inflammation regulation within a clinical decision support protocol for patients with severe COVID-19. *PLoS ONE* **2021**, *16*, e0245296. [CrossRef] [PubMed]
31. Mielnik, P.; Chwalinska-Sadowska, H.; Wiesik-Szewczyk, E.; Maslinski, W.; Olesinska, M. Serum concentration of interleukin 15, interleukin 2 receptor and TNF receptor in patients with polymyositis and dermatomyositis: Correlation to disease activity. *Rheumatol. Int.* **2012**, *32*, 639–643. [CrossRef]
32. Purzycka-Bohdan, D.; Nedoszytko, B.; Zablotna, M.; Glen, J.; Szczerkowska-Dobosz, A.; Nowicki, R.J. Chemokine Profile in Psoriasis Patients in Correlation with Disease Severity and Pruritus. *Int. J. Mol. Sci.* **2022**, *23*, 13330. [CrossRef]

33. Deshmane, S.L.; Kremlev, S.; Amini, S.; Sawaya, B.E. Monocyte chemoattractant protein-1 (MCP-1): An overview. *J. Interferon Cytokine Res.* **2009**, *29*, 313–326. [CrossRef]
34. Kerstein, A.; Schüler, S.; Cabral-Marques, O.; Fazio, J.; Häsler, R.; Müller, A.; Pitann, S.; Moosig, F.; Klapa, S.; Haas, C. Environmental factor and inflammation-driven alteration of the total peripheral T-cell compartment in granulomatosis with polyangiitis. *J. Autoimmun.* **2017**, *78*, 79–91. [CrossRef]
35. Wunderlich, T.; Frey, N.; Kähler, W.; Lutz, M.; Radermacher, P.; Klapa, S.; Koch, I.; Tillmans, F.; Witte, J.; Koch, A. Influence of hyperoxia on diastolic myocardial and arterial endothelial function. *Undersea Hyperb. Med.* **2017**, *44*, 521–533. [CrossRef]
36. Armstrong, R.A. When to use the Bonferroni correction. *Ophthalmic Physiol. Opt. J. Br. Coll. Ophthalmic Opt.* **2014**, *34*, 502–508. [CrossRef] [PubMed]
37. Bakhshipour, E.; Koiler, R.; Milla, K.; Getchell, N. Understanding the Cognitive Demands of the Purdue Pegboard Test: An fNIRs Study. In *Advances in Neuroergonomics and Cognitive Engineering*; Springer: Cham, Switzerland, 2021; pp. 55–61.
38. Al-Hakim, R.; Hedge, J.C.; Jahangiri, Y.; Kaufman, J.A.; Galuppo, R.; Farsad, K. Palmar Warming for Radial Artery Vasodilation to Facilitate Transradial Access: A Randomized Controlled Trial. *J. Vasc. Interv. Radiol. JVIR* **2019**, *30*, 421–424. [CrossRef]
39. Tanaka, H.; Katura, T.; Sato, H. Task-related oxygenation and cerebral blood volume changes estimated from NIRS signals in motor and cognitive tasks. *NeuroImage* **2014**, *94*, 107–119. [CrossRef]
40. LaManna, J.C. In situ measurements of brain tissue hemoglobin saturation and blood volume by reflectance spectrophotometry in the visible spectrum. *J. Biomed. Opt.* **2007**, *12*, 062103. [CrossRef]
41. Huppert, T.J.; Diamond, S.G.; Franceschini, M.A.; Boas, D.A. HomER: A review of time-series analysis methods for near-infrared spectroscopy of the brain. *Appl. Opt.* **2009**, *48*, D280–D298. [CrossRef] [PubMed]
42. Yücel, M.A.; Selb, J.; Cooper, R.J.; Boas, D.A. Targeted principle component analysis: A new motion artifact correction approach for near-infrared spectroscopy. *J. Innov. Opt. Health Sci.* **2013**, *7*, 1350066. [CrossRef] [PubMed]
43. Ye, J.C.; Tak, S.; Jang, K.E.; Jung, J.; Jang, J. NIRS-SPM: Statistical parametric mapping for near-infrared spectroscopy. *NeuroImage* **2009**, *44*, 428–447. [CrossRef] [PubMed]

Disclaimer/Publisher's Note: The statements, opinions and data contained in all publications are solely those of the individual author(s) and contributor(s) and not of MDPI and/or the editor(s). MDPI and/or the editor(s) disclaim responsibility for any injury to people or property resulting from any ideas, methods, instructions or products referred to in the content.

International Journal of
Molecular Sciences

MDPI

Review

Oxy-Inflammation in Humans during Underwater Activities

Alessandra Vezzoli [1,2], Simona Mrakic-Sposta [1,*], Andrea Brizzolari [2], Costantino Balestra [3,4,5], Enrico Maria Camporesi [6] and Gerardo Bosco [2]

1 Institute of Clinical Physiology-National Research Council (CNR-IFC), 20142 Milano, Italy; alessandra.vezzoli@cnr.it
2 Department of Biomedical Sciences, University of Padova, 35131 Padova, Italy; andreabrizzolari79@gmail.com (A.B.); gerardo.bosco@unipd.it (G.B.)
3 Environmental, Occupational, Aging (Integrative) Physiology Laboratory, Haute Ecole Bruxelles-Brabant (HE2B), 1160 Brussels, Belgium; cbalestra@he2b.be
4 Physical Activity Teaching Unit, Motor Sciences Department, Université Libre de Bruxelles (ULB), 1050 Brussels, Belgium
5 DAN Europe Research Division (Roseto-Brussels), 1160 Brussels, Belgium
6 TEAM Health Anaesthesia, Tampa General Hospital, Tampa, FL 33606, USA; ecampore@usf.edu
* Correspondence: simona.mrakicsposta@cnr.it

Abstract: Underwater activities are characterized by an imbalance between reactive oxygen/nitrogen species (RONS) and antioxidant mechanisms, which can be associated with an inflammatory response, depending on O_2 availability. This review explores the oxidative stress mechanisms and related inflammation status (Oxy-Inflammation) in underwater activities such as breath-hold (BH) diving, Self-Contained Underwater Breathing Apparatus (SCUBA) and Closed-Circuit Rebreather (CCR) diving, and saturation diving. Divers are exposed to hypoxic and hyperoxic conditions, amplified by environmental conditions, hyperbaric pressure, cold water, different types of breathing gases, and air/non-air mixtures. The "diving response", including physiological adaptation, cardiovascular stress, increased arterial blood pressure, peripheral vasoconstriction, altered blood gas values, and risk of bubble formation during decompression, are reported.

Keywords: breath-hold diving; SCUBA; closed-circuit rebreather; saturation diving; oxidants; reactive oxygen species; reactive nitrogen species

1. Introduction

SCUBA (Self-Contained Underwater Breathing Apparatus) and BH (breath-hold breathing) diving are breathtaking adventures that allow us to explore the world beneath the seas. However, diving comes with its own set of inherent risks and challenges. From time to time, thankfully rarely, SCUBA diving accidents or illnesses may occur. These can range from minor discomfort to life-threatening situations. One essential tool that plays a crucial role in mitigating the consequences of diving-related diseases is oxygen (O_2) [1].

Regarding diving-related diseases, time is another vital parameter in diving activities. The inhalation of O_2 (normobaric or hyperbaric, and with various types of masks, depending on whether the diver is conscious or unconscious) works after decompression sickness (DCS) by accelerating the diffusion and elimination of the excess nitrogen absorbed during SCUBA diving [2]. Diving-related activities are well known to produce partial O_2 pressure (pO_2) variations since the ambient pressure changes during underwater excursions; these changes can go from hyperoxia during hyperbaric phases and reach hypoxia on return from depths during some BH diving activities. Prolonged hyperoxia is known during SCUBA diving but does not always reach levels above 1 absolute atmosphere of O_2 in the breathing mix [3]. Prolonged hyperoxia (apart from in medical settings) is not easy to reach under physiological conditions. However, it is still possible, for instance, if people are living below sea level around the "Dead Sea" in Israel (located 402 m below sea level, where the barometric pressure reaches 800 mmHg) [4]. The other setting to achieve a prolonged hyperoxia above 1 atmosphere of pure O_2 breathing can be reached during Closed-Circuit Rebreather diving since the O_2 set point for such dives is commonly set between 1.2 and 1.4 ATA during several hours of the excursion [5–9]. A chronic, less important form of hyperoxia is encountered during other saturation diving procedures where, depending on the methods used, around 0.49 ATA of partial O_2 pressure (pO_2) levels are kept during several days of decompression needed to reach sea level [10].

This review will discuss the impact of diving activities on oxidative/inflammatory stress (Oxy-Inflammation).

2. Oxy-Inflammation-Related Mechanisms and Outcomes

Humans and most terrestrial animal organisms have adapted to live in the Earth's atmosphere, where the fraction of inspired oxygen (fiO_2) equals approximately 0.21. O_2 is the third most abundant element in the universe, after hydrogen (H_2) and helium (He) as compounds, including oxides, which constitute around 50% of Earth's crust [11]. Furthermore, O_2 is one of the main components of biological macromolecules (proteins, carbohydrates, nucleic acids) and the last acceptor of electrons in oxidative phosphorylation, providing most of the natural energy in living organisms.

2.1. Oxidative Stress in Hypoxia and Hyperoxia

The redox system plays a crucial role in maintaining cell homeostasis and balancing the generation/elimination of reactive oxygen (ROS) and nitrogen (RNS) species [12]. A continuous flux of oxidant species guarantees redox homeostasis originated by mitochondria to deal with the electron consumption during the electron chain, resulting in the release of superoxide anions (O_2^{2-}) [13]. Being O_2-derived compounds, ROS and RNS are *"double-faced"* elements because they carry out an essential function in several physiological mechanisms, including pathogen phagocytosis, modulating activities, and regulatory ability during the transduction of intercellular information [14]. On the other hand, an imbalance between ROS/RNS generation and detoxification leads to a condition of "oxidative stress" and the damage of biological macromolecules like lipids, proteins, and DNA [15] (see Figure 1). Following one of the most complete definitions, oxidative stress is "*the consequence of the failure to maintain the physiological redox steady state, which is the self-correcting physiological response to different challenges*" [16]. ROS such as O_2^{2-} act both as a signaling molecule, contributing to the release of proinflammatory cytokine [17], and inflammatory mediator, reacting with nitric oxide (NO) to give peroxynitrite ($ONOO^-$), an aggressive RNS that induces nitrosative stress, exacerbating the inflammation status [18]. Furthermore, the overproduction of ROS has been implicated in the development and progression of some diseases: cardiovascular, neurodegenerative, and metabolic diseases and cancer [19]. Elevated ROS levels contribute to stabilizing hypoxia-inducible factor-1α (HIF-1α), a key regulator of cellular responses to low oxygen. Additionally, ROS are essential messenger and signaling molecules in muscle adaptations to exercise and disuse, as documented by various studies [20]. The interplay between hypoxia-induced signaling pathways and oxidative stress is intricated [1,21].

On the other hand, an overdose of oxygen can harm cell membranes, lungs, and overall health by increasing oxidative stress and inflammation. For example, it damages the lungs, affecting surfactant proteins and mucociliary clearance, leading to lung collapse, reduced compliance, and higher infection risk [22]. Also, hyperoxemia constricts vessels, reducing coronary blood flow and cardiac output and potentially altering microvascular circulation [23].

2.2. Inflammation in Hypoxia and Hyperoxia

Inflammation may be influenced by fiO_2 level, as reported by some authors investigating subjects exposed to hypoxia that showed pulmonary edema caused by inflammatory markers release, including interleukin-6 (IL-6) and protein C-reactive (CRP) [24–26]. To adapt body tissues to hypoxia, hypoxia-inducible factors (HIFs), a family of heterodimers that constitute a transcription complex that is stabilized by hypoxia [26] or a return from hyperoxia [27–30], are activated to coordinate several transcriptional pathways to optimize metabolic and vascular functions toward low fiO_2 [31]. Furthermore, HIFs are controlled by prolyl hydroxylase domain (PHD) proteins, a class of "O_2 sensors" that are involved in HIF level regulation and O_2 homeostasis [32]. Nuclear factor κB (NF-κB) is involved in inflammation regulation and immune response [33], interacting with the PHD-HIF pathway [34], confirming the link between hypoxia and inflammation [35]. Other hypoxia–inflammation interactions involve the IκB kinase complex, an NF-κB regulatory component [31], and the regulation of HIF transcription before and during the inflammation [36]. Under inflammatory status, NF-κB activation stimulates immune defense by neutrophil release [37]. At the same time, HIF-α promotes type 2 helper T-cell (Th2) production [38] and macrophage activation with a ROS-dependent mechanism [39]. Inflammation onset against hypoxia can be clinically significant (e.g., chronic respiratory/renal/kidney/cardiovascular/neurological disease, mitochondrial/endothelial dysfunction, tumors) [21].

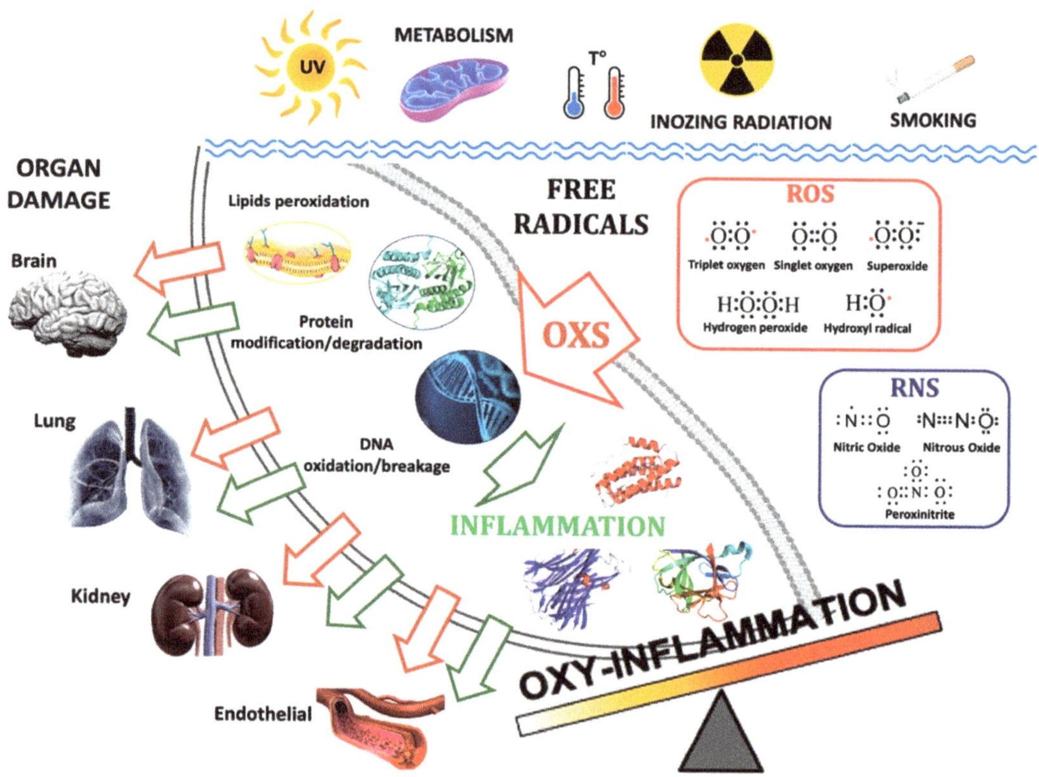

Figure 1. The main pathways of the formation of Oxy-Inflammation and organ damage. Environmental triggers such as exposure to UV and ionizing radiation, metabolism, water/body temperature, and smoking can produce free radicals: ROS (e.g., $^3O_2$, O_2, O_2^-, H_2O_2, HO·) and RNS (e.g., NO, N_2O, $ONOO^-$). Their accumulations can lead to lipids' cellular membrane degradation, misfolded proteins, and DNA oxidation/breakage. The inflammation triggered by Oxi-Inflammation is the cause of many types of organ damage and acute/chronic diseases.

Hyperoxia represents the other side of the coin of fiO_2 value. In this case, tissues are exposed to an excess supply of O_2, with the arterial partial pressure of O_2 (paO_2) value being greater than 100 mmHg [40]. As mentioned above, exposure to prolonged hyperoxia exacerbates oxidative stress, leading to cellular damage via lipid peroxidation, enzyme inactivation, biological macromolecule oxidation, and apoptosis or necrosis [41]. Exposure to high fiO_2 levels during significant time lapse results in O_2 lung toxicity, characterized by a pulmonary inflammatory response [42] and a release of proinflammatory cytokines implicated in mediating neutrophil action into hyperoxic lungs [43] in the early stages of inflammatory response [44]. On the other hand, short-term hyperoxia seems to attenuate cytokine production [45], β2-integrin expression necessary for leukocyte adhesion [46], and macrophage phagocytosis and killing [47]. In animal models, some authors found that hyperoxia could mitigate the inflammatory response after glucan intake [48,49].

2.3. Endothelial Dysfunction

Increased partial O_2 pressure (pO_2) promotes oxidative stress, which triggers endothelial dysfunction. There are two mechanisms strongly related to the decrease in nitric oxide availability (NO). First, hyperoxia-related oxidative stress leads to the generation of the superoxide anion (O_2^-), which reacts with NO to produce peroxynitrite ($ONOO^-$) [50]. ROS can also oxidize nitric oxide synthase (NOS) cofactor tetrahydrobiopterin (BH4) into dihydrobiopterin (BH2), which causes a reduced liberation of NO uncoupling endothelial NO synthase [51], leading to endothelial dysfunctions [52]. NO can be preserved by the activation of antioxidant defenses, as observed by several authors that found NO increases during the deep phases of both SCUBA and BH dives [53]. The same tendencies have been shown in SCUBA [54] or CCR diving [55]. After exiting saturation diving, endothelial recovery is fast, showing no long-term adverse effect on vascular function [56]. Furthermore, circulating bubbles may induce endothelial dysfunctions [57] through direct contact between microbubbles and endothelial cells [58] and the activation of a coagulation cascade [59,60]. However, we want to highlight that both deep and repetitive BH diving lead to endothelial dysfunction that may play an essential role in the genesis of neurological decompression sickness [61].

2.4. Hypoxia, Reoxygenation, and Hyperoxia

Redox balance/unbalance is significantly modulated by external factors such as environmental hypoxia [62–68], hyperoxia [69–73], and physical activity [74–77]. Moreover, both environmental hypoxia and physical activity have been shown to augment oxidative stress in a dose-dependent manner [77–79].

Reduced O_2 tension during ischemia–reperfusion (IRI) episodes activates cellular pathways that upregulate proinflammatory signaling and promote oxidant generation [80]. Reperfusion after ischemia recruits inflammatory cells to the vascular wall, further exacerbating oxidant production and ultimately resulting in cell death, tissue injury, and organ dysfunction. As an IRI consequence, the activation of the NF-κB pathway leads to the release of proinflammatory cytokines (IL-1, IL-6, IL-8) [81] and major histocompatibility complex (MHC) upregulation [82]. Observing the correlation of the renal expression of Toll-like receptor (TLR) 4 with IRI degree [83], a link between IRI and innate/adaptive immunity has been hypothesized, as reported by some authors in transplant models [84,85].

Physical exercise has been proposed as a model of "intermittent hypoxia" (IH) or "intermittent hyperoxia" since oxidative stress increases during exercise, which can be defined as a combination of cycles of hypoxia and normoxia, hypercapnia, and hyperoxia, depending on the training type and duration [70,86,87]. Physical exercise, mainly moderate activity, improves health by reducing the risk of obesity and cardiovascular and chronic degenerative disease onset [88], raising NO availability, decreasing oxidative stress, and fostering antioxidant defenses [89]. On the other hand, exercise at altitude exposes tissue to hypoxia, which may increase oxidative stress by reducing antioxidant defense efficacy [90].

2.5. Oxy-Inflammation Biomarkers

The simultaneous measurement of a panel of biomarkers has been frequently chosen, as this can also provide a comprehensive assessment of oxidative stress effects on vascular function. Protein biomarkers were selected to cover critical features of vascular function, i.e., inflammation, endothelial function, and fibrinolysis. CRP is a biomarker of inflammation and endothelial function [91]; its increase is associated with impaired endothelium-dependent vasodilatation [92]. IL-6 increases the adhesiveness of the endothelial cells for lymphocytes by upregulating Intercellular Adhesion Molecule-1 (ICAM-1) for a proinflammatory reaction [93].

In this review, we use the term "Oxy-Inflammation", proposed by Valacchi et al. [94], to describe *"a condition characterized by a combination of systemic oxidative stress associated with an inflammatory condition"*. This review summarizes the "Oxy-Inflammation" in underwater activities such as breath-hold (BH) and SCUBA diving.

The main mechanisms of the formation of Oxy-Inflammation and relative organ damage are illustrated in Figure 1.

3. The Oxy-Inflammation Mechanism in Underwater Activity

3.1. Breath-Hold (BH) Diving

BH diving elicits a physiological adaptation collectively termed the "diving response", which includes changes such as bradycardia, reduced cardiac output, increased arterial blood pressure, peripheral vasoconstriction, and altered blood gas values [95]. Hyperoxia occurs during descent and bottom time in BH divers due to increased environmental pressure and thorax compression [96,97]. Hypoxia-induced endothelial damage might be less pronounced because hypoxia appears in the last portion of the ascent phase of a dive [96–99].

Hyperoxia-induced changes observed in BH diving may influence arterial blood gas (ABG) parameters, especially PaO_2 and arterial pCO_2 ($PaCO_2$). At the maximum depth, PaO_2 increases due to hyperoxia-induced effects caused by the rise in environmental pressure [99–102], but this trend was not observed in all BH divers. This unexpected PaO_2 decrease is related to a lung volume reduction leading to a right-to-left shunt through lung atelectasis [101–104]. Furthermore, Bosco et al. [105] reported that BH diving-related exercise breaks down PaO_2 levels due to muscle O_2 consumption [105], which may increase the risk of injuries [106] during the ascent phase. $PaCO_2$ values do not change much, probably due to the body's capacity to store soluble CO_2 [101] and hyperventilation that decreases PaO_2 [98].

Similarly to PaO_2, $PaCO_2$ variation may be related to BH diving type, as reported by Bosco et al., who found higher $PaCO_2$ values after static apnea concerning those after a deep dive [105], which reduced from initial values. In the case of deep diving, $PaCO_2$ rises in BH divers who do muscular work when returning to the surface using fins. The muscular work contribution may be confirmed by the higher augmented lactate value that was not recorded in other conditions [105].

In BH diving, IH can be a powerful trigger for endothelial dysfunction [106,107]. More severe diving stress in repetitive BH dives could lead to strains on the cardiovascular system, vascular function, and endothelial integrity. Endothelial dysfunctions in BH diving have been investigated by Theunissen et al. [54], where the reduction in NO-dependent vascular function resulted from low NO bioavailability. The same authors also showed a decrease in this endothelial dysfunction when supplementing antioxidants to the divers [108].

High pO_2 may also promote oxidative stress due to the hyperbaric environment, increasing free O_2 that may generate ROS [109]. Oxidative stress has been investigated in BH diving [54,107–109], confirming its role in the development of endothelial dysfunction [110]. The overproduction of ROS and consequent oxidative damage to membrane lipids and total antioxidant capacity (TAC) reflects a hypoxic condition in the last few meters while ascending to the surface [109]. Neopterin and creatinine levels increase, which suggests an alteration in renal function as a physiological response to pO_2 variations during the dive [109,110].

Changes in polyunsaturated fatty acids (PUFAs) and eicosanoids after a single apnea event revealed different kinetics of pro- and anti-inflammatory regulations and changes in oxidative stress levels [111].

Adaptation to hypoxia may involve amino acid metabolism [112,113], and hypoxia might be a stimulus for amino acids' release in the bloodstream because serine and taurine may be engaged in hypoxia adaptation, especially during the ascent phase of a BH dive [113].

Furthermore, prolonged exposure to hypoxia, such as diving at high altitudes, may affect platelet activity, as reported by some authors [114], but this aspect seems to be related to pO_2 [115]. Platelet activation can be induced by exercise-related inflammation [116] engaging with leukocytes via soluble factors and physical interaction with several receptors, including platelet P-selectin (CD62P), CD40 ligand (CD40L), as well as PSGL-1, CD40, and Mac-1 (integrin $\alpha M\beta 2$, CD11b/CD18) on leukocytes [117,118]. Platelet–leukocyte interactions facilitate leukocyte recruitment and extravasation to inflammation sites, leading to leukocyte proinflammatory mediator release but, in some cases, damping inflammation [119,120]. Furthermore, some authors found a link between gene activity and immune cell activation against inflammation, observing a temporary increase in leucocytes and an upregulation of the anti-inflammatory response genes [121].

As reported by Wang et al. [122], ultrasound lung comets (ULCs) may be associated with lung inflammation and represent a tool to evaluate heart alteration [122], and some mechanical pressure changes in the chest provoked diaphragmatic spasms with a closed glottis (during the struggling phase of breath-holding), leading to lung alveolo-vascular stress [123]. Paganini et al. [101] investigated ULC during a BH dive at increasing depths, observing the onset of lung comets in some subjects; this may have been due to an altered recovery from atelectasis [103] that seemed to have been caused by the alternating closing and opening of bronchioles and alveoli during the dives [102]. As reported by Tojo et al. [124], atelectasis may lead to alveolar hypoxia-induced inflammation, releasing NF-κB-dependent CXCL-1 from epithelial cells and activating HIF-1α toward alveolar hypoxia [124].

Interestingly, cetaceans exhibit physiological adaptations that allow the transition to aquatic life, including a robust antioxidant defense system that prevents injury from repeated exposure to ischemia–reperfusion events associated with BH diving. x. Heme oxygenase (HO) activity increased in dolphin cells but not human cells. On the contrary, TNF-α expression increased in human cells but not in dolphin cells [125].

HO is a cytoprotective protein with anti-inflammatory properties, catalyzing the first step in the oxidative degradation of heme. Various stimuli, including hypoxia, oxidant stress, and inflammatory cytokines, regulate the inducible HO-1 isoform.

Some authors investigated microparticle (MP) release after a BH-diving training protocol, observing that the alterations in endothelial reactivity were coupled to increased levels of Endothelial MPs (EMPs) (CD31+/41−), markers of endothelial apoptosis [126,127]. Intermittent hypoxia could increase cellular stress [61]. An increase in CD31+/annexin+EMP level was observed in some volunteers exposed to normobaric hypoxia in a chamber with oxygen saturation (SaO_2) reduced to 73% $\pm$ 10% [3]. A similar increase in CD144 EMPs was found in some BH divers who performed single maximal dry BH (SaO_2 of 72% $\pm$ 12%). Both experiments were conducted in dry conditions but showed that short-term hypoxic situations could trigger endothelial cell stress. Nevertheless, diving stress in BH diving is only partly related to hypoxia [127].

In Figure 2A, we illustrate up–down regulation biomarkers in breath-hold diving.

3.2. Self-Contained Underwater Breathing Apparatus (SCUBA) and Closed-Circuit Rebreather (CCR) Diving

One of the most commonly known activities that leads to hyperoxia is SCUBA diving. SCUBA diving exposes the human body to environmental stress represented by increased pO_2, physical effort, and elevated breathing resistance, which alter the endothelial function [128–130]. SCUBA diving-related physical activity can induce oxidative and cardiovascular stress, amplified by environmental conditions, including hyperoxia, hyperbaric pressure, and cold water [131,132].

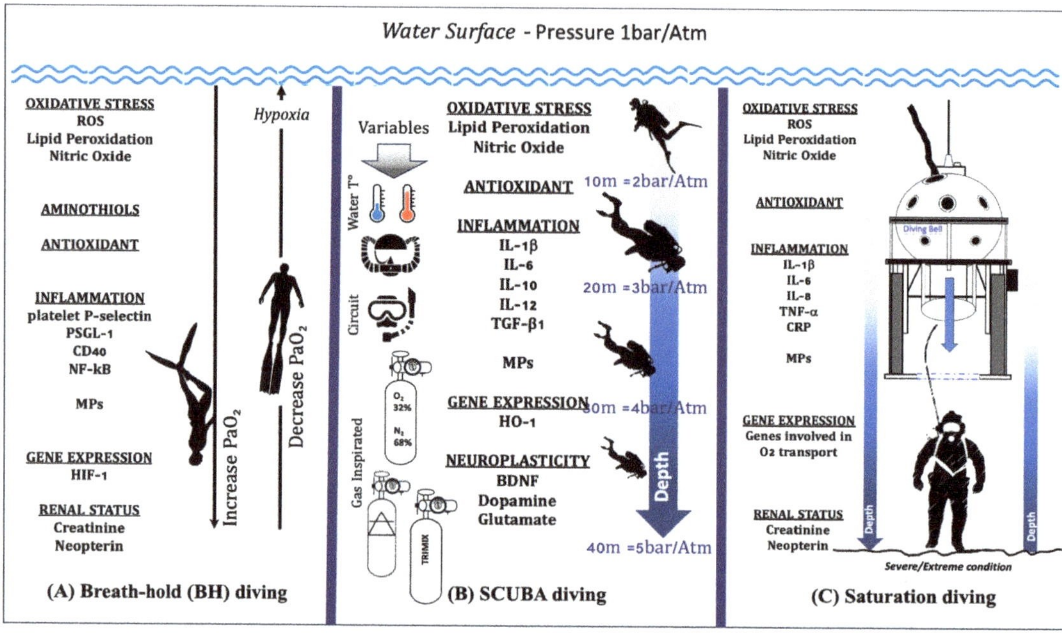

Figure 2. Illustration of up–down regulation biomarkers in different human underwater activities: (**A**) Breath-hold diving. The physiological changes in PaO_2 during the descent and ascent of a deep breath-hold dive are one of the causes of biological changes at a systemic and molecular level. (**B**) SCUBA diving. The response in SCUBA diving varies depending on number of dives carried out, depth, water temperature, type of breathing circuit (open vs. CCR), gases inspired, and exercise. (**C**) Saturation diving. In the sketch, the saturation worksite is shown. The working depth corresponds to the maximum depth reached by the divers, where the "scenario" is considered a severe/extreme condition. All these activities involve changes in levels of Oxy-Inflammation, redox states (aminothiols), gene expression, antioxidants, markers of neuroplasticity, and renal status.

The mechanisms that lead to endothelial dysfunction in SCUBA diving may result from increased hyperoxia-induced oxidative stress and peripheral vasoconstriction [129]. The hyperoxia associated with SCUBA diving results in ROS production, which activates the antioxidant defenses, leading to an increased expression of several antioxidant enzymes, such as catalase (CAT) [133], glutathione peroxidase (GPx) [134], and superoxide dismutase (SOD) [135]. As CAT activity rises in lymphocytes within a few hours after the dive, while GPx activity rises after surfacing, ROS production stimulates lymphocyte mobilization because GPx is one of the first antioxidants activated to detoxify ROS [134]. SOD activity increases to protect against $ONOO^-$ and to preserve NO generation [135]. Due to the mobilization of endogenous antioxidant systems, the total antioxidant capacity increases after surfacing to help control vascular oxidative stress, activating a signaling cascade that stimulates resistance against diving-related oxidative stress [136].

Oxidative stress may also impair cognitive functions during a dive due to brain-derived neurotrophic factor (BDNF) loss, followed by a decrease in dopamine and glutamate, especially during decompression [137]. This BDNF deficit seems to alter excitatory/inhibitory neurotransmission, including GABA receptors [138], whose interaction with N_2 has been proposed as a mechanism of nitrogen narcosis [137–143].

Pressure changes during a dive or decompression significantly influence the hematocrit component level, including leukocytes and platelets [144,145]. Some authors observed that SCUBA diving did not affect the number of lymphocytes but their functions were affected, while no changes in H_2O_2 production in lymphocytes and GPx were found. Additionally, CAT activities increased [135]. On the other hand, Morabito et al. [146] showed significantly decreased levels of H_2O_2 in lymphocytes, probably due to increased CAT activity and endogenous antioxidant enzymes.

Dumić et al. [147] reported that regular recreational SCUBA diving promotes an anti-inflammatory status, thus contributing to cardioprotection and conferring multiple health benefits. Divers who performed five dives, one per week, at a depth of 20–30 m that lasted 30 min, manifested IgG and TPP N-glycosylation alterations toward anti-inflammatory status over the whole study period with an increase in monogalyctosylated and core-fucosylated IgG N-glycans and a decrease in galactosylated TPP N-glycans. On the other hand, military combat swimmers (O_2 divers) are regularly exposed to hyperbaric hyperoxia in addition to intensive endurance training intervals and, therefore, are exposed to extreme levels of oxidative stress. Compared to controls, they exhibited a proinflammatory immune status exemplified by an elevated number of CD4+CD25+ T cells, the elevated expression of proinflammatory cytokine IL-12, and the diminished expression of anti-inflammatory TGF-β1 [148]. Supported by decreased basal gene expression and the prolonged upregulation of anti-oxidative HO-1, these data suggest that higher oxidative stress levels, as those present under intermitted hyperbaric hyperoxia conditions, e.g., through oxygen diving, promote a higher inflammatory immune status.

Breathing air in hyperbaric condition leads to the formation of venous gas emboli (VGE) that interact with the endothelium [149], leading to platelet aggregation to the bubble surface [150] and resulting in the formation of microthrombi in lung vessels after decompression in the DCS model [151,152].

In addition to a mechanical explanation for DCS, an inflammatory mechanism has been suggested [153]. In an observational study carried out on a similarly well-matched control group consisting of equally fit non-divers with identical physical training and living conditions before and after a 2-month period of daily diving, no changes in IL-6 and IL-1 receptor antagonist (IL-1ra), but an increase in IL-8 and neutrophil gelatinase-associated lipocalin (NGAL), together with a decrease in secretory leukocyte protease inhibitor (SLPI), were found [154]. The findings suggest inflammatory activation that is not severe because no changes in IL-6 or IL-1ra were found. The increase in NGAL and IL-8 levels was interpreted as a sign of leukocyte activation. The decreased SLPI levels suggest an influence on the inflammatory defense mechanism. Therefore, the compensated activation of the inflammatory defense mechanism without the loss of homeostasis of the inflammatory system was shown. The formation of bubbles during decompression may trigger this inflammatory response. It is also probable that the interplay between pro- and anti-inflammatory substances is a fine-tuned balancing act and that it is only when this balance collapses that morbidity ensues.

Different types of breathing gas are used in SCUBA diving: air and non-air mixtures [155]. The latter contains mainly oxygen, nitrogen, and helium that form nitrox (nitrogen + oxygen), heliox (helium + oxygen), and trimix (oxygen, helium, and nitrogen) with different advantages and features [9,155]. Nitrox is mainly used for shallow recreational dives, heliox for deep diving, and trimix for deep but short dives to avoid neurological side effects. The use of trimix in SCUBA diving has recently become more widespread to reduce nitrogen narcosis compared to air diving [140–142].

Some experimental studies, although conflicting, invoked a possible anti-inflammatory role of helium [156]. This gas could increase NO, induce nuclear factor erythroid 2-related factor 2 activation, and cause consequent reductions in systemic inflammation and oxidative stress. Recently, increases in extracellular vesicles and inflammatory status (IL-1) were found in CCR SCUBA divers, highlighting a decrease in plasma gelsolin (pGSN) [157]. It has been demonstrated that pGSN modulates the production of IL-1β-containing microparticles following high-pressure exposure and decompression [158].

Another study [159] found no difference in most of the inflammatory factors (including monocyte chemoattractant protein 1) measured between the trimix and air groups, casting doubt on the protective effect of helium. Following the dive, IL-6 values slightly increased, while IL-8 and epithelial growth factor (EGF) decreased in both groups without significant variation.

To reduce bubble formation and platelet activation, some authors proposed a hyperbaric pretreatment with O_2 before the dive, observing a significant decrease in decompression-induced bubbles [160,161] and the activation of antioxidant enzymes such as CAT and SOD [162]. The increased O_2 diffuses in micronuclei in substitution of N_2, which is eliminated through the lungs and then absorbed, reducing micronuclei formation [163]. Furthermore, the reduction in pN_2 and breathing enriched air nitrox (EAN) can reduce platelet activation [164], as well as breathing normobaric O_2 before a dive [115]. On the other hand, exposure to EAN mixtures and diving-related physical activity can raise ROS generation [129]; oxidative stress biomarkers including 8-isoprostane and 8-deoxyguanosine; and inflammatory markers such as IL-1β, IL-6, and TNFα [165].

Bosco et al. [165] observed oxidative stress markers' increase after a dive using close-circuit rebreather (CCR) apparatus, probably originating from increased fiO_2, amplified by additional variables such as physical exercise [166] and breathing resistance [167]. On the other hand, mild exercise during a dive may be enough to allow VGE transit, suggesting a potential benefit of exercise before a dive [168].

No association between the decompression model chosen for a 50 msw dive and the likelihood of DCS was established [169]. The dive profiles induced only minor changes in inflammatory markers. The significant increase in IL-6 and decreased IL-8 and EGF levels observed in groups following the ratio decompression strategy (RDS) or compartmental decompression models (CDMs) were within the normal range and were consistent with exercise-induced changes. However, compared to CDM, the RDS-controlled model has the disadvantage of the increased secretion of chemokines in developing vascular damage. This increased secretion of proinflammatory chemokines seems related to the decompression system rather than the more prolonged exposure to high partial pressures of oxygen that RDS divers undergo.

A short-term ketogenic diet has been observed to be effective in weight loss, decreasing inflammation, and protecting against lipid peroxidation during a dive [165].

In Figure 2B, we illustrate up–down regulation biomarkers in SCUBA diving.

3.3. Saturation Diving

A particular case of diving activity is "saturation diving", which describes a diving method that enables the diver to stay under pressure for a long time (several hours or even days), practiced by military forces and commercial divers. Saturation diving is an established way to conduct subsea operations with human intervention. Saturation divers are exposed to severe/extreme environmental conditions, exposing themselves to higher risks and accidents [170–175].

Saturation diving involves divers staying under pressure until their tissues are saturated with breathing gas, exposing them to increased oxygen pressure, potential toxic gases, and the risk of bubble formation during decompression. Prolonged exposure to hyperoxia can generate ROS, damaging cell structures like lipids, proteins, and nucleic acids. All these factors, coupled with vascular gas bubble formation, may lead to endothelial dysfunction. The diver's antioxidant status, influenced by diet and genetics, plays a crucial role in protecting against injuries caused by these conditions [174].

While working, divers must acclimatize to hyperbaric environments [175–177]. In saturation diving, hyperoxia, partial gas pressure changes, and inert gas exchange during decompression are likely sources of excess ROS [178]. Mrakic-Sposta et al. [178] found an increase in oxidative stress-related biomarkers, including 8-deoxyguanosine, 3-nitrotyrosine, and neopterin, due to prolonged exposure to higher pO_2 value. Furthermore, saturation divers showed elevated concentrations of IL-6, the first cytokine released into the circulation during inflammation response [10,178–182], and creatinine in the post-dive stage, reflecting the systemic effects induced by hyperoxia, hyperbaric pressure, and exercise at depth [150].

Moreover, Krog et al. [183] demonstrated the increase in Natural Killer (NK) cell cytotoxicity during the compression phase accompanied by alterations in the cytotoxic NK cell subsets (CD32CD16brightCD56dim) in saturation divers' peripheral blood, with a reduction in glutathione levels [184,185].

Previous studies have concluded that high oxidative stress in divers may be reversed through antioxidant vitamin supplementation [186,187]. In an earlier experiment, the supplementation of vitamin C, α-tocopherol (vitamin E), and tea catechins given to divers during a 400 msw deep saturation dive every day for 40 days prevented hepatic disturbances [188]. A more recent publication demonstrated that divers' endogenous antioxidant mechanisms counteracted the effects of hyperbaric hyperoxia after 200 msw saturation diving [184]. Sparse data showing the impact of antioxidant vitamins on vascular function in diving are available; however, Deb et al.'s [189] review on antioxidant effects in saturation diving subjects indicates that care is warranted when choosing whether and how to give antioxidant supplements [190].

The iron reserve can also be a valid aid in saturation diving. Data provided by Zwart et al. [179] showed that elevated body iron stores in a hyperoxic environment trigger a DNA damage repair response in peripheral blood mononuclear cells, excluding double-stranded DNA damage. Furthermore, folate levels decrease rapidly in this setting, suggesting higher folate requirements may be necessary when both body iron stores and DNA damage repair responses are elevated. This observation indicates potential interplay between iron status, O_2 levels, and folate in cellular responses.

Acclimatization to professional saturation diving was associated with post-saturation gene expression changes to elevated O_2 partial pressure by the extensive downregulation of factors involved in O_2 transport, including heme, hemoglobin, and erythrocytes. Primary endogenous antioxidants, such as SOD-1, CAT, and glutathione synthetase, were upregulated, and there was increased expression of genes involved in immune activity and inflammatory signaling pathways [186].

The observation that a hyperbaric and hyperoxic environment in saturation diving induces proinflammatory responses that help the body adapt to the inherent oxidative stress in maintaining homeostasis was confirmed recently by Monnoyer et al. [191]. They reported elevated salivary levels of CRP, IL-1β, IL-8, SIgA, and TNF-α during the bottom phase of the hyperbaric saturation, whereas IL-6, cortisol, and alpha-amylase were unchanged. All changes observed during saturation were abolished at the end of decompression. Figure 2C illustrates up–down regulation biomarkers in saturation diving.

4. Conclusions

Several studies encompassed the possibility of mitigating some diving-related impairments; in fact, underwater activities induce oxidative stress and inflammatory-related parameter changes depending on O_2 availability. While in SCUBA diving, these changes are related only to hyperoxia onset, in BH diving, they are a consequence of hyperoxia/hypoxia alternation. As described, the presence of ROS, RNS, and inflammation can result in organ dysfunction (e.g., endothelium, lung, kidney, brain) with complex interplay activity [192–196]. In the recreational field, several preconditioning methods have been considered which have challenged previously accepted ideas [197–200]. One direction was chosen to mitigate diving-related risks: one aiming to endothelial dysfunction, although conduit arteries and microcirculation seem not to behave in parallel [201,202], and supplementation with antioxidant agents before diving [203–207].

Future research should compare and correlate different environmental conditions (e.g., hot/cold water, sea/lake/swimming pool) in different underwater activity scenarios from BH to SCUBA diving. Furthermore, it should also consider the dose-dependent effects of the gas/mixture alongside dive time and depth, associated with decompression times and with the effects of changes in oxygen concentrations. To date, the risk/benefit ratio has not yet been clearly defined.

Author Contributions: Conceptualization, A.V., S.M.-S. and G.B.; methodology, A.V., S.M.-S. and G.B.; writing—original draft preparation, A.V. and A.B.; writing—review and editing, S.M.-S., C.B., E.M.C. and G.B.; visualization, A.B., S.M.-S., C.B., E.M.C. and G.B.; supervision, S.M.-S. and G.B. All authors have read and agreed to the published version of the manuscript.

Funding: This work was primarily supported by the Office of Naval Resource (ONR) Undersea Medicine Program (N00014-23-1-2757).

Institutional Review Board Statement: Not applicable.

Informed Consent Statement: Not applicable.

Data Availability Statement: Not applicable.

Conflicts of Interest: The authors declare no conflicts of interest.

Abbreviations

AA	Amino acid
ABG	Arterial blood gas
BH	Breath-hold diving
CAT	Catalase
CCR	Closed-Circuit Rebreather
CDM	Compartmental decompression model
CRP	Protein C-reactive
DCS	Decompression sickness
EGF	Epithelial growth factor
HIF	Hypoxia-inducible factor
IL-	Interleukin
IRI	Ischemia–reperfusion
NO	Nitric oxide
NK	Natural Killer
O_2	Oxygen
O_2^{2-}	Superoxide anion
ONOO	Peroxinitrite
OxS	Oxidative stress
$PaCO_2$	Arterial partial CO_2 pressure
pO_2	Partial O_2 pressure
pGSN	Plasma gelsolin
RDS	Ratio decompression strategy
ROS	Reactive oxygen species
RNS	Reactive nitrogen species
SCUBA	Self-Contained Underwater Breathing Apparatus
SOD	Superoxide dismutase
TAC	Total Antioxidant Capacity
8-OH-dG	8-OH-2-deoxyguanosine
8-iso-PGF2α	8-isoprostane

References

1. Wilmshurst, P. ABC of Oxygen. Diving and Oxygen. *BMJ* **1998**, *317*, 996–999. [CrossRef]
2. Lee, Y.I.; Ye, B.J. Underwater and Hyperbaric Medicine as a Branch of Occupational and Environmental Medicine. *Ann. Occup. Environ. Med.* **2013**, *25*, 39. [CrossRef]
3. Balestra, C.; Mrakic-Sposta, S.; Virgili, F. Oxygen Variations—Insights into Hypoxia, Hyperoxia and Hyperbaric Hyperoxia—Is the Dose the Clue? *Int. J. Mol. Sci.* **2023**, *24*, 13472. [CrossRef]
4. Kramer, M.R.; Godfrey, S. Dead Sea: Natural oxygen enrichment at low altitude. *Isr. J. Med. Sci.* **1996**, *32*, S20–S23.

5. Gouin, E.; Balestra, C.; Orsat, J.; Dugrenot, E.; L'Her, E. Pulmonary Effects of One Week of Repeated Recreational Closed-Circuit Rebreather Dives in Cold Water. *Medicina* **2023**, *59*, 81. [CrossRef] [PubMed]
6. Walker, J.R., III; Murphy-Lavoie, H.M. Diving Rebreathers. In *StatPearls [Internet]*; StatPearls Publishing: Treasure Island, FL, USA, 2024; Bookshelf ID: NBK430743.
7. Balestra, C.; Guerrero, F.; Theunissen, S.; Germonpre, P.; Lafere, P. Physiology of repeated mixed gas 100-m wreck dives using a closed-circuit rebreather: A field bubble study. *Eur. J. Appl. Physiol.* **2022**, *122*, 515–522. [CrossRef] [PubMed]
8. Tsur, N.; Bar, R.; Hilly, O.; Handzel, O. Balloon Eustachian tuboplasty in a professional Navy SEAL diver: Case report. *Undersea Hyperb. Med.* **2020**, *47*, 467–470. [CrossRef] [PubMed]
9. Mitchell, S.J.; Doolette, D.J. Recreational technical diving part 1: An introduction to technical diving methods and activities. *Diving Hyperb. Med.* **2013**, *43*, 86–93. [PubMed]
10. Imbert, J.P.; Egi, S.M.; Balestra, C. Vascular Function Recovery Following Saturation Diving. *Medicina* **2022**, *58*, 1476. [CrossRef] [PubMed]
11. Eisenberg, R.; Gray, H.B. Preface on making Oxygen. *Inorg. Chem.* **2008**, *47*, 1697–1699. [CrossRef] [PubMed]
12. Kamata, H.; Hirata, H. Redox regulation of cellular signaling. *Cell. Signal.* **1999**, *11*, 1–14. [CrossRef]
13. Rimessi, A.; Previati, M.; Nigro, F.; Wieckowski, M.R.; Pinton, P. Mitochondrial reactive oxygen species and inflammation: Molecular mechanisms, diseases and promising therapies. *Int. J. Biochem. Cell Biol.* **2016**, *81*, 281–293. [CrossRef]
14. Bergendi, L.; Benes, L.; Durackova, Z.; Ferencik, M. Chemistry, physiology and pathology of free radicals. *Life Sci.* **1999**, *65*, 1865–1874. [CrossRef]
15. Caliri, A.W.; Tommasi, S.; Besaratinia, A. Relationships among smoking, oxidative stress, inflammation, macromolecular damage, and cancer. *Mutat. Res. Rev. Mutat. Res.* **2021**, *787*, 108365. [CrossRef]
16. Ursini, F.; Maiorino, M.; Forman, H.J. Redox homeostasis: The Golden Mean of healthy living. *Redox Biol.* **2016**, *8*, 205–215. [CrossRef]
17. Ryter, S.W.; Nakahira, K.; Haspel, J.A.; Choi, A.M. Autophagy in pulmonary diseases. *Annu. Rev. Physiol.* **2012**, *74*, 377–401. [CrossRef] [PubMed]
18. Sunil, V.R.; Shen, J.; Patel-Vayas, K.; Gow, A.J.; Laskin, J.D.; Laskin, D.L. Role of reactive nitrogen species generated via inducible nitric oxide synthase in vesicant-induced lung injury, inflammation and altered lung functioning. *Toxicol. Appl. Pharmacol.* **2012**, *261*, 22–30. [CrossRef] [PubMed]
19. Liu, Z.; Ren, Z.; Zhang, J.; Chuang, C.-C.; Kandaswamy, E.; Zhou, T.; Zou, L. Role of ROS and Nutritional Antioxidants in Human Diseases. *Front. Physiol.* **2018**, *9*, 477. [CrossRef] [PubMed]
20. Debevec, T.; Millet, G.P.; Pialoux, V. Hypoxia-Induced Oxidative Stress Modulation with Physical Activity. *Front. Physiol.* **2017**, *8*, 84. [CrossRef] [PubMed]
21. McGarry, T.; Biniecka, M.; Veale, D.J.; Fearon, U. Hypoxia, oxidative stress and inflammation. *Free Radic. Biol. Med.* **2018**, *125*, 15–24. [CrossRef] [PubMed]
22. Cooper, J.S.; Phuyal, P.; Shah, N. Oxygen Toxicity. In *StatPearls [Internet]*; StatPearls Publishing: Treasure Island, FL, USA, 2024.
23. Smit, B.; Smulders, Y.M.; van der Wouden, J.C.; Straaten, H.M.O.-V.; Man, A.M.E.S.-D. Hemodynamic effects of acute hyperoxia: Systematic review and meta-analysis. *Crit. Care* **2018**, *22*, 45. [CrossRef]
24. Hackett, P.H.; Roach, R.C. High-altitude illness. *N. Engl. J. Med.* **2001**, *345*, 107–114. [CrossRef]
25. Hartmann, G.; Tschop, M.; Fischer, R.; Bidlingmaier, C.; Riepl, R.; Tschop, K.; Hautmann, H.; Endres, S.; Toepfer, M. High altitude increases circulating interleukin-6, interleukin-1 receptor antagonist and C-reactive protein. *Cytokine* **2000**, *12*, 246–252. [CrossRef] [PubMed]
26. Semenza, G.L.; Nejfelt, M.K.; Chi, S.M.; Antonarakis, S.E. Hypoxia-inducible nuclear factors bind to an enhancer ele-ment located 3′ to the human erythropoietin gene. *Proc. Natl. Acad. Sci. USA* **1991**, *88*, 5680–5684. [CrossRef]
27. Salvagno, M.; Coppalini, G.; Taccone, F.S.; Strapazzon, G.; Mrakic-Sposta, S.; Rocco, M.; Khalife, M.; Balestra, C. The Normobaric Oxygen Paradox-Hyperoxic Hypoxic Paradox: A Novel Expedient Strategy in Hematopoiesis Clinical Issues. *Int. J. Mol. Sci.* **2022**, *24*, 82. [CrossRef]
28. Kiboub, F.Z.; Balestra, C.; Loennechen, O.; Eftedal, I. Hemoglobin and Erythropoietin After Commercial Saturation Diving. *Front. Physiol.* **2018**, *9*, 1176. [CrossRef]
29. Koch, A.; Kähler, W.; Klapa, S.; Grams, B.; van Ooij, P.J.A.M. The conundrum of using hyperoxia in COVID-19 treatment strategies: May intermittent therapeutic hyperoxia play a helpful role in the expression of the surface receptors ACE2 and Furin in lung tissue via triggering of HIF-1α? *Intensiv. Care Med. Exp.* **2020**, *8*, 1–6. [CrossRef] [PubMed]
30. Semenza, G.L. Oxygen sensing, homeostasis, and disease. *N. Engl. J. Med.* **2011**, *365*, 537–547. [CrossRef]
31. Fong, G.H.; Takeda, K. Role and regulation of prolyl hydroxylase domain proteins. *Cell Death Differ.* **2008**, *15*, 635–641. [CrossRef] [PubMed]
32. Naugler, W.E.; Karin, M. NF-kappaB, and cancer-identifying targets and mechanisms. *Curr. Opin. Genet. Dev.* **2008**, *18*, 19–26. [CrossRef]
33. Taylor, C.T. Interdependent roles for Hypoxia-inducible factor and nuclear factor-kappaB in hypoxic inflammation. *J. Physiol.* **2008**, *586*, 4055–4059. [CrossRef] [PubMed]

34. Leveque, C.; Mrakic Sposta, S.; Theunissen, S.; Germonpré, P.; Lambrechts, K.; Vezzoli, A.; Gussoni, M.; Levenez, M.; Lafère, P.; Guerrero, F.; et al. Oxidative Stress Response Kinetics after 60 Minutes at Different Levels (10% or 15%) of Normobaric Hypoxia Exposure. *Int. J. Mol. Sci.* **2023**, *24*, 10188. [CrossRef]
35. Cummins, E.P.; Berra, E.; Comerford, K.M.; Ginouves, A.; Fitzgerald, K.T.; Seeballuck, F.; Godson, C.; Nielsen, J.E.; Moynagh, P.; Pouyssegur, J.; et al. Prolyl hydroxylase-1 negatively regulates IkappaB kinase-beta, giving in-sight into hypoxia-induced NFkappaB activity. *Proc. Natl. Acad. Sci. USA* **2006**, *103*, 18154–18159. [CrossRef] [PubMed]
36. Rius, J.; Guma, M.; Schachtrup, C.; Akassoglou, K.; Zinkernagel, A.S.; Nizet, V.; Johnson, R.S.; Haddad, G.G.; Karin, M. NF-kappaB links innate immunity to the hypoxic response through transcriptional regulation of HIF-1alpha. *Nature* **2008**, *453*, 807–811. [CrossRef] [PubMed]
37. McDonald, P.P.; Bald, A.; Cassatella, M.A. Activation of the NF-κB Pathway by Inflammatory Stimuli in Human Neutrophils. *Blood* **1997**, *89*, 3421–3433. [CrossRef]
38. Ben-Shoshan, J.; Afek, A.; Maysel-Auslender, S.; Barzelay, A.; Rubinstein, A.; Keren, G.; George, J. HIF-1alpha overex-pression and experimental murine atherosclerosis. *Arterioscler. Thromb. Vasc. Biol.* **2009**, *29*, 665–670. [CrossRef]
39. Alonso, D.; Serrano, E.; Bermejo, F.J.; Corral, R.S. HIF-1alpha-regulated MIF activation and Nox2-dependent ROS generation promote Leishmania amazonensis killing by macrophages under Hypoxia. *Cell Immunol.* **2019**, *335*, 15–21. [CrossRef]
40. Damiani, E.; Donati, A.; Girardis, M. Oxygen in the critically ill: Friend or foe? *Curr. Opin. Anaesthesiol.* **2018**, *31*, 129–135. [CrossRef]
41. Jamieson, D.; Chance, B.; Cadenas, E.; Boveris, A. The relation of free radical production to hyperoxia. *Annu. Rev. Physiol.* **1986**, *48*, 703–719. [CrossRef]
42. Jackson, R.M. Pulmonary oxygen toxicity. *Chest* **1985**, *88*, 900–905. [CrossRef]
43. Bhandari, V. Molecular mechanisms of hyperoxia-induced acute lung injury. *Front. Biosci.* **2008**, *13*, 6653–6661. [CrossRef]
44. Li, L.F.; Yang, C.T.; Huang, C.C.; Liu, Y.Y.; Kao, K.C.; Lin, H.C. Low-molecular-weight heparin reduces hyperoxia-augmented ventilator-induced lung injury via serine/threonine kinase-protein kinase B. *Respir. Res.* **2011**, *12*, 90. [CrossRef] [PubMed]
45. Qadan, M.; Battista, C.; Gardner, S.A.; Anderson, G.; Akca, O.; Polk, H.C., Jr. Oxygen and surgical site infection: A study of underlying immunologic mechanisms. *Anesthesiology* **2010**, *113*, 369–377. [CrossRef]
46. McInturff, A.M.; Cody, M.J.; Elliott, E.A.; Glenn, J.W.; Rowley, J.W.; Rondina, M.T.; Yost, C.C. Mammalian target of rapamycin regulates neutrophil extracellular trap formation via induction of hypoxia-inducible factor 1 alpha. *Blood* **2012**, *120*, 3118–3125. [CrossRef] [PubMed]
47. O'Reilly, P.J.; Hickman-Davis, J.M.; Davis, I.C.; Matalon, S. Hyperoxia impairs antibacterial function of macrophages through effects on actin. *Am. J. Respir. Cell Mol. Biol.* **2003**, *28*, 443–450. [CrossRef] [PubMed]
48. Hou, L.; Xie, K.; Li, N.; Qin, M.; Lu, Y.; Ma, S.; Ji, G.; Xiong, L. 100% oxygen inhalation protects against zymosan-induced sterile sepsis in mice: The roles of inflammatory cytokines and antioxidant enzymes. *Shock* **2009**, *32*, 451–461. [CrossRef] [PubMed]
49. Zhang, Z.; Bai, X.; Du, K.; Huang, Y.; Wang, W.; Zhao, Y.; Pei, Y.; Mu, J.; Han, H.; Hu, S.; et al. Activation of the cholinergic anti-inflammatory pathway contributes to the protective effects of 100% oxygen inhalation on zymosan-induced generalized inflammation in mice. *J. Surg. Res.* **2012**, *174*, e75–e83. [CrossRef] [PubMed]
50. Sureda, A.; Ferrer, M.D.; Batle, J.M.; Tauler, P.; Tur, J.A.; Pons, A. Scuba diving increases erythrocyte and plasma antioxidant defenses and spares NO without oxidative damage. *Med. Sci. Sport. Exerc.* **2009**, *41*, 1271–1276. [CrossRef]
51. Forstermann, U. Nitric oxide and oxidative stress in vascular disease. *Pflug. Arch.* **2010**, *459*, 923–939. [CrossRef]
52. Landmesser, U.; Dikalov, S.; Price, S.R.; McCann, L.; Fukai, T.; Holland, S.M.; Mitch, W.E.; Harrison, D.G. Oxidation of tetrahydrobiopterin leads to uncoupling of endothelial cell nitric oxide synthase in hypertension. *J. Clin. Investig.* **2003**, *111*, 1201–1209. [CrossRef]
53. Solich-Talanda, M.; Żebrowska, A.; Mikołajczyk, R.; Kostorz-Nosal, S.; Ziora, D.; Jastrzębski, D.; Siermontowski, P. Effect of Apnea-Induced Hypoxia on Cardiovascular Adaptation and Circulating Biomarkers of Oxidative Stress in Elite Breath-Hold Divers. *Front. Physiol.* **2021**, *12*, 726434. [CrossRef]
54. Theunissen, S.; Guerrero, F.; Sponsiello, N.; Cialoni, D.; Pieri, M.; Germonpre, P.; Obeid, G.; Tillmans, F.; Papadopoulou, V.; Hemelryck, W.; et al. Nitric oxide-related endothelial changes in breath-hold and scuba divers. *Undersea Hyperb. Med.* **2013**, *40*, 135–144.
55. Arya, A.K.; Balestra, C.; Bhopale, V.M.; Tuominen, L.J.; Raisanen-Sokolowski, A.; Dugrenot, E.; L'Her, E.; Bhat, A.R.; Thom, S.R. Elevations of Extracellular Vesicles and Inflammatory Biomarkers in Closed Circuit SCUBA Divers. *Int. J. Mol. Sci.* **2023**, *24*, 5969. [CrossRef]
56. Sharma, R.I.; Marcinkowska, A.B.; Mankowska, N.D.; Waśkow, M.; Kot, J.; Winklewski, P.J. Cognitive Functions in Scuba, Technical and Saturation Diving. *Biology* **2023**, *12*, 229. [CrossRef]
57. Nossum, V.; Hjelde, A.; Brubakk, A.O. Small amounts of venous gas embolism cause delayed impairment of endothelial function and increase polymorphonuclear neutrophil infiltration. *Eur. J. Appl. Physiol.* **2002**, *86*, 209–214. [CrossRef]
58. Klinger, A.L.; Pichette, B.; Sobolewski, P.; Eckmann, D.M. Mechanotransductional basis of endothelial cell response to intravascular bubbles. *Integr. Biol.* **2011**, *3*, 1033–1042. [CrossRef]
59. Pontier, J.M.; Gempp, E.; Ignatescu, M. Blood platelet-derived microparticles release and bubble formation after an open-sea air dive. *Appl. Physiol. Nutr. Metab.* **2012**, *37*, 888–892. [CrossRef]

60. Brett, K.D.; Nugent, N.Z.; Fraser, N.K.; Bhopale, V.M.; Yang, M.; Thom, S.R. Microparticle and interleukin-1β production with human simulated compressed air diving. *Sci. Rep.* **2019**, *9*, 13320. [CrossRef] [PubMed]
61. Barak, O.F.; Janjic, N.; Drvis, I.; Mijacika, T.; Mudnic, I.; Coombs, G.B.; Thom, S.R.; Madic, D.; Dujic, Z. Vascular dysfunction following breath-hold diving. *Can. J. Physiol. Pharmacol.* **2020**, *98*, 124–130. [CrossRef] [PubMed]
62. Magalhaes, J.; Ascensao, A.; Viscor, G.; Soares, J.; Oliveira, J.; Marques, F.; Duarte, J. Oxidative stress in humans during and after 4 hours of hypoxia at a simulated altitude of 5500 m. *Aviat. Space Environ. Med.* **2004**, *75*, 16–22. [PubMed]
63. Irarrázaval, S.; Allard, C.; Campodónico, J.; Pérez, D.; Strobel, P.; Vásquez, L.; Urquiaga, I.; Echeverría, G.; Leighton, F. Oxidative Stress in Acute Hypobaric Hypoxia. *High Alt. Med. Biol.* **2017**, *18*, 128–134. [CrossRef] [PubMed]
64. Mrakic-Sposta, S.; Gussoni, M.; Dellanoce, C.; Marzorati, M.; Montorsi, M.; Rasica, L.; Pratali, L.; D'Angelo, G.; Martinelli, M.; Bastiani, L.; et al. Effects of acute and sub-acute hypobaric hypoxia on oxidative stress: A field study in the Alps. *Eur. J. Appl. Physiol.* **2021**, *121*, 297–306. [CrossRef] [PubMed]
65. Li, X.; Zhang, J.; Liu, G.; Wu, G.; Wang, R.; Zhang, J. High altitude hypoxia and oxidative stress: The new hope brought by free radical scavengers. *Life Sci.* **2023**, *336*, 122319. [CrossRef] [PubMed]
66. Burtscher, J.; Mallet, R.T.; Pialoux, V.; Millet, G.P.; Burtscher, M. Adaptive Responses to Hypoxia and/or Hyperoxia in Humans. *Antioxid. Redox Signal.* **2022**, *37*, 887–912. [CrossRef] [PubMed]
67. Mrakic Sposta, S.; Montorsi, M.; Porcelli, S.; Marzorati, M.; Healey, B.; Dellanoce, C.; Vezzoli, A. Effects of Prolonged Exposure to Hypobaric Hypoxia on Oxidative Stress: Overwintering in Antarctic Concordia Station. *Oxid. Med. Cell Longev.* **2022**, *2022*, 4430032. [CrossRef]
68. Rathor, R.; Suryakumar, G.; Singh, S.N. Diet and redox state in maintaining skeletal muscle health and performance at high altitude. *Free. Radic. Biol. Med.* **2021**, *174*, 305–320. [CrossRef]
69. Verratti, V.; Bondi, D.; Jandova, T.; Camporesi, E.; Paoli, A.; Bosco, G. Sex Hormones Response to Physical Hyperoxic and Hyperbaric Stress in Male Scuba Divers: A Pilot Study. *Adv. Exp. Med. Biol.* **2019**, *1176*, 53–62. [CrossRef]
70. Balestra, C.; Lambrechts, K.; Mrakic-Sposta, S.; Vezzoli, A.; Levenez, M.; Germonpré, P.; Virgili, F.; Bosco, G.; Lafère, P. Hypoxic and Hyperoxic Breathing as a Complement to Low-Intensity Physical Exercise Programs: A Proof-of-Principle Study. *Int. J. Mol. Sci.* **2021**, *22*, 9600. [CrossRef]
71. Leveque, C.; Mrakic-Sposta, S.; Theunissen, S.; Germonpr, P.; Lambrechts, K.; Vezzoli, A.; Bosco, G.; Lévenéz, M.; Lafèvre, P.; Guerrero, F.; et al. Oxidative Stress Response Kinetics after 60 Minutes at Different (1.4 ATA and 2.5 ATA) Hyperbaric Hyperoxia Exposures. *Int. J. Mol. Sci.* **2023**, *24*, 12361. [CrossRef] [PubMed]
72. Brugniaux, J.V.; Coombs, G.B.; Barak, O.F.; Dujic, Z.; Sekhon, M.S.; Ainslie, P.N. Highs and lows of hyperoxia: Physiological, performance, and clinical aspects. *Am. J. Physiol. Regul. Integr. Comp. Physiol.* **2018**, *315*, R1–R27. [CrossRef] [PubMed]
73. Modun, D.; Krnic, M.; Vukovic, J.; Kokic, V.; Kukoc-Modun, L.; Tsikas, D.; Dujic, Z. Plasma nitrite concentration decreases after hyperoxia-induced oxidative stress in healthy humans. *Clin. Physiol. Funct. Imaging* **2012**, *32*, 404–408. [CrossRef]
74. Thom, S.R.; Bhopale, V.; Fisher, D.; Manevich, Y.; Huang, P.L.; Buerk, D.G. Stimulation of nitric oxide synthase in cerebral cortex due to elevated partial pressures of oxygen: An oxidative stress response. *J. Neurobiol.* **2002**, *51*, 85–100. [CrossRef]
75. Mrakic-Sposta, S.; Gussoni, M.; Porcelli, S.; Pugliese, L.; Pavei, G.; Bellistri, G.; Montorsi, M.; Tacchini, P.; Vezzoli, A. Training effects on ROS production determined by electron paramagnetic resonance in master swimmers. *Oxid. Med. Cell. Longev.* **2015**, *2015*, 804794. [CrossRef] [PubMed]
76. Thirupathi, A.; Pinho, R.A.; Ugbolue, U.C.; He, Y.; Meng, Y.; Gu, Y. Effect of Running Exercise on Oxidative Stress Biomarkers: A Systematic Review. *Front. Physiol.* **2021**, *11*, 610112. [CrossRef]
77. Brizzolari, A.; Bosco, G.; Vezzoli, A.; Dellanoce, C.; Barassi, A.; Paganini, M.; Cialoni, D.; Mrakic-Sposta, S. Seasonal Oxy-Inflammation and Hydration Status in Non-Elite Freeskiing Racer: A Pilot Study by Non-Invasive Analytic Method. *Int. J. Environ. Res. Public Health* **2023**, *20*, 3157. [CrossRef]
78. Goto, C.; Higashi, Y.; Kimura, M.; Noma, K.; Hara, K.; Nakagawa, K.; Kawamura, M.; Chayama, K.; Yoshizumi, M.; Nara, I. Effect of different intensities of exercise on endothelium-dependent vasodilation in humans: Role of endothelium-dependent nitric oxide and oxidative stress. *Circulation* **2003**, *108*, 530–535. [CrossRef]
79. Vezzoli, A.; Dellanoce, C.; Mrakic-Sposta, S.; Montorsi, M.; Moretti, S.; Tonini, A.; Pratali, L.; Accinni, R. Oxidative Stress Assessment in Response to Ultraendurance Exercise: Thiols Redox Status and ROS Production according to Duration of a Competitive Race. *Oxid. Med. Cell. Longev.* **2016**, *2016*, 6439037. [CrossRef]
80. Granger, D.N.; Kvietysb, P.R. Reperfusion injury, and reactive oxygen species: The evolution of a concept. *Redox Biol.* **2015**, *6*, 524–551. [CrossRef] [PubMed]
81. Chen, G.Y.; Nunez, G. Sterile inflammation: Sensing and reacting to damage. *Nat. Rev. Immunol.* **2010**, *10*, 826–837. [CrossRef]
82. Mills, K.H. TLR-dependent T cell activation in autoimmunity. *Nat. Rev. Immunol.* **2011**, *11*, 807–822. [CrossRef] [PubMed]
83. Kruger, B.; Krick, S.; Dhillon, N.; Lerner, S.M.; Ames, S.; Bromberg, J.S.; Lin, M.; Walsh, L.; Vella, J.; Fischereder, M.; et al. Donor Toll-like receptor 4 contributes to ischemia and reperfusion injury following human kidney transplantation. *Proc. Natl. Acad. Sci. USA* **2009**, *106*, 3390–3395. [CrossRef] [PubMed]
84. Huang, Y.; Yin, H.; Han, J.; Huang, B.; Xu, J.; Zheng, F.; Tan, Z.; Fang, M.; Rui, L.; Chen, D.; et al. Extracellular hmgb1 functions as an innate immune mediator implicated in murine cardiac allograft acute rejection. *Am. J. Transplant.* **2007**, *7*, 799–808. [CrossRef] [PubMed]

85. Moser, B.; Szabolcs, M.J.; Ankersmit, H.J.; Lu, Y.; Qu, W.; Weinberg, A.; Herold, K.C.; Schmidt, A.M. Blockade of RAGE suppresses alloimmune reactions in vitro and delays allograft rejection in murine heart transplantation. *Am. J. Transplant.* **2007**, *7*, 293–302. [CrossRef]
86. Rybnikova, E.A.; Nalivaeva, N.N.; Zenko, M.Y.; Baranova, K.A. Intermittent Hypoxic Training as an Effective Tool for Increasing the Adaptive Potential, Endurance and Working Capacity of the Brain. *Front. Neurosci.* **2022**, *16*, 941740. [CrossRef] [PubMed]
87. Lakka, T.A.; Venalainen, J.M.; Rauramaa, R.; Salonen, R.; Tuomilehto, J.; Salonen, J.T. Relation of leisure-time physical activity and cardiorespiratory fitness to the risk of acute myocardial infarction. *N. Engl. J. Med.* **1994**, *330*, 1549–1554. [CrossRef] [PubMed]
88. Briones, A.M.; Touyz, R.M. Moderate exercise decreases inflammation and oxidative stress in hypertension: But what are the mechanisms? *Hypertension* **2009**, *54*, 1206–1208. [CrossRef] [PubMed]
89. Moller, P.; Loft, S.; Lundby, C.; Olsen, N.V. Acute hypoxia and hypoxic exercise induce DNA strand breaks and oxidative DNA damage in humans. *FASEB J.* **2001**, *15*, 1181–1186. [CrossRef]
90. Wozniak, A.; Drewa, G.; Chesy, G.; Rakowski, A.; Rozwodowska, M.; Olszewska, D. Effect of altitude training on sportsmen's peroxidation and antioxidant enzymes. *Med. Sci. Sport. Exerc.* **2001**, *33*, 1109–1113. [CrossRef]
91. Ridker, P.M.; Cushman, M.; Stampfer, M.J.; Tracy, R.P.; Hennekens, C.H. Inflammation, aspirin, and the risk of cardiovascular disease in apparently healthy men. *N. Engl. J. Med.* **1997**, *336*, 973–979. [CrossRef]
92. Verma, S.; Buchanan, M.R.; Anderson, T.J. Endothelial function testing as a biomarker of vascular disease. *Circulation* **2003**, *108*, 2054–2059. [CrossRef]
93. Watson, C.; Whittaker, S.; Smith, N.; Vora, A.J.; Dumonde, D.C.; Brown, K.A. IL-6 acts on endothelial cells to preferentially increase their lymphocyte adherence. *Clin. Exp. Immunol.* **1996**, *105*, 112–119. [CrossRef] [PubMed]
94. Valacchi, G.; Virgili, F.; Cervellati, C.; Pecorelli, A. OxInflammation: From Subclinical Condition to Pathological Biomarker. *Front. Physiol.* **2018**, *9*, 858. [CrossRef] [PubMed]
95. Heusser, K.; Dzamonja, G.; Tank, J.; Palada, I.; Valic, Z.; Bakovic, D.; Obad, A.; Ivancev, V.; Breskovic, T.; Diedrich, A.; et al. Cardiovascular regulation during apnea in elite divers. *Hypertension* **2009**, *53*, 719–724. [CrossRef] [PubMed]
96. Bosco, G.; Rizzato, A.; Moon, R.E.; Camporesi, E.M. Environmental Physiology and Diving Medicine. *Front. Psychol.* **2018**, *9*, 72. [CrossRef] [PubMed]
97. Ferretti, G. Extreme human breath-hold diving. *Eur. J. Appl. Physiol.* **2001**, *84*, 254–271. [CrossRef] [PubMed]
98. Muth, C.M.; Radermacher, P.; Pittner, A.; Steinacker, J.; Schabana, R.; Hamich, S.; Paulat, K.; Calzia, E. Arterial blood gases during diving in elite apnea divers. *Int. J. Sport. Med.* **2003**, *24*, 104–107. [CrossRef]
99. Garbella, E.; Piarulli, A.; Fornai, E.; Pingitore, A.; Prediletto, R. Preliminary observations on the effect of hypoxic and hyperbaric stress on pulmonary gas exchange in breath-hold divers. *Diving Hyperb. Med.* **2011**, *41*, 97–100.
100. Bosco, G.; Rizzato, A.; Martani, L.; Schiavo, S.; Talamonti, E.; Garetto, G.; Paganini, M.; Camporesi, E.M.; Moon, R.E. Arterial Blood Gas Analysis in Breath-Hold Divers at Depth. *Front. Physiol.* **2018**, *9*, 1558. [CrossRef]
101. Paganini, M.; Moon, R.E.; Giacon, T.A.; Cialoni, D.; Martani, L.; Zucchi, L.; Garetto, G.; Talamonti, E.; Camporesi, E.M.; Bosco, G. Relative hypoxemia at depth during breath-hold diving investigated through arterial blood gas analysis and lung ultrasound. *J. Appl. Physiol.* **2023**, *135*, 863–871. [CrossRef]
102. Barković, I.; Jurilj, Z.; Marinelli, F.; Maričić, V.; Pavlović, M.; Wensveen, T.T.; Peršić, V. Arterial blood gases' analysis in elite breath-hold divers at extreme depths. *Eur. J. Appl Physiol.* **2023**, *123*, 857–865. [CrossRef]
103. Scott, T.; van Waart, H.; Vrijdag, X.C.E.; Mullins, D.; Mesley, P.; Mitchell, S.J. Arterial blood gas measurements during deep open-water breath-hold dives. *J. Appl. Physiol.* **2021**, *130*, 1490–1495. [CrossRef]
104. Fitz-Clarke, J.R. Mechanics of airway and alveolar collapse in human breath-hold diving. *Respir. Physiol. Neurobiol.* **2007**, *159*, 202–210. [CrossRef]
105. Bosco, G.; Paganini, M.; Rizzato, A.; Martani, L.; Garetto, G.; Lion, J.; Camporesi, E.M.; Moon, R.E. Arterial blood gases in divers at the surface after prolonged breath-hold. *Eur. J. Appl. Physiol.* **2020**, *120*, 505–512. [CrossRef]
106. Patrician, A.; Dujić, Z.; Spajić, B.; Drviš, I.; Ainslie, P.N. Breath-Hold Diving—The Physiology of Diving Deep and Returning. *Front. Physiol.* **2021**, *12*, 639377. [CrossRef]
107. Barlow, M.J.; Elia, A.; Shannon, O.M.; Zacharogianni, A.; Lodin-Sundstrom, A. The Effect of a Dietary Nitrate Supplementation in the Form of a Single Shot of Beetroot Juice on Static and Dynamic Apnea Performance. *Int. J. Sport Nutr. Exerc. Metab.* **2018**, *28*, 497–501. [CrossRef] [PubMed]
108. Theunissen, S.; Schumacker, J.; Guerrero, F.; Tillmans, F.; Boutros, A.; Lambrechts, K.; Mazur, A.; Pieri, M.; Germonpre, P.; Balestra, C. Dark chocolate reduces endothelial dysfunction after successive breath-hold dives in cool water. *Eur. J. Appl. Physiol.* **2013**, *113*, 2967–2975. [CrossRef] [PubMed]
109. Mrakic-Sposta, S.; Vezzoli, A.; Rizzato, A.; Della Noce, C.; Malacrida, S.; Montorsi, M.; Paganini, M.; Cancellara, P.; Bosco, G. Oxidative stress assessment in breath-hold diving. *Eur. J. Appl. Physiol.* **2019**, *119*, 2449–2456. [CrossRef] [PubMed]
110. Cai, H.; Harrison, D.G. Endothelial dysfunction in cardiovascular diseases: The role of oxidant stress. *Circ. Res.* **2000**, *87*, 840–844. [CrossRef] [PubMed]
111. Dolscheid-Pommerich, R.C.; Weikert, J.; Reinicke, M.; Fimmers, R.; Stoffel-Wagner, B.; Erdfelder, F.; Ceglarek, U.; Eichhorn, L. Changes in PUFA and eicosanoid metabolism during/after apnea diving: A prospective single-center study. *Undersea Hyperb. Med.* **2020**, *47*, 539–549. [CrossRef]

112. Data, P.G.; Di Tano, G.; Arborelius, M., Jr.; Polidoro, G.; Arduini, A. Change in plasma amino acid concentrations during breath-hold diving at high altitude. *Clin. Physiol. Biochem.* **1988**, *6*, 327–333.
113. Cialoni, D.; Brizzolari, A.; Sponsiello, N.; Lancellotti, V.; Bosco, G.; Marroni, A.; Barassi, A. Serum Amino Acid Profile Changes After Repetitive Breath-Hold Dives: A Preliminary Study. *Sport. Med. Open* **2022**, *8*, 80. [CrossRef]
114. Zaccaria, M.; Borea, P.A.; Opocher, G.; Ponchia, A.; Varani, K.; Fraccarollo, D.; Scandellari, C. Effects of high-altitude chronic Hypoxia on platelet alpha 2-receptors in man. *Eur. J. Clin. Investig.* **1997**, *27*, 316–321. [CrossRef]
115. Bosco, G.; Yang, Z.J.; Savini, F.; Nubile, G.; Data, P.G.; Wang, J.P.; Camporesi, E.M. Environmental stress on diving-induced platelet activation. *Undersea Hyperb. Med.* **2001**, *28*, 207–211.
116. Goebel, M.U.; Mills, P.J.; Irwin, M.R.; Ziegler, M.G. Interleukin-6 and tumor necrosis factor-alpha production after acute psychological stress, exercise, and infused isoproterenol: Differential effects and pathways. *Psychosom. Med.* **2000**, *62*, 591–598. [CrossRef] [PubMed]
117. Kurose, I.; Anderson, D.C.; Miyasaka, M.; Tamatani, T.; Paulson, J.C.; Todd, R.F.; Rusche, J.R.; Granger, D.N. Molecular determinants of reperfusion-induced leukocyte adhesion and vascular protein leakage. *Circ. Res.* **1994**, *74*, 336–343. [CrossRef] [PubMed]
118. Lievens, D.; Zernecke, A.; Seijkens, T.; Soehnlein, O.; Beckers, L.; Munnix, I.C.; Wijnands, E.; Goossens, P.; van Kruchten, R.; Thevissen, L.; et al. Platelet CD40L mediates thrombotic and inflammatory processes in atherosclerosis. *Blood* **2010**, *116*, 4317–4327. [CrossRef] [PubMed]
119. Ando, Y.; Oku, T.; Tsuji, T. Platelets attenuate production of cytokines and nitric oxide by macrophages in response to bacterial endotoxin. *Platelets* **2016**, *27*, 344–350. [CrossRef] [PubMed]
120. Gudbrandsdottir, S.; Hasselbalch, H.C.; Nielsen, C.H. Activated platelets enhance IL-10 secretion and reduce TNF-alpha secretion by monocytes. *J. Immunol.* **2013**, *191*, 4059–4067. [CrossRef] [PubMed]
121. Eftedal, I.; Flatberg, A.; Davis, I.; Dujic, Z. Immune and inflammatory responses to freediving calculated from leukocyte gene expression profiles. *Physiol. Genom.* **2016**, *48*, 795–802. [CrossRef]
122. Wang, Z.L.; Liu, J.Y.; Zhou, C.J.; Wang, M.B.; Wang, H.Y.; Xu, Y. Risk factors and impacts on prognosis of ultrasound lung comets in patients undergoing hemodialysis. *Zhonghua Yi Xue Za Zhi* **2017**, *97*, 3796–3801. [CrossRef]
123. Boussuges, A.; Coulange, M.; Bessereau, J.; Gargne, O.; Ayme, K.; Gavarry, O.; Fontanari, P.; Joulia, F. Ultrasound lung comets induced by repeated breath-hold diving, a study in underwater fishermen. *Scand. J. Med. Sci. Sports* **2011**, *21*, e384–e392. [CrossRef] [PubMed]
124. Tojo, K.; Nagamine, Y.; Yazawa, T.; Mihara, T.; Baba, Y.; Ota, S.; Goto, T.; Kurahashi, K. Atelectasis causes alveolar hypoxia-induced inflammation during uneven mechanical ventilation in rats. *Intensive Care Med. Exp.* **2015**, *3*, 56. [CrossRef] [PubMed]
125. Reyes-Ramos, C.A.; Ramírez-Jirano, L.J.; Bitzer-Quintero, O.K.; Vázquez-Medina, J.P.; Gaxiola-Robles, R.; Zenteno-Savín, T. Dolphin leukocytes exhibit an attenuated cytokine response and increase heme oxygenase activity upon exposure to lipopolysaccharides. *Comp. Biochem. Physiol. A Mol. Integr. Physiol.* **2023**, *281*, 111438. [CrossRef] [PubMed]
126. Eichhorn, L.; Dolscheid-Pommerich, R.; Erdfelder, F.; Ayub, M.A.; Schmitz, T.; Werner, N.; Jansen, F. Sustained apnea induces endothelial activation. *Clin. Cardiol.* **2017**, *40*, 704–709. [CrossRef] [PubMed]
127. Lichtenauer, M.; Goebel, B.; Fritzenwanger, M.; Foster, M.; Betge, S.; Laute, A.; Figulla, H.-R.; Jung, C. Simulated temporary hypoxia triggers the release of CD31+/Annexin+ endothelial microparticles: A prospective pilot study in humans. *Clin. Hemorheol. Microcirc.* **2015**, *61*, 83–90. [CrossRef] [PubMed]
128. Brubakk, A.O.; Duplancic, D.; Valic, Z.; Palada, I.; Obad, A.; Bakovic, D.; Wisloff, U.; Dujic, Z. A single air dive reduces arterial endothelial function in man. *J. Physiol.* **2005**, *566*, 901–906. [CrossRef] [PubMed]
129. Obad, A.; Marinovic, J.; Ljubkovic, M.; Breskovic, T.; Modun, D.; Boban, M.; Dujic, Z. Successive deep dives impair endothelial function and enhance oxidative stress in man. *Clin. Physiol. Funct. Imaging* **2010**, *30*, 432–438. [CrossRef]
130. Perovic, A.; Nikolac, N.; Braticevic, M.N.; Milcic, A.; Sobocanec, S.; Balog, T.; Dabelic, S.; Dumic, J. Does recreational scuba diving have clinically significant effect on routine haematological parameters? *Biochem. Med.* **2017**, *27*, 325–331. [CrossRef]
131. Sureda, A.; Batle, J.M.; Ferrer, M.D.; Cases, N.; Aguiló, A.; Pons, A. Neutrophil tolerance to oxidative stress induced by hypoxia/reoxygenation. *Free Radic. Res.* **2004**, *38*, 1003–1009. [CrossRef]
132. Bosco, G.; Yang, Z.J.; Di Tano, G.; Camporesi, E.M.; Faralli, F.; Savini, F.; Landolfi, A.; Doria, C.; Fano, G. Effect of in-water Oxygen prebreathing at different depths on decompression-induced bubble formation and platelet activation. *J. Appl. Physiol.* **2010**, *108*, 1077–1083. [CrossRef]
133. Ferrer, M.D.; Sureda, A.; Batle, J.M.; Tauler, P.; Tur, J.A.; Pons, A. Scuba diving enhances endogenous antioxidant defenses in lymphocytes and neutrophils. *Free Radic. Res.* **2007**, *41*, 274–281. [CrossRef]
134. Perovic, A.; Sobocanec, S.; Dabelic, S.; Balog, T.; Dumic, J. Effect of scuba diving on the oxidant/antioxidant status, SIRT1 and SIRT3 expression in recreational divers after a winter nondive period. *Free Radic. Res.* **2018**, *52*, 188–197. [CrossRef]
135. Faraci, F.M.; Didion, S.P. Vascular protection: Superoxide dismutase isoforms in the vessel wall. *Arterioscler. Thromb. Vasc. Biol.* **2004**, *24*, 1367–1373. [CrossRef] [PubMed]
136. Sureda, A.; Batle, J.M.; Ferrer, M.D.; Mestre-Alfaro, A.; Tur, J.A.; Pons, A. Scuba diving activates vascular antioxidant system. *Int. J. Sport. Med.* **2012**, *33*, 531–536. [CrossRef]

137. Bosco, G.; Giacon, T.A.; Paolocci, N.; Vezzoli, A.; Noce, C.D.; Paganini, M.; Agrimi, J.; Garetto, G.; Cialoni, D.; D'Alessandro, N.; et al. Dopamine/BDNF loss underscores narcosis cognitive impairment in divers: A proof of concept in a dry condition. *Eur. J. Appl. Physiol.* **2022**, *123*, 143–158. [CrossRef] [PubMed]
138. Kim, J.; Lee, S.; Kang, S.; Kim, S.H.; Kim, J.C.; Yang, M.; Moon, C. Brain-derived neurotropic factor and GABAergic transmission in neurodegeneration and neuroregeneration. *Neural. Regen. Res.* **2017**, *12*, 1733–1741. [CrossRef] [PubMed]
139. Lavoute, C.; Weiss, M.; Rostain, J.C. Alterations in nigral NMDA and GABAA receptor control of the striatal dopamine level after repetitive exposures to nitrogen narcosis. *Exp. Neurol.* **2008**, *212*, 63–70. [CrossRef] [PubMed]
140. Lemaitre, F.; Costalat, G.; Allinger, J.; Balestra, C. Possible causes of narcosis-like symptoms in freedivers. *Undersea Hyperb. Med.* **2023**, *50*, 85–93. [CrossRef]
141. Di Pumpo, F.; Gualtiero, M.; Paganini, M.; Cialoni, D.; Giacomo, G.; Alessandro Cipriano, A.; Giacon, T.A.; Martani, L.; Camporesi, E.; Bosco, G. Comparison between Arterial Blood Gases and Oxygen Reserve Index™ in a SCUBA Diver: A Case Report. *Healthcare* **2023**, *11*, 1102. [CrossRef]
142. Rocco, M.; Pelaia, P.; Di Benedetto, P.; Conte, G.; Maggi, L.; Fiorelli, S.; Mercieri, M.; Balestra, C.; De Blasi, R.A.; on behalf of ROAD Project Investigators. Inert gas narcosis in scuba diving, different gases different reactions. *Eur. J. Appl. Physiol.* **2019**, *119*, 247–255. [CrossRef]
143. Lafere, P.; Balestra, C.; Hemelryck, W.; Guerrero, F.; Germonpre, P. Do Environmental Conditions Contribute to Narcosis Onset and Symptom Severity? *Int. J. Sport. Med.* **2016**, *37*, 1124–1128. [CrossRef] [PubMed]
144. Ersoz, G.; Ocakcioglu, B.; Bastug, M.; Ficicilar, H.; Yavuzer, S. Platelet aggregation and release function in hyperbaric oxygenation. *Undersea Hyperb. Med.* **1998**, *25*, 229–232. [PubMed]
145. Hjelde, A.; Bergh, K.; Brubakk, A.O.; Iversen, O.J. Complement activation in divers after repeated air/heliox dives and its possible relevance to DCS. *J. Appl. Physiol.* **1995**, *78*, 1140–1144. [CrossRef]
146. Morabito, C.; Bosco, G.; Pilla, R.; Corona, C.; Mancinelli, R.; Yang, Z.; Camporesi, E.M.; Fano, G.; Mariggio, M.A. Effect of pre-breathing Oxygen at different depth on oxidative status and calcium concentration in lymphocytes of scuba divers. *Acta Physiol.* **2011**, *202*, 69–78. [CrossRef]
147. Dumić, J.; Cvetko, A.; Abramović, I.; Goreta, S.S.; Perović, A.; Bratičević, M.N.; Kifer, D.; Sinčić, N.; Gornik, O.; Žarak, M. Changes in Specific Biomarkers Indicate Cardiac Adaptive and Anti-inflammatory Response of Repeated Recreational SCUBA Diving. *Front. Cardiovasc. Med.* **2022**, *9*, 855682. [CrossRef]
148. Tillmans, F.; Sharghi, R.; Noy, T.; Kähler, W.; Klapa, S.; Sartisohn, S.; Sebensm, S.; Kochm, A. Effect of Hyperoxia on the immune status of oxygen divers and endurance athletes. *Free Radic. Res.* **2019**, *53*, 522–534. [CrossRef]
149. Eckmann, D.M.; Armstead, S.C. Influence of endothelial glycocalyx degradation and surfactants on air embolism adhesion. *Anesthesiology* **2006**, *105*, 1220–1227. [CrossRef] [PubMed]
150. Philp, R.B.; Inwood, M.J.; Warren, B.A. Interactions between gas bubbles and components of the blood: Implications in decompression sickness. *Aerosp. Med.* **1972**, *43*, 946–953.
151. Philp, R.B.; Schacham, P.; Gowdey, C.W. Involvement of platelets and microthrombi in experimental decompression sickness: Similarities with disseminated intravascular coagulation. *Aerosp. Med.* **1971**, *42*, 494–502.
152. Kuroiwa, K. The functional and biochemical changes of platelets in experimental decompression sickness of rabbits. *Bull. Tokyo Med. Dent. Univ.* **1984**, *31*, 73–84.
153. Bennett, M.; Mitchell, S.; Dominguez, A. Adjunctive treatment of decompression illness with a non-steroidal anti-inflammatory drug (tenoxicam) reduces compression requirement. *Undersea Hyperb. Med.* **2003**, *30*, 195–205. [PubMed]
154. Ersson, A.; Walles, M.; Ohlsson, K.; Ekholm, A. Chronic hyperbaric exposure activates proinflammatory mediators in humans. *J. Appl. Physiol.* **2002**, *92*, 2375–2380. [CrossRef] [PubMed]
155. Kelly, K.R.; Palombo, L.J.; Jensen, A.E.; Bernards, J.R. Efficacy of closed cell wet-suit at various depths and gas mixtures for thermoprotection during military training dives. *Front. Physiol.* **2023**, *14*, 1165196. [CrossRef]
156. Li, Y.; Liu, K.; Kang, Z.M.; Sun, X.J.; Liu, W.W.; Mao, Y.F. Helium preconditioning protects against neonatal hypoxia-ischemia via nitric oxide-mediated up-regulation of antioxidants in a rat model. *Behav. Brain Res.* **2016**, *300*, 31–37. [CrossRef] [PubMed]
157. Bhopale, V.M.; Ruhela, D.; Brett, K.D.; Nugent, N.Z.; Fraser, N.K.; Levinson, S.L.; DiNubile, M.J.; Thom, S.R. Plasma gelsolin modulates the production and fate of IL-1β-containing microparticles following high-pressure exposure and decompression. *J. Appl. Physiol.* **2021**, *130*, 1604–1613. [CrossRef] [PubMed]
158. Balestra, C.; Arya, A.K.; Leveque, C.; Virgili, F.; Germonpre, P.; Lambrechts, K.; Lafere, P.; Thom, S.R. Varying Oxygen Partial Pressure Elicits Blood-Borne Microparticles Expressing Different Cell-Specific Proteins-Toward a Targeted Use of Oxygen? *Int. J. Mol. Sci.* **2022**, *23*, 7888. [CrossRef]
159. Rocco, M.; Maggi, L.; Loffredo, C.; Pelli, M.; Di Benedetto, P.; Fiorelli, S.; Simmaco, M.; De Blasi, R.A. The impact of different gas mixtures on inflammatory responses in advanced recreational divers. *Diving Hyperb. Med.* **2021**, *51*, 140–146. [CrossRef]
160. Yang, M.; Milovanova, T.N.; Bogush, M.; Uzun, G.; Bhopale, V.M.; Thom, S.R. Microparticle enlargement and altered surface proteins after air decompression are associated with inflammatory vascular injuries. *J. Appl. Physiol.* **2012**, *112*, 204–211. [CrossRef]
161. Landolfi, A.; Yang, Z.J.; Savini, F.; Camporesi, E.M.; Faralli, F.; Bosco, G. Pretreatment with hyperbaric oxygenation reduces bubble formation and platelet activation. *Sport Sci. Health* **2006**, *1*, 122–128. [CrossRef]
162. Camporesi, E.M.; Bosco, G. Hyperbaric oxygen pretreatment and preconditioning. *Undersea Hyperb. Med.* **2014**, *41*, 259–263.

163. Dreyer, S.; Schneppendahl, J.; Moeller, F.; Koch, A.; Muth, T.; Schipke, J.D. An Updated Narrative Review on Er-gometric Systems Applied to Date in Assessing Divers' Fitness. *Healthcare* **2021**, *9*, 1044. [CrossRef]
164. Baj, Z.; Olszanski, R.; Majewska, E.; Konarski, M. The effect of air and nitrox divings on platelet activation tested by flow cytometry. *Aviat. Space Environ. Med.* **2000**, *71*, 925–928.
165. Bosco, G.; Rizzato, A.; Quartesan, S.; Camporesi, E.; Mangar, D.; Paganini, M.; Cenci, L.; Malacrida, S.; Mrakic-Sposta, S.; Moretti, S.; et al. Effects of the Ketogenic diet in overweight divers breathing Enriched Air Nitrox. *Sci. Rep.* **2018**, *8*, 2655. [CrossRef]
166. Gronow, G.; Kahler, W.; Koch, A.; Klause, N. Benzoate hydroxylation: A measure of oxidative stress in divers. *Adv. Exp. Med. Biol.* **2005**, *566*, 223–229. [CrossRef]
167. Doubt, T.J. Cardiovascular and thermal responses to SCUBA diving. *Med. Sci. Sport. Exerc.* **1996**, *28*, 581–586. [CrossRef]
168. Madden, D.; Thom, S.R.; Milovanova, T.N.; Yang, M.; Bhopale, V.M.; Ljubkovic, M.; Dujic, Z. Exercise before SCUBA diving ameliorates decompression-induced neutrophil activation. *Med. Sci. Sports Exerc.* **2014**, *46*, 1928–1935. [CrossRef] [PubMed]
169. Spisni, E.; Marabotti, C.; De Fazio, L.; Valerii, M.C.; Cavazza, E.; Brambilla, S.; Hoxha, K.; L'Abbate, A.; Longobardi, P. A comparative evaluation of two decompression procedures for technical diving using inflammatory responses: Compartmental versus ratio deco. *Diving Hyperb. Med.* **2017**, *47*, 9–16. [CrossRef]
170. Romsbotn, S.; Eftedal, I.; Vaag, J.R. A Work Environment Under Pressure: Psychosocial Job Demands and Resources Among Saturation Divers. *Front. Public Health* **2022**, *10*, 765197. [CrossRef] [PubMed]
171. Dreyer, S.; Deussen, A.; Berndt, D.; Schipke, J.D. How to Survive 33 min after the Umbilical of a Saturation Diver Severed at a Depth of 90 msw? *Healthcare* **2022**, *10*, 453. [CrossRef] [PubMed]
172. Kulkarni, A.C. Rescue of a saturation diver, unconscious due to an explosion underwater. *Int. Marit. Health* **2021**, *72*, 46–48. [CrossRef]
173. Gjerde, K.Ø.; Ryggvik, H. *On the Edge, Under Water: Offshore Diving in Norway*, 2nd ed.; Wigestrand Forlag: Stavanger, Norway, 2014.
174. Ramnefjell, M.P.; Morild, I.; Mørk, S.J.; Lilleng, P.K. Fatal diving accidents in western Norway 1983–2007. *Forensic Sci. Int.* **2012**, *223*, e22–e26. [CrossRef]
175. Keatinge, W.R.; Hayward, M.G.; McIver, N.K. Hypothermia during saturation diving in the North Sea. *Br. Med. J.* **1980**, *280*, 291. [CrossRef]
176. Beyerstein, G.; Lang, M.A.; Smith, N.E. Commercial Diving: Surface-Mixed Gas, Sur-D-O_2, Bell Bounce, Saturation. In Proceedings of the Advanced Scientific Diving Workshop, Washington, DC, USA, 23–24 February 2006.
177. Brubakk, A.O.; Ross, J.A.; Thom, S.R. Saturation diving; physiology and pathophysiology. *Compr. Physiol.* **2014**, *4*, 1229–1272. [CrossRef]
178. Mrakic-Sposta, S.; Vezzoli, A.; D'Alessandro, F.; Paganini, M.; Dellanoce, C.; Cialoni, D.; Bosco, G. Change in Oxidative Stress Biomarkers During 30 Days in Saturation Dive: A Pilot Study. *Int. J. Environ. Res. Public Health* **2020**, *17*, 7118. [CrossRef] [PubMed]
179. Zwart, S.R.; Jessup, J.M.; Ji, J.; Smith, S.M. Saturation Diving Alters Folate Status and Biomarkers of DNA Damage and Repair. *PLoS ONE* **2012**, *7*, e31058. [CrossRef]
180. Imbert, J.P.; Balestra, C.; Kiboub, F.Z.; Loennechen, Ø.; Eftedal, I. Commercial Divers' Subjective Evaluation of Saturation. *Front. Psychol.* **2019**, *9*, 2774. [CrossRef]
181. Monnoyer, R.; Eftedal, I.; Hjelde, A.; Deb, S.; Haugum, K.; Lautridou, J. Functional Profiling Reveals Altered Metabolic Activity in Divers' Oral Microbiota During Commercial Heliox Saturation Diving. *Front. Physiol.* **2021**, *12*, 702634. [CrossRef]
182. Sureda, A.; Batle, J.M.; Capo, X.; Martorell, M.; Cordova, A.; Tur, J.A.; Pons, A. Scuba diving induces nitric oxide synthesis and the expression of inflammatory and regulatory genes of the immune response in neutrophils. *Physiol. Genom.* **2014**, *46*, 647–654. [CrossRef]
183. Krog, J.; Tønnesen, E.K.; Jepsen, C.F.; Parner, E.; Segadal, K.; Hope, A.; Ulvik, R.J.; Holland, M.E. Nural killer cells as biomarkers of hyperbaric stress during a dry heliox saturation dive. *Aviat. Space Environ. Med.* **2010**, *81*, 467–474. [CrossRef] [PubMed]
184. Domoto, H.; Iwaya, K.; Ikomi, F.; Matsuo, H.; Tadano, Y.; Fujii, S.; Tachi, K.; Itoh, Y.; Sato, M.; Inoue, K.; et al. Upregulation of antioxidant proteins in the plasma proteome during saturation diving: Unique coincidence under hypobaric Hypoxia. *PLoS ONE* **2016**, *11*, e0163804. [CrossRef] [PubMed]
185. Djurhuus, R.; Segadal, K.; Svardal, A.M. Glutathione in blood cells decreases without DNA breaks after a simulated saturation dive to 250 msw. *Aviat. Space Environ. Med.* **2006**, *77*, 597–604.
186. Kiboub, F.Z.; Møllerløkken, A.; Hjelde, A.; Flatberg, A.; Loennechen, Ø.; Eftedal, I. Blood Gene Expression and Vascular Function Biomarkers in Professional Saturation Diving. *Front. Physiol.* **2018**, *9*, 937. [CrossRef]
187. Smith, S.M.; Davis-Street, J.E.; Fesperman, J.V.; Smith, M.D.; Rice, B.L.; Zwart, S.R. Nutritional assessment during a 14-d saturation dive: The NASA Extreme Environment Mission Operations V Project. *J. Nutr.* **2004**, *134*, 1765–1771. [CrossRef]
188. Ikeda, M.; Nakabayashi, K.; Shinkai, M.; Hara, Y.; Kizaki, T.; Oh-Ishi, S.; Ohno, H. Supplementation of antioxidants prevents oxidative stress during a deep saturation dive. *Tohoku J. Exp. Med.* **2004**, *203*, 353–357. [CrossRef]
189. Deb, S.K.; Swinton, P.A.; Dolan, E. Nutritional considerations during prolonged exposure to a confined, hyperbaric, hyperoxic environment: Recommendations for saturation divers. *Extrem. Physiol. Med.* **2016**, *5*, 1. [CrossRef]
190. Deb, S.K.; Dolan, E.; Hambly, C.; Speakman, J.R.; Eftedal, O.; Zariwala, M.G.; Eftedal, I. The Assessment of Daily Energy Expenditure of Commercial Saturation Divers Using Doubly Labelled Water. *Front. Physiol.* **2021**, *12*, 687605. [CrossRef]

191. Monnoyer, R.; Lautridou, J.; Deb, S.; Hjelde, A.; Eftedal, I. Using Salivary Biomarkers for Stress Assessment in Offshore Saturation Diving: A Pilot Study. *Front. Physiol.* **2021**, *12*, 791525. [CrossRef] [PubMed]
192. Mittal, M.; Siddiqui, M.R.; Tran, K.; Reddy, S.P.; Malik, A.B. Oxygen Species in Inflammation and Tissue Injury. *Antioxid. Redox Signal.* **2014**, *20*, 7. [CrossRef] [PubMed]
193. Alhayaza, R.; Haque, E.; Karbasiafshar, C.; Sellke, F.W.; Abid, M.R. The Relationship Between Reactive Oxygen Species and Endothelial Cell Metabolism. *Front. Chem.* **2020**, *8*, 592688. [CrossRef] [PubMed]
194. Teleanu, D.M.; Niculescu, A.-G.; Lungu, I.I.; Radu, C.I.; Vladâcenco, O.; Roza, E.; Costăchescu, B.; Grumezescu, A.M.; Teleanu, R.I. An Overview of Oxidative Stress, Neuroinflammation, and Neurodegenerative Diseases. *Int. J. Mol. Sci.* **2022**, *23*, 5938. [CrossRef] [PubMed]
195. Georgieva, E.; Ananiev, J.; Yovchev, Y.; Arabadzhiev, G.; Abrashev, H.; Abrasheva, D.; Atanasov, V.; Kostandieva, R.; Mitev, M.; Petkova-Parlapanska, K.; et al. COVID-19 Complications: Oxidative Stress, Inflammation, and Mitochondrial and Endothelial Dysfunction. *Int. J. Mol. Sci.* **2023**, *24*, 14876. [CrossRef]
196. Comhair, S.A.; Erzurum, S.C. Antioxidant responses to oxidant-mediated lung diseases. *Am. J. Physiol. Lung Cell. Mol. Physiol.* **2002**, *283*, 246–255. [CrossRef]
197. Gempp, E.; Blatteau, J.E. Preconditioning Methods and Mechanisms for Preventing the Risk of Decompression Sickness in Scuba Divers: A Review. *Res. Sports Med.* **2010**, *18*, 205–218. [CrossRef]
198. Winkler, B.; Muth, C.M.; Piepho, T. Hyperbare Therapie und Tauchmedizin—Tauchmedizin: Status quo und Ausblick. *Anästhesiol Intensivmed Notfallmed Schmerzther* **2015**, *50*, 638–646. [CrossRef]
199. Madden, D.; Thom, S.R.; Dujic, Z. Exercise before and after SCUBA diving and the role of cellular microparticles in decompression stress. *Med. Hypotheses* **2016**, *86*, 80–84. [CrossRef]
200. Held, H.E.; Pendergast, D.R. The effects of respiratory muscle training on respiratory mechanics and energy cost. *Respir. Physiol. Neurobiol.* **2014**, *200*, 7–17. [CrossRef] [PubMed]
201. Germonpré, P.; Balestra, C. Preconditioning to Reduce Decompression Stress in Scuba Divers. *Aerosp. Med. Hum. Perform.* **2017**, *88*, 114–120. [CrossRef] [PubMed]
202. Šegrt Ribičić, I.; Valić, M.; Lušić Kalcina, L.; Božić, J.; Obad, A.; Glavaš, D.; Glavičić, I.; Valić, Z. Effects of Oxygen Prebreathing on Bubble Formation, Flow-Mediated Dilatation, and Psychomotor Performance during Trimix Dives. *Sports* **2024**, *12*, 35. [CrossRef] [PubMed]
203. Barak, O.F.; Caljkusic, K.; Hoiland, R.L.; Ainslie, P.N.; Thom, S.R.; Yang, M.; Jovanov, P.; Dujic, Z. Differential influence of vitamin C on the peripheral and cerebral circulation after diving and exposure to hyperoxia. *Am. J. Physiol. Regul. Integr. Comp. Physiol.* **2018**, *315*, R759–R767. [CrossRef]
204. Thiele, R.H. Subcellular Energetics and Metabolism: Potential Therapeutic Applications. *Obstet. Anesthesia Dig.* **2017**, *124*, 1872–1885. [CrossRef]
205. Arieli, R. Nanobubbles Form at Active Hydrophobic Spots on the Luminal Aspect of Blood Vessels: Consequences for Decompression Illness in Diving and Possible Implications for Autoimmune Disease—An Overview. *Front. Physiol.* **2017**, *8*, 591. [CrossRef] [PubMed]
206. Yang, M.; Barak, O.F.; Dujic, Z.; Madden, D.; Bhopale, V.M.; Bhullar, J.; Thom, S.R. Ascorbic acid supplementation diminishes microparticle elevations and neutrophil activation following SCUBA diving. *Am. J. Physiol. Regul. Integr. Comp. Physiol.* **2015**, *309*, R338–R344. [CrossRef] [PubMed]
207. Obad, A.; Valic, Z.; Palada, I.; Brubakk, A.O.; Modun, D.; Dujić, Z. Antioxidant Pretreatment and Reduced Arterial Endothelial Dysfunction After Diving. *Aviat. Space Environ. Med.* **2007**, *78*, 1114–1120. [CrossRef] [PubMed]

Disclaimer/Publisher's Note: The statements, opinions and data contained in all publications are solely those of the individual author(s) and contributor(s) and not of MDPI and/or the editor(s). MDPI and/or the editor(s) disclaim responsibility for any injury to people or property resulting from any ideas, methods, instructions or products referred to in the content.

International Journal of
Molecular Sciences

MDPI

Review

Hyperoxia: Effective Mechanism of Hyperbaric Treatment at Mild-Pressure

Mariana Cannellotto [1], Ali Yasells García [2] and María Silvina Landa [1,*]

[1] Research Department, International Hyperbaric Medicine and Research Association (IHMERA), Buenos Aires 1429, Argentina
[2] UniVida Medical Centers, Miami, FL 33126, USA
* Correspondence: silvina.landal@ihmera.com

Abstract: HBOT increases the proportion of dissolved oxygen in the blood, generating hyperoxia. This increased oxygen diffuses into the mitochondria, which consume the majority of inhaled oxygen and constitute the epicenter of HBOT effects. In this way, the oxygen entering the mitochondria can reverse tissue hypoxia, activating the electron transport chain to generate energy. Furthermore, intermittent HBOT is sensed by the cell as relative hypoxia, inducing cellular responses such as the activation of the HIF-1α pathway, which in turn, activates numerous cellular processes, including angiogenesis and inflammation, among others. These effects are harnessed for the treatment of various pathologies. This review summarizes the evidence indicating that the use of medium-pressure HBOT generates hyperoxia and activates cellular pathways capable of producing the mentioned effects. The possibility of using medium-pressure HBOT as a direct or adjunctive treatment in different pathologies may yield benefits, potentially leading to transformative therapeutic advancements in the future.

Keywords: hyperbaric oxygen treatment (HBOT); hyperoxia; mild pressure; PO_2; reactive oxygen species (ROS)

1. Introduction

Oxygen is the essential component of cellular aerobic metabolism. It enters the respiratory pathways and blood vessels through convection, then diffuses through the capillary wall to the interstitium, with its ultimate destination being the mitochondria, where it plays a role in cellular respiration.

Oxygen is utilized as a therapeutic agent, not only for treating patients in need of oxygen supplementation, but it is also considered a drug capable of inducing targeted clinical responses, such as hyperbaric oxygen therapy (HBOT) [1] or therapies utilizing the "Normobaric Oxygen Paradox" or the "Hyperoxia-Hypoxia Paradox" [2,3]. These effects may vary in response to different pressures used, oxygen exposure durations, and the number of sessions for various pathologies. Therefore, it is necessary to standardize these parameters and characterize the responses based on the patient's specific needs.

The aim of this review is to demonstrate that hyperbaric treatment using 1.5 atm generates an oxygen increase in blood and tissues, impacting cellular metabolism and producing beneficial effects for the therapy of various pathologies.

2. Hyperoxia

Hyperoxia is defined as an increase in the presence of tissue and plasma oxygen at concentrations higher than normal. The term "hyperoxia" is widely used in scientific language, and the word "HYPEROXIA" is documented in 23,957 articles on Pubmed Central (PMC)-nih.gov and in 9541 publications on PubMed-nih.gov. Given its clinical relevance, this concept is also extensively employed in the 243 clinical studies reported on ClinicalTrials.gov.

Hyperoxia can be achieved in situations where individuals are provided with oxygen supplementation (oxygen therapy) under normobaric or hyperbaric conditions. Normobaric oxygen supplementation, delivered through a mask, is used as a therapy for various medical conditions. Hyperbaric oxygen therapy (HBOT) involves breathing high concentrations of oxygen (O_2) (~100%) within a pressurized chamber set above normal atmospheric pressure (at sea level, 1.0 absolute atmospheres or atm). For clinical usage, the pressure must be at least 1.4 atm according to the UHMS (Undersea and Hyperbaric Medical Society) guidelines, as stated in the 14th Edition 2019-Hyperbaric Oxygen Therapy Indications. Hyperoxia is the causal factor behind the beneficial effects achieved through these treatments [4].

3. Oxygen Homeostasis

Oxygen is essential for all aerobic organisms. Normoxia is defined as the normal oxygenation conditions necessary for the proper execution of physiological processes.

The oxygen level within the mitochondria [2] is very low, so even small variations act as potent triggers for metabolic signaling. Mitochondria play a central role in oxygen utilization, as cellular respiration occurs there. ATP, the cell's energy source, is produced from glucose, with oxygen acting as the final electron acceptor in the respiratory chain. During this process, small amounts of reactive oxygen species (ROS) are generated, which are molecules capable of reacting with other molecules.

The hyperoxic state during hyperbaric oxygen therapy can elevate ROS production. Recently, it has been demonstrated that HBOT induces an increase in ROS with a kinetic profile similar to that of plasma reactive oxygen species at 1.4 ATA and 2.5 ATA. The peak production is attained around 2 h and persists above the baseline level for 48 h [5] (See Figure 1).

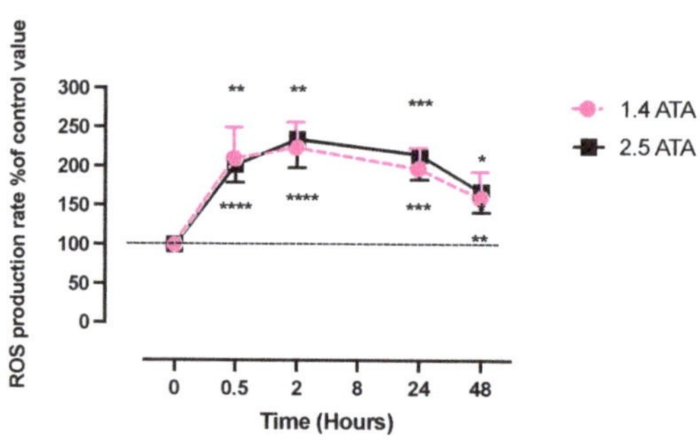

Figure 1. Percentual variations in ROS (plasma) production after 60 min of oxygen breathing of mild (1.4 ATA, n = 6) or high hyperbaric exposure (2.5 ATA, n = 8). Levels of oxygen are shown in the figure legend. Results are expressed as mean percentage change of control values (*: $p < 0.05$, **: $p < 0.01$, ***: $p < 0.001$, ****: $p < 0.0001$; RM-ANOVA and Dunnet's post hoc test).

The effects of ROS can be counterbalanced by the action of NRF2, a transcription factor that regulates the antioxidant response [3] (See Figure 2).

Its response magnitude and duration are also dependent on the oxygen dose applied as proposed by Fratantonio et al. (Fratantonio et al., 2021) [6].

When there is an excess of oxygen in the cell, and the endogenous antioxidant system is disrupted, oxidative stress is triggered. This can result in damage to lipids, proteins, and DNA. Furthermore, it is known that oxidative stress, inflammation, the immune system, and metabolism are interconnected. In this context, ROS is used as part of the signaling cascades of certain inflammatory cytokines, contributing to the development and/or progression of chronic inflammatory diseases [7].

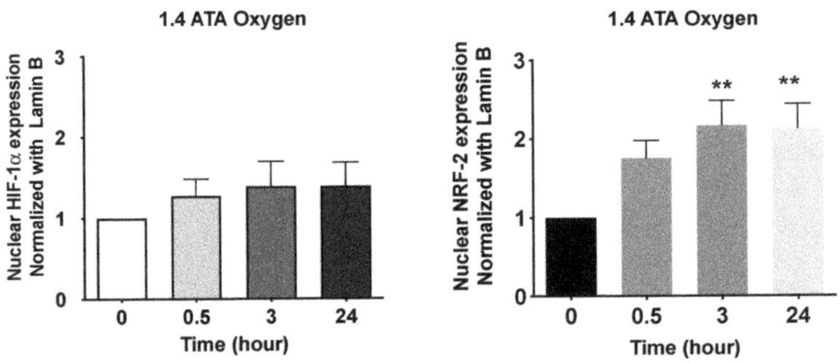

Figure 2. HIF-1α and NRF-2 nuclear translocation following 1 h of hyperbaric hyperoxia at 1.4 ATA hyperoxia in human subjects (N = 6) before and after the recovery to normoxic conditions. Results are expressed as fold change (mean ± SEM) in comparison to baseline (0), which was set at 1. ** $p < 0.01$; for one-way ANOVA followed by Dunnett's post hoc test (Modified from Fratantonio et al. (2021) [6].

On the contrary, in the case of persistent tissue hypoxia (oxygen deficiency), tissues can develop hypoxemic stress, which can lead to organ dysfunction and permanent functional impairment, as seen in conditions such as acute mountain sickness [8,9]. To prevent such damage, hypoxia serves as a key inducer of cellular gene expression, promoting various processes such as cellular protection and repair, angiogenesis, stem cell proliferation and differentiation, and more. Most of the induced gene expression is guided by transcription factors known as HIF-1 (hypoxia-inducible factors 1). Under normoxic conditions, HIF-1 levels are reduced since the reactive oxygen species (ROS) in the cell, products of cellular metabolism, promote their degradation. In a hypoxic situation, fewer ROS are produced, causing HIF-1 to stabilize, translocate to the nucleus, and promote the expression of approximately 200 genes essential for adapting to low-oxygen conditions. These genes include glycolytic enzymes for ATP synthesis, VEGF to induce angiogenesis, iNOS (inducible nitric oxide synthase), and other factors to enhance tissue oxygenation. HIF-1 is also associated with other processes such as mitochondrial biogenesis and aging through SIRT1 [2].

4. HBOT (Hyperbaric Oxygen Therapy)

In certain circumstances, hyperbaric oxygen therapy represents the primary treatment modality, while in others, it serves as a complement to surgical or pharmacological interventions [10].

Hyperbaric oxygen therapy is conducted using various types of chambers. Multiplace chambers are employed to simultaneously treat up to approximately 20 patients. These chambers are pressurized with compressed air, and 100% oxygen is administered via masks covering the nose and mouth or hoods that envelop the entire head. The atmosphere is carefully regulated and controlled concerning air and temperature. These chambers allow for the entry of equipment from intensive care units and the presence of medical personnel.

Monoplace Chambers are the most used type. These chambers can be pressurized with nearly 100% oxygen, and the patient directly breathes the oxygen from the chamber environment. They can also be pressurized with compressed air while the patient breathes oxygen (close to 100%) through masks, head hoods, or endotracheal tubes. This type of chamber offers individual patient management (isolation, useful for infections), making patients easy to observe. No special decompression procedures are required. More cost-effective than multiplace chambers. Requires less space than multiplace chambers. Fewer operators are needed. The design of monoplace chambers is ideal for caring for patients who do not require the presence of personnel within the chamber. Most bodily functions can be monitored externally, including the ventilator, which can be controlled from outside the chamber.

4.1. Fundamentals of Hyperoxic Treatment

The primary physiological effect of HBOT is the generation of hyperoxia, which allows for greater oxygen dilution in the blood plasma, and this process is independent of hemoglobin [11]. The oxygen supply chain begins in the lungs, where it is delivered through convection in the respiratory passages and blood vessels. It then diffuses through the capillary wall to the interstitium, with its ultimate destination being the mitochondria [2].

In the blood, oxygen is transported in two forms: a fraction bound to hemoglobin and a free fraction dissolved in the plasma. The amount of dissolved oxygen is proportional to the partial pressure of oxygen at a specific temperature, according to Henry's Law [12]. Therefore, at a higher partial gas pressure, it tends to shift from a gaseous to a liquid state, with the reverse occurring when the pressure of the gas dissolved in the plasma decreases.

Furthermore, we should consider that the air we normally breathe is composed of 78% nitrogen, 21% oxygen, and the rest is made up of trace gases. According to Dalton's Law, the total pressure exerted by a mixture of gases is equal to the sum of the partial pressures of the gases. This means that at sea level, 1 ATA (absolute pressure), the partial pressure of oxygen in the atmosphere is 159.6 mmHg. Exposure to pure oxygen at 1.5 ATA (absolute atmospheres) entails an oxygen pressure of 1140 mmHg. An increase in inspired oxygen pressure leads to an increase in alveolar oxygen pressure, which reaches 1053 mmHg when breathing 100% oxygen in a hyperbaric chamber at 1.5 ATA, compared to 102 mmHg when breathing air at 1 ATA, meaning it increases by a factor of 10.

At normal atmospheric pressures, only a limited portion of inspired oxygen is dissolved in the blood, but at higher pressures, as used in HBOT, it becomes possible to dissolve enough oxygen to meet the body's usual needs. In line with this, Jain et al. described that arterial oxygen pressure increases with pressure, such that ideally, breathing 100% oxygen at 1.5 ATA results in a 10-fold increase in arterial oxygen compared to arterial oxygen under normal conditions (breathing air at 1 ATA), demonstrating the hyperoxia generated in HBOT at 1.5 ATA [13]. Ishihara et al. also reported an increase in dissolved oxygen using mid-pressure HBOT [14].

Breathing 100% oxygen in a high-pressure environment increases tissue oxygen tension. The diffusion of dissolved oxygen into tissues follows the mathematical model described by Krogh [15]. Using the Krogh model, the existence of radial and longitudinal pressure gradients (PpO_2) is explained, based on the capillary radius and the arterial and venous endpoints, respectively. Combining these variables, the model allows the prediction of PpO_2 in tissues. By administering O_2 at close to 100% concentration in an environment at 1.45 atm, the oxygen penetration radius from capillaries to tissues is approximately ~75 μm, enabling the attainment of an arteriolar PpO_2 of about 950 mmHg. This pressure is more than sufficient to ensure adequate oxygen supply to all tissues in the body through the diffusion and penetration of oxygen from plasma to all cells. Therefore, at 1.5 ATA, the minimum required PpO_2 (20 mmHg) is achieved and considerably exceeded to cover the minimum average penetration radius needed to support cellular functions (~40 μm). Holbach et al. demonstrated that HBOT al 1.5 ATA increased arterial PO_2 and cerebrospinal fluid oxygen pressure [16].

The increase in tissue oxygen levels after subjecting a patient to HBOT treatment has been widely demonstrated [17,18]. This increase persists even after the vasoconstriction generated by HBOT, as it does not impede the elevation of tissue partial oxygen pressure [18].

In addition, tissue hyperoxia has been demonstrated in the brains of rats exposed to hyperbaric therapy at 1.5 ATA [19]. These results were confirmed in clinical studies by Rockwold and colleagues, showing a significant increase in tissue oxygenation induced by HBOT at 1.5 ATA in the brains of patients [20]. These findings were also replicated in a phase II clinical trial, demonstrating hyperoxia generated at that pressure [21]. Moreover, the increase in tissue oxygenation achieved by HBOT at 1.5 ATA is capable of elevating ATP and NAD+ levels in brain tissue following a brain injury, meaning that hyperbaric oxygen supply can restore mitochondrial function after one hour of treatment. These effects were accompanied by a reduced loss of neuronal cells in the hippocampus, contributing to improved cognitive recovery [19].

Niza et al. observed that exposure to HBOT increases blood flow in peripheral tissue capillaries through parasympathetic activation induced by hyperoxia at 1.4 ATA [22].

It has been demonstrated that the increase in tissue oxygen induced by HBOT at 1.5 ATA using a monoplace chamber generates cellular responses, as described by Fratantonio et al. They reported that hyperoxia induced in healthy individuals at 1.5 ATA led to an increase in the expression of transcription factors that regulate cellular responses related to oxygen fluctuations. Additionally, an increase in glutathione and MMP9 (metalloproteinase 9) was observed, indicating that the treatment induces oxidative stress. These observations highlight a cellular response mediated by transcription factors induced by hyperoxia generated at 1.5 ATA [6].

Leveque et al. described the kinetics of ROS in healthy patients after 1 h of exposure to hyperbaric oxygen at 1.5 ATA and 2.5 ATA, up to 48 h following the treatment. The work demonstrated a significant increase in ROS due to hyperoxia generated at 1.5 ATA and the activation of antioxidant mechanisms. Both the ROS kinetics and the levels reached were comparable to the group that received HBOT at 2.5 ATA. Similarly, it was observed that the kinetics and levels of antioxidants were comparable at both pressures, while the immunomodulatory effects varied depending on the dosage [5].

The increase in ROS and antioxidants after HBOT was also described in the study by Bosco et al. They observed that these parameters remained elevated during the 20 daily sessions of HBOT conducted at the same pressures. At 1.5 ATA, ROS levels remained comparable between the two pressures until day 7 and returned to normal after completing the 20 sessions, while they continued to be elevated at 2.5 ATA. This was accompanied by an increase in antioxidant compounds with the same kinetics at both pressures, even up to one month after completing the treatment, indicating a shift in the redox balance toward the reduced state [23]. This allows us to conclude that at 1.5 ATA, there is a clear antioxidant effect that predominates over oxidative stress, which remains elevated one month after completing the 20 sessions tested. Furthermore, an anti-inflammatory effect was observed, evidenced by a decrease in IL-6 and miRNA expression, consistent with findings from other studies showing a decrease in proinflammatory cytokines and an increase in hemoglobin. These results demonstrate that intermittent hyperoxia generated at 1.5 ATA leads to an increase in ROS due to increased tissue oxygen, as well as cellular responses that contribute to an antioxidant, anti-inflammatory, and hemoglobin-increasing effect in a safer context without renal damage [24,25].

The effects of intermittent hyperoxia on processes such as inflammation, oxidative stress, and others can be explained through the phenomenon known as the "normobaric oxygen paradox" or "hypoxia-hyperoxia paradox" [2,26] depending on the pressure used. However, it is important to consider that both normobaric and hyperbaric intermittent exposures generate the same reactions. This paradox was proposed in 2006 when the authors observed that intermittent hyperoxia/normoxia exposure induced the synthesis of EPO (Erythropoietin). Essentially in a hyperoxic environment, there is more dissolved oxygen, leading to an increase in ROS. The adaptive response induces an increase in antioxidant proteins (scavengers) to counteract the increased ROS, preventing reactive species from causing damage to DNA and other cellular processes. When returning to normoxia, oxygen and ROS levels normalize, but the scavenger activity remains high for an extended period. When the hyperoxic exposure is repeated, the ROS/scavenger ratio is low because the half-life of scavengers is longer than that of ROS. This results in fewer ROS and, consequently, less degradation of HIF (Hypoxia-Inducible Factor) in the proteasome and more active HIF entering the nucleus to promote the transcription of EPO, VEGF, sirtuins, among others, leading to effects like hypoxia (angiogenesis, cell regeneration, etc.). In other words, the cell perceives intermittent hyperoxia as a state of hypoxia, promoting cellular processes induced by HIF but under normoxic conditions.

The effect of hyperbaric oxygen at 1.5 ATA on the immune system has been addressed by various authors who observed an increase in blood flow in capillaries [22]. As previously mentioned, U Nisa and colleagues recently demonstrated that IL-6 does not change, nor does IL-12, suggesting that the treatment would have an anti-inflammatory effect on healthy women exposed to HBOT at half-pressure. The authors also reported an increase in parasympathetic activity and an increase in natural killer cells (NKC), indicating an increase in the mobilization and proliferation of these cells involved in early immunity [27]. In other words, hyperoxia generated at 1.5 ATA in healthy women has an anti-inflammatory effect.

4.2. Physiological Effects of Hyperoxia Generated by HBOT

4.2.1. Reversal of Hypoxia

Hyperbaric oxygen restores mitochondrial functionality and cellular respiration. Hyperoxia maintains the mitochondrial membrane potential and increases ATP production [28,29]. HBOT provides tissue perfusion exchange capability due to the increased instance of oxygen diffusion, distinguishing it from all other oxygen therapy methods. In this regard, HBOT treatments at 1.4–2.0 ATA for hypoxemia in critical COVID-19 patients continue to be a promising avenue [30]. Cannellotto et al. demonstrate that hyperbaric oxygen therapy at 1.45 atmospheres of pressure among patients with COVID-19 resulted in significantly faster resolution of hypoxia in those who received HBOT compared to control patients [31].

4.2.2. Non-Hypoxemic Vasoconstriction

The increased oxygen available generated by HBOT induces vasoconstriction in small arteries and capillaries in healthy tissues, without impairing oxygenation, favoring the redistribution of blood flow to underperfused areas. The vasoconstriction produced is called "non-hypoxemic" because it does not counteract the effect of hyperoxia or deepen hypoxia in ischemic or poorly perfused tissues. Vasoconstriction, mediated by the central nervous system through α-adrenergic receptors, reduces blood flow by up to 20% without altering venous return, resulting in benefits for edema reduction at any level and a reduction in the inflammatory response. Additionally, HBOT can increase vascular tone, raising blood pressure and reducing heart rate [32,33].

4.2.3. Angiogenesis

Hyperoxia stimulates neo-vascularization or the formation of new blood vessels through two processes: angiogenesis and vasculogenesis [1]. Numerous growth factors, transcription factors, hormones, and chemical mediators are involved in these mechanisms, including Hypoxia-Inducible Factor 1 (HIF-1), Vascular Endothelial Growth Factor (VEGF), Epidermal Growth Factor (EGF), Platelet-Derived Growth Factor (PDGF), interleukins (IL) [34]. Particularly, the pro-angiogenic effect triggered by HBOT is mediated by an increase in VEGF production, promoting the formation of new blood vessels after several sessions [35]. In bone marrow, HBOT affects the activity of medullary nitric oxide synthase (NOS) enzyme, which synthesizes nitric oxide (NO) and plays a role in the mobilization of stem cells, promoting neovascularization and healing [36].

4.2.4. Proliferation and Stimulation of Stem Cells

HBOT generates the hyperoxia necessary for oxidative stress via nitric oxide synthase to release pluripotent stem cells from the bone marrow stroma [37]. The mobilization of progenitor stem cells (SPCs) due to has been demonstrated in healthy individuals and in patients receiving treatment for radionecrosis. Hyperbaric oxygen mobilizes endothelial progenitor cells (EPCs), which have been associated with endothelial cell generation and demonstrated vasculogenesis [38]. It also promotes the differentiation of neural stem cells into neurons and oligodendrocytes, and reduces the number of astrocytes in vitro, possibly by regulating the Wnt3 protein signaling pathway, beta-catenin, and bone morphogenetic protein 2 (BMP2). An up-regulation of neural cell proliferation is also observed within neurogenic niches in the adult brain [39].

4.2.5. Collagen Synthesis

HBOT has been shown to increase the expression of type I pro-collagen genes in tendon and ligament healing and inhibits the expression of metalloproteinases [40]. Hyperoxia induced by HBOT activates the expression of growth factors for fibroblast activation, resulting in a significant increase in type I and type III collagen synthesis related to local nitric oxide production at the wound site during healing. Oxygen is not only important in collagen maturation, necessary for stable collagen formation, but it also increases collagen precursor synthesis, favoring the synthesis and repair of various types of tissues [41].

4.2.6. Osteogenesis

Hyperbaric oxygenation increases oxygen perfusion even in inflamed or infected bone, promoting angiogenesis that nourishes bone tissue and subsequently osteogenesis. Hyperoxia also promotes bone tissue differentiation. In this regard, it has been demonstrated that HBOT at 1.5 ATA and 2.4 ATA HBO treatments stimulates early osteogenic differentiation increasing the number of osteoblasts, calcium deposition, alkaline phosphatase activity and bone nodule [42]. Osteogenesis is accelerated compared to osteoblasts that did not receive hyperbaric oxygen [43]. Increased oxidative stress triggers the bone resorption process associated with aging and osteoporosis [44].

4.2.7. Antimicrobial Effect

Hyperoxia generated by HBOT reverses tissue hypoxia, which is a conducive environment for the development and proliferation of anaerobic and microaerophilic bacteria. It enhances the bactericidal effectiveness of antimicrobials against biofilm-producing bacteria, such as *Pseudomonas aeruginosa*, demonstrating a synergistic bactericidal action with antimicrobials in biofilm-producing bacteria [45]. It increases the concentration of reactive oxygen species (which have intrinsic bactericidal activity against bacteria), promotes innate and adaptive immune responses, enhances the phagocytosis of bacteria like *Staphylococcus aureus*, supports mitochondrial function, reverses mitochondrial damage, and provides oxygen for metabolism and reactive oxygen species production. This provides the necessary elements to promote cellular immunity and increase defenses against various pathogens. It inhibits the action of bacterial toxins that are important in infectious diseases [46].

4.2.8. Neural Function and Neuroprotection

Hyperoxia generated by HBOT increases Hypoxia-Inducible Factor 1 alpha (HIF-1alpha) and the subsequent synthesis of the cytokine erythropoietin (EPO), resulting in significant neuroprotective effects [47,48]. Hyperbaric oxygen, as a preconditioning method, also confers hypoxia tolerance by providing neuroprotection in the cerebral cortex, hippocampus, and spinal cord. It promotes the inhibition of neuronal apoptosis, reduces Caspase-3 expression, preventing DNA fragmentation and preserving cellular integrity [49].

4.2.9. Mitochondrial Function, Oxidative Stress, and Inflammatory Response

HBOT induces the production of reactive oxygen species (ROS), which can act as signals measuring physiological responses in mitochondria. Hyperbaric oxygen preserves mitochondrial integrity by maintaining the mitochondrial membrane potential and reducing the mitochondrial apoptosis pathway. It restores cellular respiration in cases of poisoning [50]. Additionally, hyperbaric oxygen treatment induces mitophagy [51]. Mitophagy activation is associated with a significant decrease in neuropathic pain [52]. Increased dissolved oxygen leads to a significant reduction in neuropathic pain. Hyperoxia can simultaneously stimulate an increase in ROS levels and antioxidant species, both enzymatic and non-enzymatic [53]. It can induce protection against oxidative stimuli in endothelial cells by overexpressing antioxidant genes following multiple hyperbaric oxygenation sessions in some tissues [23]. The short-term effect of HBOT generates stress and causes mitochondria to decrease their activity, partially reducing ROS production. However, in the long term, antioxidant activity increases, helping mitochondria function without altering the redox balance and even improving their activity [54]. The anti-inflammatory action mediated by HBOT leads to vasoconstriction, reducing edema and the inflammatory response. It also reduces the production and release of pro-inflammatory cytokines by neutrophils and monocytes [1,55]. HBOT has effects on cytokine production, reducing interleukin 1 (IL-1), interleukin 6 (IL-6), and tumor necrosis factor alpha (TNF-alpha), which are pro-inflammatory. VEGF (Vascular Endothelial Growth Factor), TGF-beta1 (Transforming Growth Factor Beta 1), and PDGF-beta (Platelet-Derived Growth Factor) exhibit biphasic release patterns. This means that they are released under both hypoxic and hyperoxic conditions. However, hyperoxia-stimulated release is greater, facilitating the healing process [56].

4.2.10. Regeneration

Studies have reported that hyperoxia generated by HBOT promotes regeneration mechanisms in various tissues, including the brain, spinal cord, bone, cartilage, cardiovascular tissue, and muscle. The observed regeneration can be explained by the effects of HBOT on the following processes: apoptosis, stem cell mobilization, oxidative stress response, inflammation, tissue remodeling, angiogenesis, cell–cell adhesion mechanisms, tissue regeneration, differentiation, and proliferation [57]. HBOT promotes axon regeneration, as hyperoxia-induced accumulation of anti-inflammatory cytokines and macrophage accumulation.

5. Safety

Hyperbaric oxygen therapy is an important complementary treatment for various pathologies, as mentioned earlier, and is currently a safe and available therapy with some reported adverse effects primarily at high pressures. The incidence of adverse events associated with HBOT is rare and generally not severe, encompassing conditions such as otic/sinus barotrauma, confinement anxiety, hypoglycemia, oxygen toxicity, ocular side effects, pneumothorax, seizure, and shortness of breath [58]. Absolute contraindications have been defined, such as untreated pneumothorax, and relative contraindications include the use of certain medications, asthma, pregnancy, claustrophobia, Chronic Obstructive Pulmonary Disease (COPD), insulin-dependent diabetes mellitus, or acute hypoglycemia, among others [59]. It is imperative to systematically assess the risk and benefit profiles at various treatment pressures and durations to standardize treatment protocols and enhance patient care.

Monge et al. demonstrated that HBOT at 1.45 atm using a portable chamber increases blood oxygen saturation, demonstrating hyperoxia, and was safer than other reported chambers, as adverse effects were milder, and no barotrauma was reported [60]. Similarly, Jaim and colleagues did not report adverse effects [13].

Other studies have shown the safety of treatment at 1.5 atm. Ilni and colleagues reported in healthy volunteers that at half-pressure, there were no observed changes in lung capacity [61]. Furthermore, there was no increase in IL6 and IL-8 in bronchoalveolar lavage, and no pulmonary or cerebral oxygen toxicity was observed [62]. Laboratory parameters studied in healthy individuals receiving HBOT at 1.45 atm showed no changes in hematological or hemostatic parameters, as well as in markers of inflammation and acute phase [63].

6. Methods

A literature search was performed in Pubmed to identify studies, conducted in the las 20 years that explore the use of HBOT at pressure above 1.45–1.5 ATA. The following search string was used: ("hyperbaric oxygenation" AND "hyperoxia" AND; "mild pressure") OR ("Hyperbaric Oxygen Therapy effects" AND "oxidative stress and HBOT" AND "1.5

ATA"). The review was focus on clinical approach in adult healthy subject or subjects with any pathology to whom tissue oxygen levels were measured. The search was restricted to articles published in English in peer-reviewed journals. No restriction on study design was imposed. Abstract presentations and conference proceedings were excluded.

Studies were manually selected based on the title and abstract. (See Table 1). Selected studies were read thoroughly to identify those suitable for inclusion in this review. We extracted the demographic and experimental data from the selected studies. For each study, the following relevant information was extracted and summarized: characteristics of the investigated population; oxygen administration protocols the experimental and/or clinical settings of application; and the main results of the studies in terms of level of oxygen and/or level of ROS enhancing effect on HIF-1α pathway.

Table 1. A summary of the main human studies demonstrating hyperoxia with hyperbaric oxygen treatment at mild pressure.

Author	Type of Study	Sample Size	Intervention	Main Results
Bosco et al. (2021) [23]	Randomized, patient-blinded, controlled trial (NCT04366427)	22 healthy humans.	100% O_2, HBOT 1.5 ATA, 60 min. 20 treatments	In plasmatic samples: Increase in ROS levels until day 14, followed by a decrease at the end of the treatment. Increase in total antioxidant capacity. Increase in glutathione and reduced cysteine. Decrease in IL-6 and IL-10.
Leveque et al. (2023) [5]	Human experimental study	47 healthy non-smoking Caucasian subjects	100% O_2, HBOT 1.4 ATA, 60 min. 1 treatment.	Increase of plasmatic ROS production similar kinetic respect 2.5 ATA. Increase in cysteinylglycine. Plasmatic Nitric oxide metabolites decrease after 2 h and return normal level al 24 h
Fratantorio et al. (2021) [6]	Human experimental study	20 healthy humans	1 h exposure to normobaric oxygen FiO_2 0.3 vs. normobaric oxygen FiO_2 1.0 vs. hyperbaric oxygen 1.4 bar FiO_2 1.4	Increase in NRF2 nuclear level and not significative changes in HIF after the first session in peripheral blood mononuclear cells. Increase glutathione and matrix metalloproteinase (MMPs) in plasma.
Niza et al. (2023) [27]	Clinical Trial (crossover randomized experimental study)	16 healthy women	1.4 ATA, with 35.0–39.5% oxygen concentration and 18 L of oxygen per minute injected into the hyperbaric chamber for 70 min.	Parasympathetic activity (Electrocardiography Analysis) was significantly increased. NK cells were increased without changes IL-6 and IL-12p70 protein levels in blood samples.
Rockswold et al. (2010) [20]	Randomized clinical trial	24 patients	100% FiO_2 (fraction of inspired oxygen) delivered for 60 min at 1.5 ATA. The NBH treatment consisted of 100% FiO_2 given for 3 h at 1.0 ATA	Mean brain tissue PO_2 levels were significantly increased after HBO_2 therapy.
Rockswold et al. (2013) [21]	Prospective randomized Phase II clinical trial (NCT00170352)	45 patients treated for severe TBI	100% FiO_2 delivered for 60 min at 1.5 ATA followed by 3 h at 1.0 ATA	Brain tissue PO_2 in both the noninjured and pericontusional brain rose during the treatment sessions to approximately 600% of the control group value. Decrease of microdialysate lactate in the pericontusional brain without change in the noninjured brain.

7. Conclusions

Hyperbaric oxygen treatment at 1.5 ATA increases dissolved oxygen levels, generating tissue hyperoxia and counteracting the effects of hypoxia by supplying the necessary oxygen to restore cellular respiration and mitochondrial function. The effect of HBOT also involves cellular responses that counteract oxidative stress effects by activating antioxidant mechanisms, and it acts on multiple processes such as angiogenesis and inflammation, among others, producing beneficial effects on various pathologies. These beneficial effects have been reported in a wide range of protocols, including various pressures, exposure times, and session numbers. Therefore, it will be necessary to conduct rigorous studies to adjust these variables for HBO therapy, whether as an independent or adjuvant treatment, in the numerous pathologies in which it may yield benefits, potentially leading to transformative therapeutic advancements in the future.

Author Contributions: Conceptualization, M.S.L.; Writing—Original Draft Preparation, M.S.L.; Writing—Review and Editing, M.C., M.S.L. and A.Y.G. All authors have read and agreed to the published version of the manuscript.

Funding: This research received no external funding.

Institutional Review Board Statement: Not applicable.

Informed Consent Statement: Not applicable.

Data Availability Statement: Not applicable.

Conflicts of Interest: M.C. is medical director and M.S.L. is scientific director in clinical research of Biobarica Hyperbaric Medical Centers. A.Y.G. declare no conflict of interest.

References

1. De Wolde, S.D.; Hulskes, R.H.; Weenink, R.P.; Hollmann, M.W.; Van Hulst, R.A. The Effects of Hyperbaric Oxygenation on Oxidative Stress, Inflammation and Angiogenesis. *Biomolecules* **2021**, *11*, 1210. [CrossRef] [PubMed]
2. Hadanny, A.; Efrati, S. The Hyperoxic-Hypoxic Paradox. *Biomolecules* **2020**, *10*, 958. [CrossRef] [PubMed]
3. Salvagno, M.; Coppalini, G.; Taccone, F.S.; Strapazzon, G.; Mrakic-Sposta, S.; Rocco, M.; Khalife, M.; Balestra, C. The Normobaric Oxygen Paradox—Hyperoxic Hypoxic Paradox: A Novel Expedient Strategy in Hematopoiesis Clinical Issues. *Int. J. Mol. Sci.* **2022**, *24*, 82. [CrossRef] [PubMed]
4. Moon, R.E. *Hyperbaric Oxygen Therapy Indications*, 14th ed.; Best Pub. Co.: North Palm Beach, FL, USA, 2019; ISBN 978-1-947239-16-6.
5. Leveque, C.; Mrakic Sposta, S.; Theunissen, S.; Germonpré, P.; Lambrechts, K.; Vezzoli, A.; Bosco, G.; Lévénez, M.; Lafère, P.; Guerrero, F.; et al. Oxidative Stress Response Kinetics after 60 Minutes at Different (1.4 ATA and 2.5 ATA) Hyperbaric Hyperoxia Exposures. *Int. J. Mol. Sci.* **2023**, *24*, 12361. [CrossRef]
6. Fratantonio, D.; Virgili, F.; Zucchi, A.; Lambrechts, K.; Latronico, T.; Lafère, P.; Germonpré, P.; Balestra, C. Increasing Oxygen Partial Pressures Induce a Distinct Transcriptional Response in Human PBMC: A Pilot Study on the "Normobaric Oxygen Paradox". *Int. J. Mol. Sci.* **2021**, *22*, 458. [CrossRef] [PubMed]
7. Chelombitko, M.A. Role of Reactive Oxygen Species in Inflammation: A Minireview. *Mosc. Univ. Biol. Sci. Bull.* **2018**, *73*, 199–202. [CrossRef]
8. Imray, C.; Wright, A.; Subudhi, A.; Roach, R. Acute Mountain Sickness: Pathophysiology, Prevention, and Treatment. *Prog. Cardiovasc. Dis.* **2010**, *52*, 467–484. [CrossRef]
9. Smedley, T.; Grocott, M.P. Acute High-Altitude Illness: A Clinically Orientated Review. *Br. J. Pain* **2013**, *7*, 85–94. [CrossRef]
10. Hafner, S.; Beloncle, F.; Koch, A.; Radermacher, P.; Asfar, P. Hyperoxia in Intensive Care, Emergency, and Peri-Operative Medicine: Dr. Jekyll or Mr. Hyde? A 2015 Update. *Ann. Intensive Care* **2015**, *5*, 42. [CrossRef]
11. Brugniaux, J.V.; Coombs, G.B.; Barak, O.F.; Dujic, Z.; Sekhon, M.S.; Ainslie, P.N. Highs and Lows of Hyperoxia: Physiological, Performance, and Clinical Aspects. *Am. J. Physiol. Regul. Integr. Comp. Physiol.* **2018**, *315*, R1–R27. [CrossRef]
12. Avishay, D.M.; Tenny, K.M. Henry's Law. In *StatPearls*; StatPearls Publishing: Treasure Island, FL, USA, 2023.
13. Jain, K.K. *Textbook of Hyperbaric Medicine*; Springer International Publishing: Cham, Switzerland, 2017; ISBN 978-3-319-47138-9.
14. Ishihara, A. Mild Hyperbaric Oxygen: Mechanisms and Effects. *J. Physiol. Sci.* **2019**, *69*, 573–580. [CrossRef] [PubMed]
15. Krogh, A. The Number and Distribution of Capillaries in Muscles with Calculations of the Oxygen Pressure Head Necessary for Supplying the Tissue. *J. Physiol.* **1919**, *52*, 409–415. [CrossRef] [PubMed]
16. Holbach, K.-H.; Wassmann, H.; Linke, D. The Use of Hyperbaric Oxygenation in the Treatment of Spinal Cord Lesions. *Eur. Neurol.* **1977**, *16*, 213–221. [CrossRef] [PubMed]
17. Singer, M.; Young, P.J.; Laffey, J.G.; Asfar, P.; Taccone, F.S.; Skrifvars, M.B.; Meyhoff, C.S.; Radermacher, P. Dangers of Hyperoxia. *Crit. Care* **2021**, *25*, 440. [CrossRef] [PubMed]

18. Yamamoto, N.; Takada, R.; Maeda, T.; Yoshii, T.; Okawa, A.; Yagishita, K. Microcirculation and Tissue Oxygenation in the Head and Limbs during Hyperbaric Oxygen Treatment. *Diving Hyperb. Med.* **2021**, *51*, 338–344. [CrossRef] [PubMed]
19. Zhou, Z.; Daugherty, W.P.; Sun, D.; Levasseur, J.E.; Altememi, N.; Hamm, R.J.; Rockswold, G.L.; Bullock, M.R. Protection of Mitochondrial Function and Improvement in Cognitive Recovery in Rats Treated with Hyperbaric Oxygen Following Lateral Fluid-Percussion Injury. *J. Neurosurg.* **2007**, *106*, 687–694. [CrossRef]
20. Rockswold, S.B.; Rockswold, G.L.; Zaun, D.A.; Zhang, X.; Cerra, C.E.; Bergman, T.A.; Liu, J. A Prospective, Randomized Clinical Trial to Compare the Effect of Hyperbaric to Normobaric Hyperoxia on Cerebral Metabolism, Intracranial Pressure, and Oxygen Toxicity in Severe Traumatic Brain Injury: Clinical Article. *J. Neurosurg.* **2010**, *112*, 1080–1094. [CrossRef]
21. Rockswold, S.B.; Rockswold, G.L.; Zaun, D.A.; Liu, J. A Prospective, Randomized Phase II Clinical Trial to Evaluate the Effect of Combined Hyperbaric and Normobaric Hyperoxia on Cerebral Metabolism, Intracranial Pressure, Oxygen Toxicity, and Clinical Outcome in Severe Traumatic Brain Injury. *J. Neurosurg.* **2013**, *118*, 1317–1328. [CrossRef]
22. un Nisa, B.; Kondo, H.; Ishihara, A.; Hidemi, F. Beneficial Effects Of Exposure to Mild Hyperbaric Oxygen on Microcirculation in Peripheral Tissues: 857 May 27 4:05 PM–4:15 PM. *Med. Sci. Sports Exerc.* **2020**, *52*, 208. [CrossRef]
23. Bosco, G.; Paganini, M.; Giacon, T.A.; Oppio, A.; Vezzoli, A.; Dellanoce, C.; Moro, T.; Paoli, A.; Zanotti, F.; Zavan, B.; et al. Oxidative Stress and Inflammation, MicroRNA, and Hemoglobin Variations after Administration of Oxygen at Different Pressures and Concentrations: A Randomized Trial. *Int. J. Environ. Res. Public Health* **2021**, *18*, 9755. [CrossRef]
24. Woo, J.; Min, J.-H.; Lee, Y.-H.; Roh, H.-T. Effects of Hyperbaric Oxygen Therapy on Inflammation, Oxidative/Antioxidant Balance, and Muscle Damage after Acute Exercise in Normobaric, Normoxic and Hypobaric, Hypoxic Environments: A Pilot Study. *Int. J. Environ. Res. Public Health* **2020**, *17*, 7377. [CrossRef] [PubMed]
25. Benson, R.M.; Minter, L.M.; Osborne, B.A.; Granowitz, E.V. Hyperbaric Oxygen Inhibits Stimulus-Induced Proinflammatory Cytokine Synthesis by Human Blood-Derived Monocyte-Macrophages. *Clin. Exp. Immunol.* **2003**, *134*, 57–62. [CrossRef] [PubMed]
26. Balestra, C.; Germonpré, P.; Poortmans, J.R.; Marroni, A. Serum Erythropoietin Levels in Healthy Humans after a Short Period of Normobaric and Hyperbaric Oxygen Breathing: The "Normobaric Oxygen Paradox". *J. Appl. Physiol.* **2006**, *100*, 512–518. [CrossRef] [PubMed]
27. Nisa, B.U.; Nakanishi, R.; Tanaka, M.; Lin, H.; Hirabayashi, T.; Maeshige, N.; Kondo, H.; Fujino, H. Mild Hyperbaric Oxygen Exposure Enhances Peripheral Circulatory Natural Killer Cells in Healthy Young Women. *Life* **2023**, *13*, 408. [CrossRef] [PubMed]
28. LL TA—Hyperbaric Oxygen Therapy in Treatment of Hypoxic Wounds. Available online: https://www.cms.gov/medicare-coverage-database/view/technology-assessments.aspx?taid=12 (accessed on 20 September 2023).
29. Choudhury, R. Hypoxia and Hyperbaric Oxygen Therapy: A Review. *Int. J. Gen. Med.* **2018**, *11*, 431–442. [CrossRef] [PubMed]
30. Oliaei, S.; SeyedAlinaghi, S.; Mehrtak, M.; Karimi, A.; Noori, T.; Mirzapour, P.; Shojaei, A.; MohsseniPour, M.; Mirghaderi, S.P.; Alilou, S.; et al. The Effects of Hyperbaric Oxygen Therapy (HBOT) on Coronavirus Disease-2019 (COVID-19): A Systematic Review. *Eur. J. Med. Res.* **2021**, *26*, 96. [CrossRef]
31. Cannellotto, M.; Duarte, M.; Keller, G.; Larrea, R.; Cunto, E.; Chediack, V.; Mansur, M.; Brito, D.M.; García, E.; Di Salvo, H.E.; et al. Hyperbaric Oxygen as an Adjuvant Treatment for Patients with COVID-19 Severe Hypoxaemia: A Randomised Controlled Trial. *Emerg. Med. J.* **2022**, *39*, 88–93. [CrossRef]
32. Schipke, J.D.; Muth, T.; Pepper, C.; Schneppendahl, J.; Hoffmanns, M.; Dreyer, S. Hyperoxia and the Cardiovascular System: Experiences with Hyperbaric Oxygen Therapy. *Med. Gas Res.* **2022**, *12*, 153–157. [CrossRef]
33. Whalen, R.E.; Saltzman, H.A.; Holloway, D.H.; Mcintosh, H.D.; Sieker, H.O.; Brown, I.W. Cardiovascular and blood gas responses to hyperbaric oxygenation. *Am. J. Cardiol.* **1965**, *15*, 638–646. [CrossRef]
34. Sunkari, V.G.; Lind, F.; Botusan, I.R.; Kashif, A.; Liu, Z.-J.; Ylä-Herttuala, S.; Brismar, K.; Velazquez, O.; Catrina, S.-B. Hyperbaric Oxygen Therapy Activates Hypoxia-Inducible Factor 1 (HIF-1), Which Contributes to Improved Wound Healing in Diabetic Mice. *Wound Repair Regen.* **2015**, *23*, 98–103. [CrossRef]
35. Buckley, C.J.; Cooper, J.S. Hyperbaric Oxygen Effects On Angiogenesis. In *StatPearls*; StatPearls Publishing: Treasure Island, FL, USA, 2023.
36. Liu, Z.-J.; Velazquez, O.C. Hyperoxia, Endothelial Progenitor Cell Mobilization, and Diabetic Wound Healing. *Antioxid. Redox Signal.* **2008**, *10*, 1869–1882. [CrossRef] [PubMed]
37. Thom, S.R.; Bhopale, V.M.; Velazquez, O.C.; Goldstein, L.J.; Thom, L.H.; Buerk, D.G. Stem Cell Mobilization by Hyperbaric Oxygen. *Am. J. Physiol. Heart Circ. Physiol.* **2006**, *290*, H1378–H1386. [CrossRef] [PubMed]
38. Goldstein, L.J.; Gallagher, K.A.; Bauer, S.M.; Bauer, R.J.; Baireddy, V.; Liu, Z.-J.; Buerk, D.G.; Thom, S.R.; Velazquez, O.C. Endothelial Progenitor Cell Release into Circulation Is Triggered by Hyperoxia-Induced Increases in Bone Marrow Nitric Oxide. *Stem Cells* **2006**, *24*, 2309–2318. [CrossRef] [PubMed]
39. Chen, C.; Yang, Y.; Yao, Y. HBO Promotes the Differentiation of Neural Stem Cells via Interactions Between the Wnt3/β-Catenin and BMP2 Signaling Pathways. *Cell Transpl.* **2019**, *28*, 1686–1699. [CrossRef]
40. Ishii, Y.; Miyanaga, Y.; Shimojo, H.; Ushida, T.; Tateishi, T. Effects of Hyperbaric Oxygen on Procollagen Messenger RNA Levels and Collagen Synthesis in the Healing of Rat Tendon Laceration. *Tissue Eng.* **1999**, *5*, 279–286. [CrossRef]
41. Gajendrareddy, P.K.; Junges, R.; Cygan, G.; Zhao, Y.; Marucha, P.T.; Engeland, C.G. Increased Oxygen Exposure Alters Collagen Expression and Tissue Architecture during Ligature-Induced Periodontitis. *J. Periodontal. Res.* **2017**, *52*, 644–649. [CrossRef] [PubMed]

42. Wu, D.; Malda, J.; Crawford, R.; Xiao, Y. Effects of Hyperbaric Oxygen on Proliferation and Differentiation of Osteoblasts from Human Alveolar Bone. *Connect. Tissue Res.* **2007**, *48*, 206–213. [CrossRef] [PubMed]
43. Al Hadi, H.; Smerdon, G.R.; Fox, S.W. Hyperbaric Oxygen Therapy Accelerates Osteoblast Differentiation and Promotes Bone Formation. *J. Dent.* **2015**, *43*, 382–388. [CrossRef]
44. Wang, J.; Zhao, B.; Che, J.; Shang, P. Hypoxia Pathway in Osteoporosis: Laboratory Data for Clinical Prospects. *Int. J. Environ. Res. Public Health* **2023**, *20*, 3129. [CrossRef]
45. Lima, F.L.; Joazeiro, P.P.; Lancellotti, M.; de Hollanda, L.M.; de Araújo Lima, B.; Linares, E.; Augusto, O.; Brocchi, M.; Giorgio, S. Effects of Hyperbaric Oxygen on Pseudomonas Aeruginosa Susceptibility to Imipenem and Macrophages. *Future Microbiol.* **2015**, *10*, 179–189. [CrossRef]
46. Memar, M.Y.; Yekani, M.; Alizadeh, N.; Baghi, H.B. Hyperbaric Oxygen Therapy: Antimicrobial Mechanisms and Clinical Application for Infections. *Biomed. Pharmacother.* **2019**, *109*, 440–447. [CrossRef] [PubMed]
47. Sun, L.; Marti, H.H.; Veltkamp, R. Hyperbaric Oxygen Reduces Tissue Hypoxia and Hypoxia-Inducible Factor-1 Alpha Expression in Focal Cerebral Ischemia. *Stroke* **2008**, *39*, 1000–1006. [CrossRef] [PubMed]
48. Gu, G.-J.; Li, Y.-P.; Peng, Z.-Y.; Xu, J.-J.; Kang, Z.-M.; Xu, W.-G.; Tao, H.-Y.; Ostrowski, R.P.; Zhang, J.H.; Sun, X.-J. Mechanism of Ischemic Tolerance Induced by Hyperbaric Oxygen Preconditioning Involves Upregulation of Hypoxia-Inducible Factor-1alpha and Erythropoietin in Rats. *J. Appl. Physiol.* **2008**, *104*, 1185–1191. [CrossRef] [PubMed]
49. Yang, C.; Yang, Q.; Xiang, Y.; Zeng, X.-R.; Xiao, J.; Le, W.-D. The Neuroprotective Effects of Oxygen Therapy in Alzheimer's Disease: A Narrative Review. *Neural Regen. Res.* **2022**, *18*, 57–63. [CrossRef]
50. Tezgin, D.; Giardina, C.; Perdrizet, G.A.; Hightower, L.E. The Effect of Hyperbaric Oxygen on Mitochondrial and Glycolytic Energy Metabolism: The Caloristasis Concept. *Cell Stress Chaperones* **2020**, *25*, 667–677. [CrossRef] [PubMed]
51. Han, G.; Liu, K.; Li, L.; Li, X.; Zhao, P. The Effects of Hyperbaric Oxygen Therapy on Neuropathic Pain via Mitophagy in Microglia. *Mol. Pain* **2017**, *13*, 1744806917710862. [CrossRef]
52. Kun, L.; Lu, L.; Yongda, L.; Xingyue, L.; Guang, H. Hyperbaric Oxygen Promotes Mitophagy by Activating CaMKKβ/AMPK Signal Pathway in Rats of Neuropathic Pain. *Mol. Pain* **2019**, *15*, 1744806919871381. [CrossRef] [PubMed]
53. Godman, C.A.; Joshi, R.; Giardina, C.; Perdrizet, G.; Hightower, L.E. Hyperbaric Oxygen Treatment Induces Antioxidant Gene Expression. *Ann. N. Y. Acad. Sci.* **2010**, *1197*, 178–183. [CrossRef]
54. Schottlender, N.; Gottfried, I.; Ashery, U. Hyperbaric Oxygen Treatment: Effects on Mitochondrial Function and Oxidative Stress. *Biomolecules* **2021**, *11*, 1827. [CrossRef]
55. de Wolde, S.D.; Hulskes, R.H.; de Jonge, S.W.; Hollmann, M.W.; van Hulst, R.A.; Weenink, R.P.; Kox, M. The Effect of Hyperbaric Oxygen Therapy on Markers of Oxidative Stress and the Immune Response in Healthy Volunteers. *Front. Physiol.* **2022**, *13*, 826163. [CrossRef]
56. Capó, X.; Monserrat-Mesquida, M.; Quetglas-Llabrés, M.; Batle, J.M.; Tur, J.A.; Pons, A.; Sureda, A.; Tejada, S. Hyperbaric Oxygen Therapy Reduces Oxidative Stress and Inflammation, and Increases Growth Factors Favouring the Healing Process of Diabetic Wounds. *Int. J. Mol. Sci.* **2023**, *24*, 7040. [CrossRef] [PubMed]
57. Lindenmann, J.; Kamolz, L.; Graier, W.; Smolle, J.; Smolle-Juettner, F.-M. Hyperbaric Oxygen Therapy and Tissue Regeneration: A Literature Survey. *Biomedicines* **2022**, *10*, 3145. [CrossRef] [PubMed]
58. Zhang, Y.; Zhou, Y.; Jia, Y.; Wang, T.; Meng, D. Adverse Effects of Hyperbaric Oxygen Therapy: A Systematic Review and Meta-Analysis. *Front. Med.* **2023**, *10*, 1160774. [CrossRef] [PubMed]
59. Gawdi, R.; Cooper, J.S. Hyperbaric Contraindications. In *StatPearls*; StatPearls Publishing: Treasure Island, FL, USA, 2023.
60. Monge, G.; Otto, M.; Norambuena, N.; Martínez, V.; Retamales, D.; Torres-Castro, R. Safety of Hyperbaric Oxygenation Treatment and Evaluation of Associated Clinical Parameters: A Single-Institutional Prospective Cohort Study. *Int. J. Transl. Med. Res. Public Health* **2023**, *7*. [CrossRef]
61. Ilmi, M.I.; Yunus, F.; Guritno, M.; Damayanti, T.; Samoedro, E.; Nazaruddin, A.M.; Nurwidya, F. Comparison of Lung Function Values of Trained Divers in 1.5 ATA Hyperbaric Chamber after Inhaling 100% Oxygen and Regular Air: A Crossover Study. *Adv. Respir. Med.* **2017**, *85*, 233–238. [CrossRef]
62. Daly, S.; Thorpe, M.; Rockswold, S.; Hubbard, M.; Bergman, T.; Samadani, U.; Rockswold, G. Hyperbaric Oxygen Therapy in the Treatment of Acute Severe Traumatic Brain Injury: A Systematic Review. *J. Neurotrauma* **2018**, *35*, 623–629. [CrossRef]
63. Jordá-Vargas, L.; Cannellotto, M. Terapia de oxigenación hiperbárica en individuos sanos: Efecto en algunos parámetros bioquímicos. *Acta Bioquím. Clín. Latinoam.* **2019**, *53*, 15–23.

Disclaimer/Publisher's Note: The statements, opinions and data contained in all publications are solely those of the individual author(s) and contributor(s) and not of MDPI and/or the editor(s). MDPI and/or the editor(s) disclaim responsibility for any injury to people or property resulting from any ideas, methods, instructions or products referred to in the content.

International Journal of
Molecular Sciences

MDPI

Article

Hyperbaric Oxygen Reduces Oxidative Stress Impairment and DNA Damage and Simultaneously Increases HIF-1α in Ischemia–Reperfusion Acute Kidney Injury

Jelena Nesovic Ostojic [1,*,†], Sanjin Kovacevic [1,†], Milan Ivanov [2], Predrag Brkic [3], Maja Zivotic [4], Nevena Mihailovic-Stanojevic [2], Danijela Karanovic [2], Una Jovana Vajic [2], Rada Jeremic [3], Djurdjica Jovovic [2] and Zoran Miloradovic [2]

1 Department of Pathological Physiology, Faculty of Medicine, University of Belgrade, 11000 Belgrade, Serbia; sanjin.kovacevic@med.bg.ac.rs

2 Department of Cardiovascular Physiology, Institute for Medical Research, National Institute of Republic of Serbia, University of Belgrade, 11000 Belgrade, Serbia; ivmilan@imi.bg.ac.rs (M.I.); nevena@imi.bg.ac.rs (N.M.-S.); danijela.karanovic@imi.bg.ac.rs (D.K.); unajovana@imi.bg.ac.rs (U.J.V.); djurdjica@imi.bg.ac.rs (D.J.); zokim@imi.bg.ac.rs (Z.M.)

3 Department of Medical Physiology, Faculty of Medicine, University of Belgrade, 11000 Belgrade, Serbia; predrag.brkic@med.bg.ac.rs (P.B.); rada.jeremic@med.bg.ac.rs (R.J.)

4 Institute of Pathology, Faculty of Medicine, University of Belgrade, 11000 Belgrade, Serbia; maja.zivotic@med.bg.ac.rs

* Correspondence: jelena.nesovic-ostojic@med.bg.ac.rs; Tel./Fax: +381-11-2685340

† These authors contributed equally to this work.

Abstract: The central exacerbating factor in the pathophysiology of ischemic–reperfusion acute kidney injury (AKI) is oxidative stress. Lipid peroxidation and DNA damage in ischemia are accompanied by the formation of 3-nitrotyrosine, a biomarker for oxidative damage. DNA double-strand breaks (DSBs) may also be a result of postischemic AKI. γH2AX(S139) histone has been identified as a potentially useful biomarker of DNA DSBs. On the other hand, hypoxia-inducible factor (HIF) is the "master switch" for hypoxic adaptation in cells and tissues. The aim of this research was to evaluate the influence of hyperbaric oxygen (HBO) preconditioning on antioxidant capacity estimated by FRAP (ferric reducing antioxidant power) and ABTS (2,2′-azino-bis(3-ethylbenzothiazoline-6-sulfonic acid)) assay, as well as on oxidative stress parameter 3-nitrotyrosine, and to assess its effects on γH2AX(S139), HIF-1α, and nuclear factor-κB (NF-κB) expression, in an experimental model of postischemic AKI induced in spontaneously hypertensive rats. The animals were divided randomly into three experimental groups: sham-operated rats (SHAM, $n = 6$), rats with induced postischemic AKI (AKI, $n = 6$), and group exposed to HBO preconditioning before AKI induction (AKI + HBO, $n = 6$). A significant improvement in the estimated glomerular filtration rate, eGFR, in AKI + HBO group ($p < 0.05$ vs. AKI group) was accompanied with a significant increase in plasma antioxidant capacity estimated by FRAP ($p < 0.05$ vs. SHAM group) and a reduced immunohistochemical expression of 3-nitrotyrosine and γH2AX(S139). Also, HBO pretreatment significantly increased HIF-1α expression ($p < 0.001$ vs. AKI group), estimated by Western blot and immunohistochemical analysis in kidney tissue, and decreased immunohistochemical NF-κB renal expression ($p < 0.01$). Taking all of these results together, we may conclude that HBO preconditioning has beneficial effects on acute kidney injury induced in spontaneously hypertensive rats.

Keywords: oxidative stress; FRAP; 3-nitrotyrosine; γH2AX(S139); HIF-1α; NF-κB; spontaneously hypertensive rats; HBO preconditioning

1. Introduction

Acute kidney injury (AKI) is defined as a sudden decrease in glomerular filtration rate (GFR), which includes structural damage and loss of function [1], leading to azotemia and often oliguria or anuria. In hospital settings, AKI commonly occurs in patients who underwent cardiac and other complex surgery [2], sepsis [3], renal transplantation [4], and reparation of an aneurysm [5]. The main risk factors include diabetes, hypertension, and peripheral artery disease [6]. AKI is also recognized as an increasing healthcare challenge [3], due to its rising incidence, complex pathophysiology, and limited treatment. A large number of studies have been directed at elucidating pathogenesis and developing AKI therapeutics in animal models [7,8]. However, to date, none of these therapies have been translated into clinical practice [9].

The most common cause of AKI is renal ischemia–reperfusion injury (IRI) [10]. Several mechanisms are involved in the pathophysiology of IRI, but the literature data confirm that oxidative stress plays a crucial role in this process and is recognized as a central deleterious factor [11,12] especially in the reperfusion phase, when the most IRI damage might occur.

An increased level of reactive oxygen species (ROS) that cannot be regulated by endogenous antioxidants promotes inflammation, vascular dysfunction, and renal tubule cell cytotoxicity, all of which are observed in the pathogenesis of AKI [13]. In addition, DNA damage, including physical DNA double-strand breaks (DSBs), and oxidative base modifications may also be a result of renal IRI [14]. Gama H2AX is the phosphorylated form of the histone H2AX at serine 139 (γH2AX(S139)), [15] and because of its sensitivity and utility for the detection of DNA double-strand breaks, γH2AX(S139) has been identified as a potentially useful biomarker with clinical implications [16]. Previously, in our investigation, we showed that γH2AX(S139) may be used to indicate DNA damage that follows ischemia–reperfusion AKI [17]. On the other hand, lipid peroxidation and DNA damage in ischemia are associated with the formation of 3-nitrotyrosine, a biomarker for ROS/reactive nitrogen species (RNS), suggesting that $NO^{\bullet}$, $O_2^{\bullet-}$, and/or peroxynitrite, contribute to renal oxidative damage [18,19]. In addition, postischemic AKI is accompanied by inflammation [20], and nuclear factor κB (NF-κB) serves as a central mediator of inflammatory response [21].

At the same time, cellular hypoxia is one of the most powerful inducers of gene expression, metabolic changes, and regenerative processes [22] in order to survive unfavorable hypoxic conditions. Hypoxia-inducible factor (HIF) is the "master switch" for hypoxic adaptation in cells and tissues. In kidneys, as in other organs, HIF improves the tolerance to conditions of hypoxia or ischemia in vivo, but HIF is often suboptimal under these conditions. Thus, there is a great therapeutic potential to activate or target HIF [23].

The therapeutical basis of hyperbaric oxygenation (HBO) is to create a hyperbaric environment with pure oxygen that allows for a significant increase in the oxygen supply to blood and to the tissues even without the Hb involvement [24], so it could be used to fix tissue hypoxia and chronic hypoxemia and to help in the clinical approach to reperfusion injuries [25]. In contrast to hypoxia, the human body has not developed specific adaptative mechanisms to hyperoxia. Moreover, the exposure to intermittent hyperoxia activates cellular mechanisms and mediators which are induced by hypoxia [22]. Actually, similar with intermittent hypoxia, the exposure to short-term hyperoxia may provoke favorable outcomes in the cell. This led us to the idea that hyperbaric oxygenation preconditioning may be beneficial in cases with a high risk of developing postischemic AKI. High PO_2 in the tissues during HBO also leads to an increased production of ROS and RNS that may have important implications in the cellular signaling, resulting in the synthesis of different growth factors, thus improving neovascularization and showing immunomodulatory properties [26,27], which contribute to clinical efficacy of hyperbaric oxygenation. Moreover, HBO therapy upregulates HIF via ROS/RNS and Extracellular Regulated Kinases (ERK1/ERK2) pathways [22,28].

In our previous studies performed on the same experimental model of postischemic AKI, we showed that hyperbaric oxygen used for preconditioning may be beneficial on the pathogenesis of acute kidney injury [29–31], and now we wanted to go further into elucidating these protective effects with the aim of this research to evaluate the influence of hyperbaric oxygen (HBO) preconditioning on antioxidant capacity estimated via a FRAP (ferric reducing antioxidant power) and ABTS (2,2′-azino-bis(3-ethylbenzothiazoline-6-sulfonic acid) assay, as well as on oxidative stress parameter 3-nitrotyrosine, and to gain more insights into the mechanisms of HBO preconditioning by assessing its effects on γH2AX histone, HIF-1α, and NF-κB expression in an experimental model of postischemic AKI induced in spontaneously hypertensive rats.

2. Results

2.1. Estimated Glomerular Filtration Rate (eGFR)

In order to evaluate the experimental procedure, the eGFR was calculated. In the group with induced postischemic AKI, a significantly decreased eGFR was noticed in comparison to the sham-operated rats ($p < 0.001$, Figure 1), while in group with HBO preconditioning, eGFR was significantly increased in comparison to the AKI group ($p < 0.05$, Figure 1).

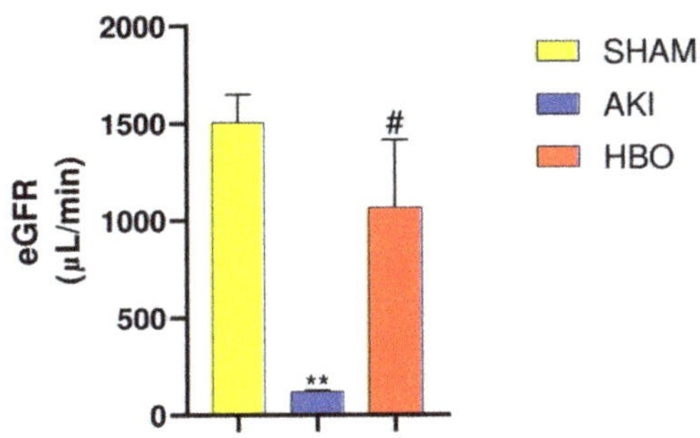

Figure 1. Estimated glomerular filtration rate in different experimental groups. One-way ANOVA with Tukey's post hoc test: ** $p < 0.01$ vs. SHAM group; # $p < 0.05$ vs. AKI group.

2.2. Antioxidant Capacity of Plasma

Regarding the antioxidant capacity of plasma, estimated with a FRAP assay (Figure 2A) and ABTS assay (Figure 2B), no significant difference was found among the groups in this experimental setting, with the exception that the group with HBO preconditioning had a significantly increased antioxidant capacity, when considering the FRAP assay in comparison to SHAM-operated rats.

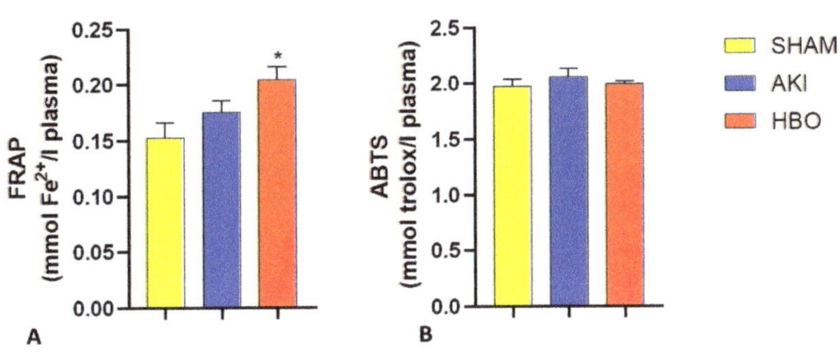

Figure 2. Antioxidant capacity of plasma, estimated via FRAP (**A**) and ABTS (**B**) assay in different experimental groups. One-way ANOVA with Tukey's post hoc test: * $p < 0.05$ vs. SHAM group.

2.3. Immunohistochemical Analysis

2.3.1. 3-Nitrotyrosine (3-NT) Expression

In SHAM-operated rats (Figure 3A), 3-NT expression was minimal, only focally present in peritubular capillaries and glomeruli, without tubular expression. In the AKI group, strong and abundant tubular expression of 3-NT, along with expression in glomeruli and peritubular capillaries, was noticed (Figure 3B). HBO preconditioning led to an evident decrease in 3-NT intensity and the extent of expression in all of the aforementioned structures (Figure 3C).

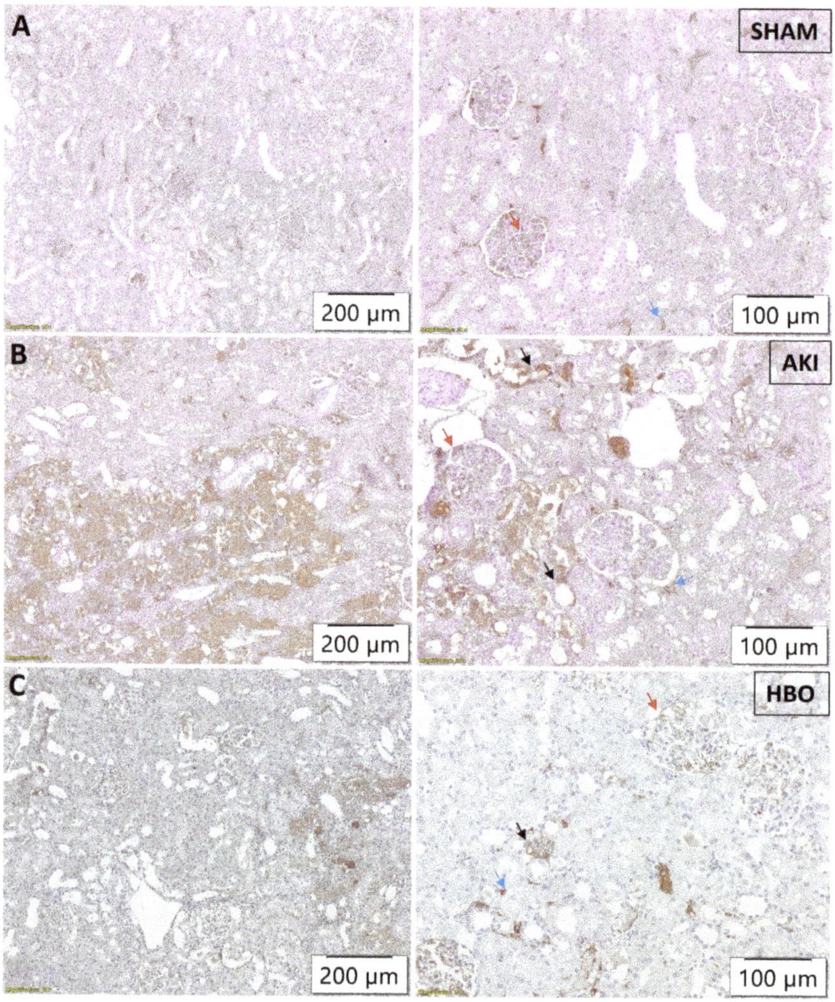

Figure 3. Immunohistochemical 3-NT expression in glomeruli (red arrows), tubules (black arrows), and peritubular capillaries (blue arrows) in representative kidney samples collected in different experimental groups: SHAM (**A**), AKI (**B**), and HBO (**C**).

2.3.2. Histone γH2AX(S139) Expression

In the SHAM-operated group, histone γH2AX(S139) was expressed in the nuclei of proximal tubular epithelial cells in cortical kidney parenchyma to varying extents, mostly pronounced in subcapsular cortical area, with decreased expression in the middle cortical zone, and even more decreased in the juxtamedullary cortical zone. Since the medulla does not contain proximal tubules, this kidney zone did not express γH2AX(S139) (Figure 4A). In the AKI group, an evidently higher extent of expression was detected in the nuclei of cortical proximal tubular cells, with more pronounced expression in the subcapsular region, middle cortex, and juxtamedullary cortical zone (Figure 4B) in comparison to the control group. HBO preconditioning led to an evident decrease in γH2AX(S139) expression in all observed cortical structures (Figure 4C), with expression more pronounced in comparison to the SHAM-operated rats, but less abundant and present in less proximal tubular epithelial cells in comparison to the AKI group.

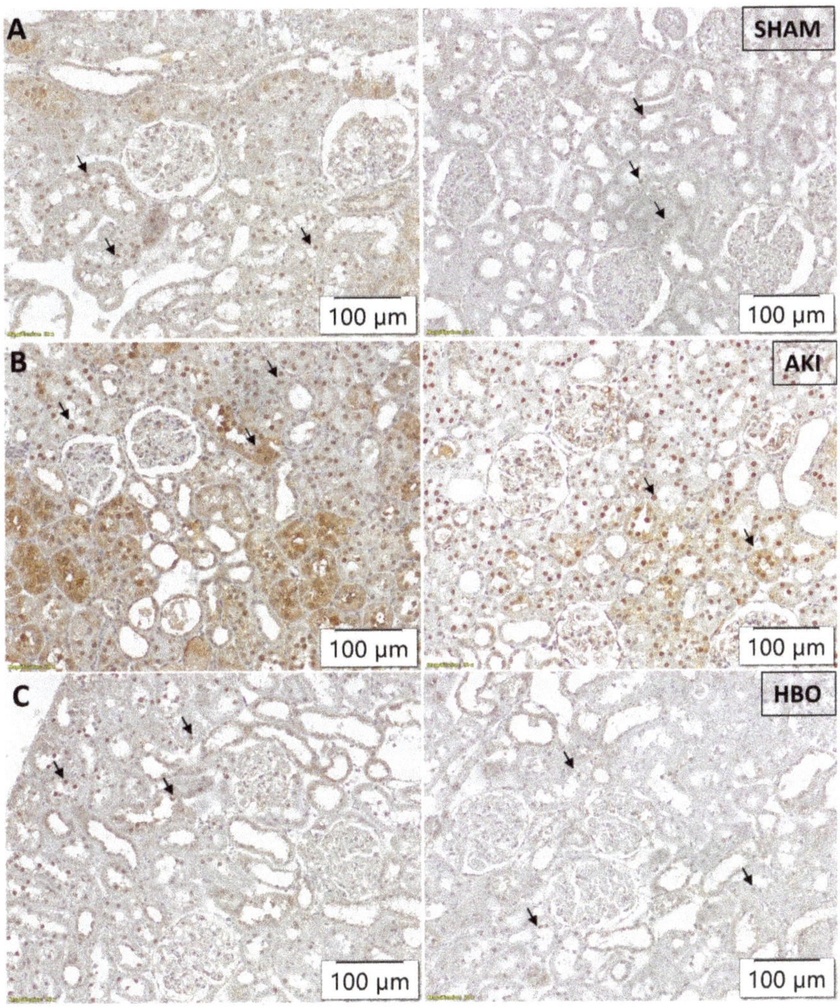

Figure 4. Immunohistochemical histone γH2AX(S139) expression in the nuclei of proximal tubular epithelial cells (arrows) in subcortical and middle cortical area of representative kidney samples collected in different experimental groups: SHAM (**A**), AKI (**B**), and HBO (**C**).

2.3.3. NF-κB Expression

In SHAM-operated rats (Figure 5A), NF-κB expression was minimal, only focally present in peritubular capillaries and glomeruli, without tubular expression. In the AKI group, strong and abundant nuclear and cytoplasmatic tubular expression, along with expression in glomeruli and peritubular capillaries, was noticed (Figure 5B). In the group with HBO preconditioning evident, decreases in the intensity and extent of expression in all of the aforementioned structures were noticed (Figure 5C).

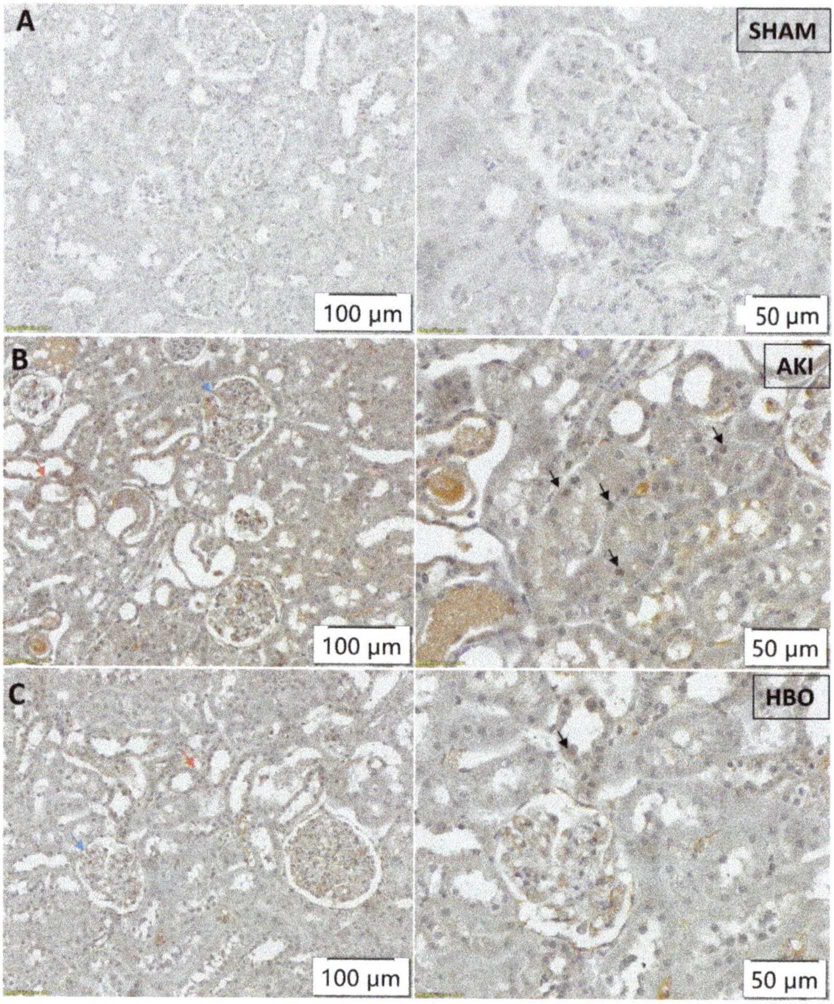

Figure 5. Immunohistochemical NF-κB expression in glomeruli (blue arrows), tubules (red arrows), and nuclei of tubular epithelial cells (black arrows) in representative kidney samples collected in different experimental groups: SHAM (**A**), AKI (**B**), and HBO (**C**).

In order to evaluate the obtained results, a semi-quantitative analysis was performed. The immunohistochemical score of 3-NT (Figure 6A), histone γH2AX(S139) (Figure 6B), and NF-κB (Figure 6C) expression was significantly higher in the AKI group compared to control group (3-NT, $p < 0.001$; γH2AX(S139), $p < 0.001$; NF-κB, $p < 0.001$). In comparison with the AKI group, the immunohistochemical scores for both parameters were significantly lower for the group with hyperbaric oxygen preconditioning (3-NT, $p < 0.01$; γH2AX(S139), $p < 0.05$; NF-κB, $p < 0.01$).

2.3.4. Hypoxia-Inducible Factor 1α (HIF-1α) Expression

In the SHAM group, the expression of HIF-1α was of moderate intensity, mostly in the cytoplasm of the tubular epithelial cells, with minimal expression in other kidney structures (Figure 7A). In response to hypoxic conditions after AKI induction, the expression pattern was different considering that previously noticed in the SHAM group, with HIF-1α translocation, and we observed both nuclear and cytoplasmatic expressions in tubular cells (Figure 7B). By observing the results of the immunohistochemical HIF-1 expression in the AKI + HBO group (Figure 7C) and comparing them with those of the AKI group, it was not clear if HBO preconditioning affected HIF-1 tissue expression, and in order to evaluate those results, we also performed a Western blot analysis to quantify the HIF-1α expression.

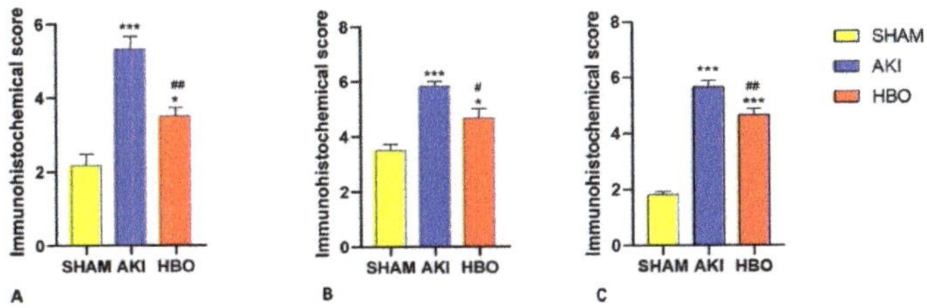

Figure 6. Immunohistochemical score of 3-nitrotyrosine (3-NT) (**A**), histone γH2AX(S139) (**B**), and NF-κB (**C**) expression in different experimental groups. One-way ANOVA with Tukey's post hoc test: *** $p < 0.001$; * $p < 0.05$ vs. SHAM group; ## $p < 0.01$; # $p < 0.05$ vs. AKI group.

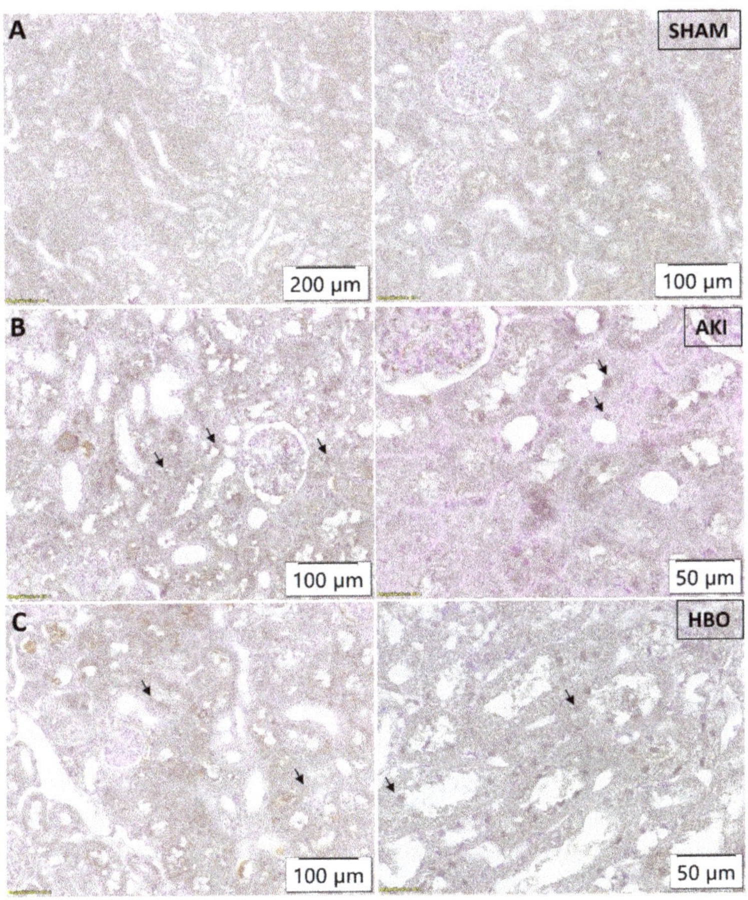

Figure 7. Immunohistochemical HIF-1α expression in representative kidney samples collected in different experimental groups: SHAM (**A**), AKI (**B**), HBO (**C**), and tubular nuclear expression (arrows).

2.4. Western Blot Analysis of Hypoxia-Inducible Factor 1α (HIF-1α) Expression

The Western blot analysis showed significantly increased HIF-1α expression after AKI induction in comparison to the SHAM-operated rats ($p < 0.001$). Nevertheless, the expression was even more pronounced in the group with hyperbaric oxygen preconditioning compared to the AKI group ($p < 0.001$; Figure 8).

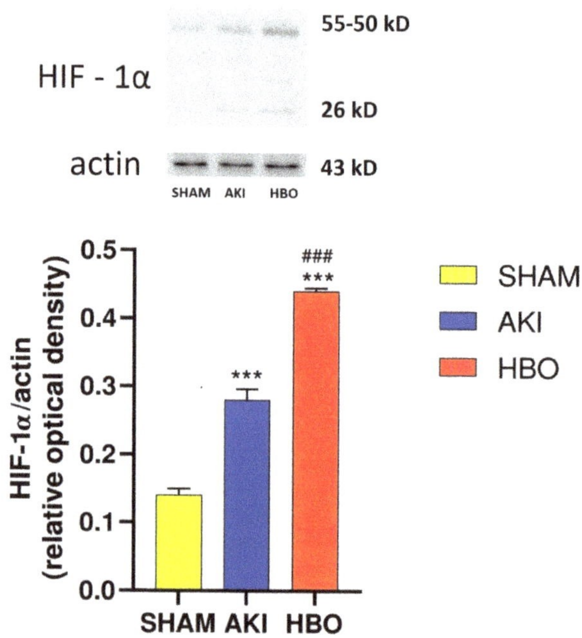

Figure 8. HIF-1α expression in different experimental groups: SHAM, AKI, and HBO. One-way ANOVA with Tukey's post hoc test: *** $p < 0.001$ vs. SHAM group; ### $p < 0.001$ vs. AKI group.

3. Discussion

In animals with induced postischemic AKI, we registered a drastic drop in eGFR, which was also a confirmation that the experimental model was adequately performed. In the group of animals exposed to HBO preconditioning, we noted a significant improvement in eGFR, indicating a general protective effect of this pretreatment in postischemic AKI. Previously, we showed that HBO used before AKI induction improved the renal hemodynamic by increasing renal blood flow and decreasing renal vascular resistance [29], and this result is in the line with the improvement in eGFR that we observed in the present study. Reduced renal blood flow accompanied by tissue hypoxia has been proposed as an important factor in the pathogenesis of postischemic AKI by initiating the activation of multiple mechanisms, including increased oxidative stress, inflammation, apoptosis, DNA damage, and necrosis [14,20]. In this research, we focused on tissue oxidative stress and systemic antioxidant capacity during AKI by evaluating the effects of HBO preconditioning on 3-NT immunohistochemical expression and plasma FRAP and ABTS levels.

In the SHAM group, we detected 3-NT expression only focally in peritubular capillaries and glomeruli. It is not surprising, considering that our experimental animals were spontaneously hypertensive rats, and hypertension is accompanied with oxidative stress [32]. But in AKI, strong and abundant tubular immunohistochemical expression of 3-NT was presented, along with expression in glomeruli and peritubular capillaries, which can be related to the increase in oxidative stress during acute kidney injury. In the kidney, NADPH oxidase and the mitochondrial respiratory chain are considered to be the main sources of ROS production [33]. As the level of oxidative stress increases, ROS and RNS promote oxidative damage and cellular death [6,13], playing a very important role in pathogenesis of postischemic AKI. These molecules directly and indirectly affect all aspects of the renal function, including vascular reactivity, renal hemodynamics, glomerular filtration, tubular reabsorption, and secretion [13]. Also, oxidative stress exerts harmful effects on biomolecules, such as proteins, DNA, RNA, enzymes, and lipids. Actually, the changes that reactive species (RS) make upon these molecules could be added up and used as biomarkers of oxidative stress [34]. The nitration of tyrosine residues to 3-nitrotyrosine in proteins represents an oxidative posttranslational modification. Indeed, high levels of ROS in the presence of NO or NO-derived metabolites lead to the formation of nitrating species such as peroxynitrite [35]. As nitrotyrosine represents a specific peroxynitrite-mediated protein modification, the detection of nitrotyrosine in proteins is considered to be a biomarker of cell, tissue, and systemic "nitroxidative stress" [35,36]. Quin et al. documented that increased plasma 3-NT level was associated with the mortality of AKI patients independent of the severity of illness [37].

Our results showed that HBO preconditioning reduced both the intensity and the extent of 3-NT immunohistochemical expression in all kidney structures compared to AKI. This finding was accompanied by increased plasma antioxidant capacity, as estimated by FRAP. These data may be interpreted as a helpful effect of HBO preconditioning, as it, at the same time, decreased oxidative stress in renal tissue and increased plasma antioxidant defense. These results are in accordance with our previous studies, obtained on the same experimental model, in which we showed that HBO used as pretreatment decreased other parameters of oxidative stress, plasma TBARS level, marker of lipid peroxidation in plasma [29], and renal tissue expression of 4-hydroxynonenal (4-HNE) compared to AKI group [31]. At the same time, plasma glutathione reductase activity, an enzyme that is involved in antioxidant response, was increased [29]. As it was discussed above, increased oxidative stress, accompanied by high levels of ROS and RNS, induces many damaging effects, but, on the other hand, ROS and RNS are able to trigger signaling processes at low levels of oxidative stress [13]. It was shown that hyperbaric oxygen is also an important stimulus to upregulate antioxidant enzymes in response to a greater production of ROS [38, 39]. We can assume that intermittent hyperoxia, induced by HBO preconditioning, in our study, provokes a "suptile increase" in ROS that further activated signaling pathways, including upregulating antioxidant enzymes. This can contribute to decreased oxidative stress in postischemic AKI upon HBO preconditioning, which we observed in present study. It may sound paradoxical that HBO decreases oxidative stress by inducing ROS formation, but ROS may have both a physiological and pathophysiological role, depending on the level of ROS that is produced. In addition, increased ROS is associated with enhanced renal vascular resistance [40], so we can presume that decreased oxidative stress and increased antioxidant capacity after HBO preconditioning may decrease renal vascular resistance that would further improve the renal hemodynamic [29] and glomerular filtration rate, as we showed in our research by evaluating eGFR.

DNA damage, including double-strand breaks, may be the major result of oxidative stress [41]. The immunohistochemical pattern of γH2AX(S139) histone expression in the SHAM group can be explained by the literature data indicating that the cells in aging organisms and senescing cells in culture display an increased γH2AX(139) signal even if there is no intentional damage [42,43]. This immunohistochemical pattern was maintained in the AKI group, but a much higher extent and intensity of γH2AX(S139) was observed. However, HBO preconditioning led to an evident reduction in γH2AX(S139) tissue expression, highlighting, again, its beneficial effect on AKI.

We observed a low expression of HIF-1α in SHAM operated animals, but in response to hypoxic conditions after AKI induction, we detected increased nuclear and cytoplasmatic expression in tubular cells, in contrast to the SHAM, where HIF-1α was observed mostly in the cytoplasm. These results are in accordance with previously published data. HIF-1α is a key player in the transcriptional response to hypoxia. It was shown that the HIF-1α

gene is constitutively active with weak expression under normoxic conditions [22], but in response to hypoxia, it is significantly increased [44]. Furthermore, HIF-1α is ubiquitously expressed [45,46]. In the kidney, HIF-1α is found in most renal epithelial cells, also detected in endothelial and interstitial cells of the papilla and inner medulla, but not in the outer medulla and cortex [47].

It should be noted that, when an ischemic tissue that overexpresses HIF is exposed to HBO therapy, tissue hypoxia is corrected and reversed, and, consequently, the overexpressed HIF is reduced towards the baseline [48–52]. In this study, we showed that hyperbaric oxygenation preconditioning significantly increased HIF-1α. This result can be explained by the already known hyperoxic–hypoxic paradox, actually with the fact that, in the cellular environment, variations in free oxygen levels rather than the absolute value of oxygen are interpreted as a deficiency of oxygen [22]. Duan et al. and Gu and colleagues showed, in their studies, separately, that when HBO is used as preconditioning, by HIF induction, the tissue will tolerate the ischemic insult better, harmful effects induced by ischemia will be alleviated, and the overall post-insult HIF expression will be higher than expected for the insult itself [53,54]. Hypoxia and inflammation are closely related [55]. The literature data indicate crosstalk between NF-κB and HIF-1α. Various studies have shown that NF-κB upregulates HIF-1α [56–58], but whether HIF-1α can directly regulate NF-κB in AKI is a matter of debate [59]. Activation of NF-κB may be induced as a protective compensatory tissue response, but increased and prolonged NF-κB activation is followed by abundant proinflammatory cytokines and can significantly contribute to tissue damage. In this study, we presented that increased HIF-1α renal expression detected in AKI + HBO group was followed by reduced NF-κB expression compared to animals with induced postischemic AKI but without HBO preconditioning. These results are in accordance with some preclinical and cell cultured studies that evaluated the effects of hyperbaric oxygen on NF-κB pathways. Bandarra et al. demonstrated that HIF-1α could limit NF-κB transcriptional activity in vivo and in vitro under inflammatory conditions [55]. In 2018, Liu and colleagues found that hyperbaric oxygen inhibits neuroinflammation through the inhibition of the lipopolysaccharide-induced NF-κB/mitogen-activated protein kinases–CCL2/CXCL1 signaling pathways [60]. Yu et al. observed that hyperbaric oxygen reduced the inflammatory response in acute pancreatitis by inhibiting NF-κB activation [61]. Vinkel and coworkers, in their review, summarized that, during normoxic homeostatic conditions, hyperbaric oxygenation increases both HIF-1α and NF-κB levels. On the contrary, during hypoxia, HBO exposure decreases HIF-1α and NF-κB signaling. They also pointed out that, in cases of inflammation followed by relative hypoxia, the effects on HIF-1α depend on the number of HBO sessions, whereas the effect on NF-κB expression, primary decreases, which indicates that multiple mechanisms impact NF-κB signaling during inflammation [62]. In our study, we used HBO as a preconditioning over a period of two days; more precisely, the experimental animals were exposed to HBO in normoxic homeostatic conditions, twice a day, 12 h apart; and 24 h after their last HBO session, they were exposed to severe hypoxic conditions by inducing postischemic AKI. So, decreased NF-κB renal expression, as we observed in the present study, is a result of net effects induced by multiple normoxic/hypoxic interactions on the NF-κB signaling pathway. Despite the fact that many researchers have investigated the effect of HBO on NF-κB activation, the precise mechanism by which oxygen sensing regulates the NF-κB pathway remains unclear [62]. On the other hand, there is a fine interplay between NF-κB and nuclear factor erythroid 2-related factor 2 (Nrf2). Nrf2 is a transcriptional regulator of cellular defense against oxidative stress that has been shown to improve renal damage by eliminating ROS [63], and it is also considered to be a therapeutic target for AKI [64]. It is documented in several papers that HBO's protective effect is mediated by the activation of Nrf2 signaling pathways [65–67]. In addition, it was confirmed that the return to normoxia after 100% O_2 hyperoxia exposure induces a shift towards an oxidative stress response followed by an Nrf2 and NF-κB increase in the first 24 h post-exposure [68,69]. In our study, the same exposure dose of oxygen led to an NF-κB decrease, but in the hyperbaric condition.

Balestra et al. [69] illustrated that variations in ROS production were not directly dependent on the oxygen dose up to 48 h following 60 min of exposure and emphasized that "the dose seems to not be the only clue". Later, in another publication, it was also pointed out that pulsed high oxygen treatment provokes specific cellular response according to its partial pressure and time of administration [70]. Nrf2 controls the expression of cytoprotective genes, including heme oxygenase-1 (HO-1), [71]. Previously, we showed that HBO preconditioning upregulates HO-1 expression in experimental model of postischemic AKI [30], but we need further study to evaluate is this HO-1 upregulation accompanied with increased Nrf2 expression itself.

Upregulation of HIF-1α during hyperbaric oxygenation preconditioning can be considered as its protective and useful effect on postischemic AKI. HIF-1 and HIF-2 stimulate multiple cellular and tissue responses that are involved in cellular adaptation to hypoxia, including anaerobic glucose metabolism, iron metabolism, erythropoiesis, angiogenesis, NO and adenosine metabolism [72,73]. Besides this, many studies on experimental models suggest HIFs take part in kidney repair. Appropriate kidney repair depends on a precise balance between renal tubular cell death and proliferation [74]. HIF-1α affects cell death by regulating Bcl-2 family genes, interacting with p53, and/or targeting mitochondria enzymes [75]. A large amount of work in different kinds of AKI models has demonstrated that HIF activation decreases renal apoptosis [76–78]. As we have already showed that HBO preconditioning in experimental model of postischemic AKI induction increases renal HO-1 and antiapoptotic Bcl-2 protein expression [30], we may say that there are multiply mechanisms that are responsible for helpful effects of HBO on pathogenesis of AKI, besides physical increase in free oxygen in blood and tissues. We also want to underline the importance that in this research we showed protective effects of HBO preconditioning in spontaneously hypertensive rats, considering high incidence of hypertension worldwide, as well as the fact that hypertension is risk factor for many other acute and chronic disease, including acute kidney injury.

Pharmacological activation of HIF-1α, by inhibition of prolyl hydroxylase domain-containing protein (PHD), which mediates degradation of HIF, applied as a pretreatment, significantly alleviates ischemic kidney injury by upregulating HIF target genes, followed by reducing apoptosis, macrophage infiltration, and vascular cell adhesion molecule 1 (VCAM1) expression [76,77,79–81]. Thus, upregulation of HIF abundance by PHD inhibitors is an attractive potential therapeutic target [82]. However, the effect of pharmacological activation of HIF-1α and HIF-2α as a postischemic treatment is controversial [23]. In remnant kidney model, pharmacological activating HIF ameliorated tubulointerstitial injury and decreased fibrosis [83,84].

Insufficient repair post-AKI leads to renal interstitial fibrosis [85]. Besides, HIF signaling may promote renal fibrosis via different mechanisms including epigenetic regulation, transcriptional regulation of fibrogenic genes, but also can crosstalk with other pro-fibrotic signaling pathways such as TGF-β, NF-κB, Notch, and PI3K/Akt pathways [86]. Taken together, these studies indicate that HIF takes part in renal fibrogenesis as a regulatory molecule. However, whether HIF is pro- or anti-fibrotic may depend on which, where, and when HIF is activated [23]. In addition, excessive activation of HIF may sometimes have adverse effects. It is therefore important to optimize the degree, timing, and duration of HIF activation [23].

At the end of this discussion, we would like to mention certain limitations of this study. Oxidative stress damage was evaluated through plasma FRAP and ABTS parameters and 3-NT renal expression. In order to obtain a more comprehensive analysis and assessment of the effects of hyperbaric oxygen preconditioning on the oxidative stress in postischemic acute kidney injury, it is necessary to analyze more parameters related to oxidative stress and antioxidant defense, and their potential interplay in this experimental setting.

4. Materials and Methods

4.1. Animals

For the purposes of this experiment, we used male spontaneously hypertensive rats (SHR), 24 weeks old and about 300 g an average weight, raised at the Institute for Medical Research, University of Belgrade. The animals were kept in controlled laboratory conditions (constant temperature, 22 ± 10 °C; humidity, 65 ± 1%; 12 h light/dark cycle) and fed with standard food for laboratory rats (Veterinary Institute Subotica, Subotica, Serbia), with free access to food and water.

4.2. Experimental Design

Before the animals were classified into experimental groups, hypertension was confirmed by indirect blood pressure measurements on a Physiograph Four device (Narco Bio Systems INC, Houston, TX, USA). After that, the animals were randomly divided into 3 experimental groups: sham-operated animals (SHAM, $n = 6$), a group of animals in which postischemic acute kidney injury was induced (AKI, $n = 6$), and a group of animals that after pretreatment with hyperbaric oxygen underwent postischemic AKI (AKI + HBO, $n = 6$).

Animals in AKI + HBO group were placed in a chamber specially adapted to the experimental conditions (Holywell Neopren, Belgrade, Serbia), where they were exposed to 100% oxygen, over a period of two days, according to the following protocol: 10 min of slow compression, exposure to values of 2.0 absolute atmospheres (ATA) during 60 min and 10 min of slow decompression, twice a day, 12 h apart. This protocol corresponds to the hyperbaric oxygenation treatment that is standardly applied in clinical conditions at the Center for Hyperbaric Medicine in Belgrade, Serbia [87], and is in the line with the recommendations of a relevant international organization, The Committee of the Undersea and Hyperbaric Medical Society [88].

Each exposure took place at the same time in order to exclude possible variations caused by changes in the biological rhythm. After pretreatment with hyperbaric oxygenation, the animals' body temperature was measured, and no significant change was observed after the HBO pretreatment. Acute kidney injury was induced in the AKI + HBO group 12 h after the last hyperbaric oxygenation exposure.

Before surgical procedures, rats were anesthetized by injecting 35 mg/kg body weight of sodium pentobarbital (Sigma Aldrich, St. Louis, MS, USA), intraperitoneally. After the laparotomy, which was performed through an abdominal incision, AKI was induced by removing the right kidney and occluding by atraumatic clamping of the left renal artery for 45 min with an atraumatic clamp. In the group of SHAM-operated animals, the same surgical procedure was performed, but without occlusion of the left renal artery. After the surgical procedure was completed, the abdominal incision was closed with a suture, and the animals were treated with the analgesic diclofenac. After that, the animals were placed in metabolic cages for 24 h, with free access to food and water.

4.3. Collection of Samples

Blood samples were taken (by abdominal aortic puncture), 24 h after AKI induction, and collected in tubes containing lithium heparin (Sigma-Aldrich, St. Louis, MO, USA) for further analysis. The collected blood was centrifuged for 20 min at 4000 revolutions per minute (Heraeus Megafuge 1.0 R, Heraeus, Hanau, Germany) in order to separate the plasma. The obtained plasma sample was stored at −20 °C until the moment of analysis.

Animals were sacrificed using pentobarbital (Sigma-Aldrich, St. Louis, MO, USA). For the determination of structural changes and immunohistochemical analysis, kidney tissue was taken immediately after sacrifice and then prepared for histological examination.

4.4. Glomerular Filtration Rate

All biochemical parameters for the estimation of glomerular filtration rate (eGFR), as a marker of kidney function, were measured by the automatic COBAS INTEGRA 400 plus

(Hoffmann-La Roche, Penzberg, Germany) analyzer, using commercial kits: creatinine concentration—via spectrophotometric method for plasma (CREJC test cassettes for plasma, Roche Diagnostics, Germany); urea concentration—via spectrophotometric method for plasma (UREL test cassettes for plasma, Roche Diagnostics, Germany);

In order to calculate eGFR, the following formulas [89] were used:

$$eGFR = 880 \times W^{0.695} \times C^{-0.660} \times U^{-0.391} \text{ (if plasma creatinine} < 52\ \mu\text{mol/L)},$$

$$eGFR = 5862 \times W^{0.695} \times C^{-1.150} \times U^{-0.391} \text{ (if plasma creatinine} \geq 52\ \mu\text{mol/L)},$$

where eGFR is the estimated GFR (μL/min), W is the weight (g), C is the plasma creatinine concentration (μmol/L), and U is the plasma urea concentration (mmol/L).

4.5. Determination of Parameters of Antioxidant Protection

4.5.1. Ferric Reducing Antioxidant Capacity of Plasma

We used ferric reducing antioxidant power (FRAP) assay to determine the antioxidant capacity of plasma [90]. In order to prepare FRAP reagent, 25 mL of 300 mM acetate buffer (pH 3.6), 2.5 mL of 10 mM TPTZ (2,4,6-tri(2-pyridyl)-s-triazine) dissolved in 40 mM HCl, and 2.5 mL of 20 mM $FeCl_3$ were mixed. Then, 70 μL of plasma was added to prepared FRAP reagent and incubated for 5 min, at 25 °C. We measured absorbance at a 593 nm wavelength. Results were expressed in mmol/L (millimoles of Fe^{2+} per liter of plasma). Vitamin C and butylated hydroxytoluene (BHT) were used as positive controls.

4.5.2. Trolox Equivalent Antioxidant Capacity of Plasma

Antioxidant capacity of plasma was also determined via a Trolox equivalent antioxidant capacity (TEAC) assay (also known as ABTS assay), according to the previously described method [91]. In short, 5 mL of 7 mM ABTS (2,2′-azino-bis(3-ethylbenzothiazoline-6-sulfonic acid)) solution was mixed with 0.1 mL of 125 mM $K_2S_2O_8$ (potassium persulfate) solution and left to stand in the dark for 12–16 h. Then, 50 mM of phosphate-buffered saline (pH 7.4) was used to adjust the absorbance of the $ABTS^{\bullet+}$ solution to 0.70 at a 734 nm wavelength. After that, 2.0 mL of diluted $ABTS^{\bullet+}$ reagent was added to 20 μL of plasma and incubated at 30 °C for 6 min. The absorbance was measured at a 734 nm wavelength. Results were expressed in mmol/L (millimoles of Trolox equivalents per liter of plasma). Vitamin C and BHT were used as positive controls.

4.6. Immunohistochemical Analysis

Immunohistochemistry was applied on formalin-fixed paraffin-embedded kidney samples. Four-micrometer-thick paraffin sections proceeded to deparaffinization and hydration steps, and afterwards they were introduced to heat-induced antigen retrieval in citrate buffer (pH 6.0). Novolink™ Polymer Detection System components (Leica Biosystems, Wetzlar, Germany) were applied according to manufactural instructions for immunohistochemistry protocol. Peroxidase block (5 min incubation time) and protein blocks (5 min) were applied prior to incubation with primary antibody for 1 h at room temperature. The following primary antibodies (Abcam, Cambridge, UK) were used: anti-3-Nitrotyrosine (3-NT, 1:100), anti-gamma H2A.X (phospho S139) (1:1000), anti NF-κB (1:100), and anti-HIF-1 alpha (rabbit polyclonal, 1:100). Secondary antibodies were applied from Novolink™ Polymer Detection System Kit (Leica Biosystems, Wetzlar, Germany). This Kit Detection System supplied "ready to use" post-primary antibody, and according to its manufactural protocol, it was incubated for 30 min at room temperature, followed by application of Novolink™ Polymer for 30 min at room temperature. Visualization of antigen–antibody reaction by 3,3′-diaminobenzidine (DAB) was applied for 5 min (brown products). Subsequent counterstaining with hematoxylin (30 s) was conducted. Slides were evaluated using the light microscope BX53 with DP70 camera (Olympus, Hamburg, Germany). The evaluation was performed by two independent pathologists, who were blind to the experimental information.

For the immunohistochemical scores, the intensity and extent of expression in renal structures were observed, and the mentioned parameters were scored semiquantitatively: expression intensity, on a scale from 0 to 3 (0—no expression; 1—weak expression; 2—moderate expression; 3—strong expression); and extent of expression, also on a scale from 0 to 3 (0—no expression; 1—focal expression; 2—focal to diffuse expression; 3—diffuse expression). For each of the mentioned parameters, the sum of scored changes represented the immunohistochemical score, which was compared between groups.

4.7. Western Blot Analysis

Kidney tissue samples were taken from six rats per group and homogenized in lysis buffer [92], and with an equal amount of protein, they were separated by 10% SDS-PAGE and transferred to nitrocellulose membrane. The membranes were incubated with the primary antibodies: HIF-1 alpha (1:1000, H6536 Sigma-Aldrich) and actin (1:500, A5060 Sigma-Aldrich). This was followed by incubation with horseradish peroxidase-conjugated secondary antibodies. Protein bands were visualized using enhanced chemiluminescence reagent and quantified by Image Lab (Bio-Rad Laboratories, Hercules, CA, USA).

4.8. Statistical Analysis

All data were expressed as the mean ± standard deviation (SD). A statistical analysis of each parameter of interest was carried out in the form of an analysis of variance (one–way ANOVA). When a significant F value in the one–way ANOVA test ($p < 0.05$) was obtained, Tukey's post hoc test was used. All statistical calculations were performed using GraphPad Prism for Windows (Version 7.0, GraphPad Software, La Jolla, CA, USA).

5. Conclusions

HBO preconditioning significantly increased the plasma antioxidant capacity estimated by FRAP and reduced the immunohistochemical expression of 3-nitrotyrosine and γH2AX(S139) histone. These data were accompanied by a significant increase in HIF-1α and decrease in NF-κB expression in kidney tissue. Thus, HBO preconditioning, at the same time, decreased oxidative stress tissue impairment and DNA damage and increased antioxidant capacity and HIF-1α transcriptional factor. Taking all of these results together, we may conclude that HBO preconditioning has beneficial effects on acute kidney injury induced in spontaneously hypertensive rats. These results are promising and open pathways for further experimental and clinical studies to confirm the protective effects of HBO preconditioning.

Author Contributions: Conceptualization, J.N.O., S.K. and M.I.; methodology, M.I., Z.M., M.Z. and P.B.; software, S.K. and U.J.V.; validation, J.N.O., M.Z., M.I. and D.K.; formal analysis, D.K. and U.J.V.; investigation, S.K., R.J., M.I. and Z.M.; resources, P.B. and N.M.-S.; data curation, P.B. and R.J.; writing—original draft preparation, J.N.O. and S.K.; writing—review and editing, J.N.O., S.K.; visualization, M.Z. and S.K.; supervision, J.N.O., N.M.-S., M.I. and Z.M.; project administration, D.J. and Z.M.; funding acquisition, D.J. and Z.M. All authors have read and agreed to the published version of the manuscript.

Funding: This study was supported by grants from the Ministry of Education and Science of the Republic of Serbia (Grants No. 451-03-66/2024-03/200015 and No. 451-03-66/2024-03/200110).

Institutional Review Board Statement: The experimental protocol was approved by the Ethics Committee for the Protection of the Welfare of Experimental Animals of the Faculty of Medicine, University of Belgrade, Serbia (number 323-07-07783/2020-05/5), as well as the Ethics Committee of the Institute for Medical Research, University of Belgrade, Serbia (number 323-07-02569/2018-05/2), in accordance with the National Law on Animal Welfare ("Službeni glasnik" No. 41/09), that follows the guidelines of the European Convention for the Protection of Vertebrate Animals Used for Experimental and Other Purposes (Official Daily N. L 358/1-358/6) and Directive on the protection of animals used for scientific purposes (Directive 2010/63/EU of the European Parliament and of the Council).

Informed Consent Statement: Not applicable.

Data Availability Statement: The data presented in this study are available within the article.

Acknowledgments: The authors would like to thank the Center for Hyperbaric Medicine, Belgrade, Serbia, for its continuous support.

Conflicts of Interest: The authors declare no conflict of interest.

References

1. Markis, K.; Spanou, L. Acute kidney injury: Diagnostic approaches and controversies. *Clin. Biochem. Rev.* **2016**, *37*, 153–175.
2. O'Neal, J.B.; Shaw, A.D.; Billings, F.T., IV. Acute kidney injury following cardiac surgery: Current understanding and future directions. *Crit. Care* **2016**, *20*, 187. [CrossRef] [PubMed]
3. Bellomo, R.; Kellum, A.J.; Ronco, C. Acute kidney injury. *Lancet* **2012**, *380*, 756–766. [CrossRef] [PubMed]
4. Kosieradzki, M.; Rowiński, W. Ischemia/Reperfusion Injury in Kidney Transplantation: Mechanisms and Prevention. *Transplant. Proc.* **2008**, *40*, 3279–3288. [CrossRef] [PubMed]
5. Munshi, R.; Hsu, C.; Himmelfarb, J. Advances in understanding ischemic acute kidney injury. *BMC Med.* **2011**, *9*, 11. [CrossRef] [PubMed]
6. Dennis, J.M.; Witting, P.K. Protective role for antioxidants in acute kidney disease. *Nutrients* **2017**, *9*, 718. [CrossRef] [PubMed]
7. Ortiz, A.; Sanchez-Niño, M.D.; Izquierdo, M.C.; Martin-Cleary, C.; Garcia-Bermejo, L.; Moreno, J.A.; Ruiz-Ortega, M.; Draibe, J.; Cruzado, J.M.; Garcia-Gonzalez, M.A.; et al. Translational value of animal models of kidney failure. *Eur. J. Pharmacol.* **2015**, *759*, 205–220. [CrossRef]
8. Skrypnyk, N.I.; Siskind, L.J.; Faubel, S.; de Caestecker, M.P. Bridging translation for acute kidney injury with better preclinical modeling of human disease. *Am. J. Physiol. Physiol.* **2016**, *310*, F972–F984. [CrossRef] [PubMed]
9. Gaut, J.P.; Liapis, H. Acute kidney injury pathology and pathophysiology: A retrospective review. *Clin. Kidney J.* **2020**, *14*, 526–536. [CrossRef] [PubMed]
10. Wang, L.; Liu, X.; Chen, H.; Chen, Z.; Weng, X.; Qiu, T.; Liu, L. Effect of picroside II on apoptosis induced by renal ischemia/reperfusion injury in rats. *Exp. Ther. Med.* **2015**, *9*, 817–822. [CrossRef]
11. Tanaka, S.; Tanaka, T.; Nangaku, M. Hypoxia as a key player in the AKI-to-CKD transition. *Am. J. Physiol. Physiol.* **2014**, *307*, F1187–F1195. [CrossRef] [PubMed]
12. Ruiz, S.; Pergola, P.E.; Zager, R.A.; Vaziri, N.D. Targeting the transcription factor Nrf2 to ameliorate oxidative stress and inflammation in chronic kidney disease. *Kidney Int.* **2013**, *83*, 1029–1041. [CrossRef] [PubMed]
13. Ratliff, B.B.; Abdulmahdi, W.; Pawar, R.; Wolin, M.S. Oxidant Mechanisms in Renal Injury and Disease. *Antioxid. Redox Signal.* **2016**, *25*, 119–146. [CrossRef] [PubMed]
14. Pressly, J.D.; Park, F. DNA repair in ischemic acute kidney injury. *Am. J. Physiol. Physiol.* **2017**, *312*, F551–F555. [CrossRef] [PubMed]
15. Kuo, L.J.; Yang, L.X. γH2AX—A novel biomarker for DNA for DNA double-strand breaks. *In Vivo* **2008**, *22*, 305–310. [PubMed]
16. Dickey, J.S.; Redon, C.E.; Nakamura, A.J.; Baird, B.J.; Sedelnikova, O.A.; Bonner, W.M. H2AX: Functional roles and potential applications. *Chromosoma* **2009**, *118*, 683–692. [CrossRef] [PubMed]
17. Ostojic, J.N.; Zivotic, M.; Kovacevic, S.; Ivanov, M.; Brkic, P.; Mihailovic-Stanojevic, N.; Karanovic, D.; Vajic, U.J.; Miloradovic, Z.; Jovovic, D.; et al. Immunohistochemical Pattern of Histone H2A Variant Expression in an Experimental Model of Ischemia–Reperfusion-Induced Acute Kidney Injury. *Int. J. Mol. Sci.* **2023**, *24*, 8085. [CrossRef] [PubMed]
18. Noiri, E.; Nakao, A.; Uchida, K.; Tsukahara, H.; Ohno, M.; Fujita, T.; Brodsky, S.; Goligorsky, M.S. Oxidative and nitrosative stress in acute renal ischemia. *Am. J. Physiol. Physiol.* **2001**, *281*, F948–F957. [CrossRef] [PubMed]
19. Walker, L.M.; York, J.L.; Imam, S.Z.; Ali, S.F.; Muldrew, K.L.; Mayeux, P.R. Oxidative Stress and Reactive Nitrogen Species Generation during Renal Ischemia. *Toxicol. Sci.* **2001**, *63*, 143–148. [CrossRef]
20. Bonventre, J.V.; Yang, L. Cellular pathophysiology of ischemic acute kidney injury. *J. Clin. Investig.* **2011**, *121*, 4210–4221. [CrossRef]
21. Liu, T.; Zhang, L.; Joo, D.; Sun, S.C. NF-κB signaling and inflammation. *Signal Transduct. Target. Ther.* **2017**, *2*, 217023. [CrossRef] [PubMed]
22. Hadanny, A.; Efrati, S. The Hyperoxic-Hypoxic Paradox. *Biomolecules* **2020**, *10*, 958. [CrossRef] [PubMed]
23. Shu, S.; Wang, Y.; Zheng, M.; Liu, Z.; Cai, J.; Tang, C.; Dong, Z. Hypoxia and Hypoxia-Inducible Factors in Kidney Injury and Repair. *Cells* **2019**, *8*, 207. [CrossRef] [PubMed]
24. Leach, R.M.; Rees, P.J.; Wilmshurst, P. ABC of oxygen: Hyperbaric oxygen therapy. *BMJ* **1998**, *317*, 1140–1143. [CrossRef] [PubMed]
25. Brugniaux, J.V.; Coombs, G.B.; Barak, O.F.; Dujic, Z.; Sekhon, M.S.; Ainslie, P.N. Highs and lows of hyperoxia: Physiological, performance, and clinical aspects. *Am. J. Physiol. Integr. Comp. Physiol.* **2018**, *315*, R1–R27. [CrossRef] [PubMed]
26. Thom, S.R. Hyperbaric Oxygen: Its Mechanisms and Efficacy. *Plast. Reconstr. Surg.* **2011**, *127*, 131S–141S. [CrossRef] [PubMed]
27. Camporesi, E.M.; Bosco, G. Mechanisms of action of hyperbaric oxygen therapy. *J. Med. Sci.* **2014**, *41*, 247–252.

28. Longobardi, P.; Hoxha, K.; Perreca, F. Is Hyperbaric Oxygen an Effective Treatment for the Prevention of Complications in SARS-CoV-2 Asymptomatic Patients? *Infect. Microbes Dis.* **2021**, *3*, 109–111. [CrossRef]
29. Kovacevic, S.; Ivanov, M.; Miloradovic, Z.; Brkic, P.; Vajic, U.J.; Zivotic, M.; Mihailovic-Stanojevic, N.; Jovovic, D.; Karanovic, D.; Jeremic, R.; et al. Hyperbaric oxygen preconditioning and the role of NADPH oxidase inhibition in postischemic acute kidney injury induced in spontaneously hypertensive rats. *PLoS ONE* **2020**, *15*, e0226974. [CrossRef]
30. Ostojic, J.N.; Ivanov, M.; Mihailovic-Stanojevic, N.; Karanovic, D.; Kovacevic, S.; Brkic, P.; Zivotic, M.; Vajic, U.J.; Jovovic, D.; Jeremic, R.; et al. Hyperbaric Oxygen Preconditioning Upregulates Heme OxyGenase-1 and Anti-Apoptotic Bcl-2 Protein Expression in Spontaneously Hypertensive Rats with Induced Postischemic Acute Kidney Injury. *Int. J. Mol. Sci.* **2021**, *22*, 1382. [CrossRef]
31. Kovacevic, S.; Ivanov, M.; Zivotic, M.; Brkic, P.; Miloradovic, Z.; Jeremic, R.; Mihailovic-Stanojevic, N.; Vajic, U.J.; Karanovic, D.; Jovovic, D.; et al. Immunohistochemical Analysis of 4-HNE, NGAL, and HO-1 Tissue Expression after Apocynin Treatment and HBO Preconditioning in Postischemic Acute Kidney Injury Induced in Spontaneously Hypertensive Rats. *Antioxidants* **2021**, *10*, 1163. [CrossRef] [PubMed]
32. Rodrigo, R.; González, J.; Paoletto, F. The role of oxidative stress in the pathophysiology of hypertension. *Hypertens. Res.* **2011**, *34*, 431–440. [CrossRef] [PubMed]
33. Sureshbabu, A.; Ryter, S.W.; Choi, M.E. Oxidative stress and autophagy: Crucial modulators of kidney injury. *Redox Biol.* **2015**, *4*, 208–214. [CrossRef] [PubMed]
34. Singh, A.; Kukreti, R.; Saso, L.; Kukreti, S. Oxidative Stress: A Key Modulator in Neurodegenerative Diseases. *Molecules* **2019**, *24*, 1583. [CrossRef]
35. Radi, R. Protein Tyrosine Nitration: Biochemical Mechanisms and Structural Basis of Functional Effects. *Acc. Chem. Res.* **2013**, *46*, 550–559. [CrossRef] [PubMed]
36. Ahsan, H. 3-Nitrotyrosine: A biomarker of nitrogen free radical species modified proteins in systemic autoimmunogenic conditions. *Hum. Immunol.* **2013**, *74*, 1392–1399. [CrossRef] [PubMed]
37. Qian, J.; You, H.; Zhu, Q.; Ma, S.; Zhou, Y.; Zheng, Y.; Liu, J.; Kuang, D.; Gu, Y.; Hao, C.; et al. Nitrotyrosine Level Was Associated with Mortality in Patients with Acute Kidney Injury. *PLoS ONE* **2013**, *8*, e79962. [CrossRef] [PubMed]
38. Sureda, A.; Ferrer, M.D.; Batle, J.M.; Tauler, P.; Tur, J.A.; Pons, A. Scuba Diving Increases Erythrocyte and Plasma Antioxidant Defenses and Spares NO without Oxidative Damage. *Med. Sci. Sports Exerc.* **2009**, *41*, 1271–1276. [CrossRef] [PubMed]
39. Labrouche, S.; Javorschi, S.; Leroy, D.; Gbikpi-Benissan, G.; Freyburger, G. Influence of Hyperbaric Oxygen on Leukocyte Functions and Haemostasis in Normal Volunteer Divers. *Thromb. Res.* **1999**, *96*, 309–315. [CrossRef]
40. Welch, W.J.; Baumgärtl, H.; Lübbers, D.; Wilcox, C.S. Nephron pO2 and renal oxygen usage in the hypertensive rat kidney. *Kidney Int.* **2001**, *59*, 230–237. [CrossRef]
41. Gonzalez-Hunt, C.P.; Wadhwa, M.; Sanders, L.H. DNA damage by oxidative stress: Measurement strategies for two genomes. *Curr. Opin. Toxicol.* **2018**, *7*, 87–94. [CrossRef]
42. Jeyapalan, J.C.; Ferreira, M.; Sedivy, J.M.; Herbig, U. Accumulation of senescent cells in mitotic tissue of aging primates. *Mech. Ageing Dev.* **2007**, *128*, 36–44. [CrossRef] [PubMed]
43. Nakamura, A.J.; Chiang, Y.J.; Hathcock, K.S.; Horikawa, I.; Sedelnikova, O.A.; Hodes, R.J.; Bonner, W.M. Both telomeric and non-telomeric DNA damage are determinants of mammalian cellular senescence. *Epigenetics Chromatin* **2008**, *1*, 6–12. [CrossRef] [PubMed]
44. Minet, E.; Ernest, I.; Michel, G.; Roland, I.; Remacle, J.; Raes, M.; Michiels, C. HIF1A Gene Transcription Is Dependent on a Core Promoter Sequence Encompassing Activating and Inhibiting Sequences Located Upstream from the Transcription Initiation Site and cis Elements Located within the 5′UTR. *Biochem. Biophys. Res. Commun.* **1999**, *261*, 534–540. [CrossRef] [PubMed]
45. Minamishima, Y.A.; Kaelin, W.G., Jr. Reactivation of Hepatic EPO Synthesis in Mice After PHD Loss. *Science* **2010**, *329*, 407. [CrossRef] [PubMed]
46. Wiesener, M.S.; Jürgensen, J.S.; Rosenberger, C.; Scholze, C.; Hörstrup, J.H.; Warnecke, C.; Mandriota, S.; Bechmann, I.; Frei, U.A.; Pugh, C.W.; et al. Widespread, hypoxia-inducible expression of HIF-2α in distinct cell populations of different organs. *FASEB J.* **2002**, *17*, 271–273. [CrossRef] [PubMed]
47. Rosenberger, C.; Mandriota, S.; Jürgensen, J.S.; Wiesener, M.S.; Hörstrup, J.H.; Frei, U.; Ratcliffe, P.J.; Maxwell, P.H.; Bachmann, S.; Eckardt, K.-U. Expression of Hypoxia-Inducible Factor-1α and -2α in Hypoxic and Ischemic Rat Kidneys. *J. Am. Soc. Nephrol.* **2002**, *13*, 1721–1732. [CrossRef] [PubMed]
48. Calvert, J.W.; Cahill, J.; Yamaguchi-Okada, M.; Zhang, J.H. Oxygen treatment after experimental hypoxia-ischemia in neonatal rats alters the expression of HIF-1α and its downstream target genes. *J. Appl. Physiol.* **2006**, *101*, 853–865. [CrossRef] [PubMed]
49. Li, Z.; Li, M.; Li, X.; Zhang, M.; Zhao, Y.; Ren, W.; Cheng, J.; Wang, X. Hyperbaric oxygen inhibits venous neointimal hyperplasia following arteriovenous fistulization. *Int. J. Mol. Med.* **2017**, *39*, 1299–1306. [CrossRef]
50. Zhang, Q.; Chang, Q.; Cox, R.A.; Gong, X.; Gould, L.J. Hyperbaric Oxygen Attenuates Apoptosis and Decreases Inflammation in an Ischemic Wound Model. *J. Investig. Dermatol.* **2008**, *128*, 2102–2112. [CrossRef]
51. Sun, L.; Marti, H.H.; Veltkamp, R. Hyperbaric Oxygen Reduces Tissue Hypoxia and Hypoxia-Inducible Factor-1α Expression in Focal Cerebral Ischemia. *Stroke* **2008**, *39*, 1000–1006. [CrossRef]
52. Li, Y.; Zhou, C.; Calvert, J.W.; Colohan, A.R.; Zhang, J.H. Multiple effects of hyperbaric oxygen on the expression of HIF-1α and apoptotic genes in a global ischemia–hypotension rat model. *Exp. Neurol.* **2005**, *191*, 198–210. [CrossRef]

53. Duan, S.; Shao, G.; Yu, L.; Ren, C. Angiogenesis contributes to the neuroprotection induced by hyperbaric oxygen preconditioning against focal cerebral ischemia in rats. *Int. J. Neurosci.* **2014**, *125*, 625–634. [CrossRef] [PubMed]
54. Gu, G.-J.; Li, Y.-P.; Peng, Z.-Y.; Xu, J.-J.; Kang, Z.-M.; Xu, W.-G.; Tao, H.-Y.; Ostrowski, R.P.; Zhang, J.H.; Sun, X.-J. Mechanism of ischemic tolerance induced by hyperbaric oxygen preconditioning involves upregulation of hypoxia-inducible factor-1α and erythropoietin in rats. *J. Appl. Physiol.* **2008**, *104*, 1185–1191. [CrossRef] [PubMed]
55. Bandarra, D.; Biddlestone, J.; Mudie, S.; Muller, H.A.; Rocha, S. HIF-1alpha restricts NF-kappaB dependent gene expression to control innate immunity signals. *Dis. Model Mech.* **2015**, *8*, 169–181. [PubMed]
56. Gorlach, A.; Bonello, S. The cross-talk between NF-κB and HIF-1: Further evidence for a significant liaison. *Biochem. J.* **2008**, *412*, e17–e19. [CrossRef]
57. Van Uden, P.; Kenneth, N.S.; Rocha, S. Regulation of hypoxia-inducible factor-1 alpha by NF-kappaB. *Biochem. J.* **2008**, *412*, 477–484. [CrossRef]
58. Li, Z.L.; Ji, J.L.; Wen, Y.; Cao, J.Y.; Kharbuja, N.; Ni, W.J.; Yin, D.; Feng, S.T.; Liu, H.; Lv, L.L.; et al. HIF-1ais transcriptionally regulated by NF-κB in acute kidney injury. *Am. J. Physiol. Renal Physiol.* **2021**, *321*, F225–F235. [CrossRef]
59. Liu, Z.; Dong, Z. A cross-talk between HIF and NF-κB in AKI. *Am. J. Physiol. Renal Physiol.* **2021**, *321*, F255–F256. [CrossRef]
60. Liu, S.; Lu, C.; Liu, Y.; Zhou, X.; Sun, L.; Gu, Q.; Shen, G.; Guo, A. Hyperbaric Oxygen alleviates the inflammatory response induced by LPS through inhibition of NF-κB/MAPKs-CCL2/CXCL1 signaling pathway in cultured astrocytes. *Inflammation* **2018**, *41*, 2003–2011. [CrossRef]
61. Yu, X.; Li, Y.; He, X.; Li, X.; Din, B.; Gan, Y.; Xu, M. Hyperbaric oxygen reduces inflammatory response in acute pancreatitis by inhibiting NF-κB activation. *Eur. Surg. Res.* **2009**, *42*, 130–135. [CrossRef]
62. Vinkel, J.; Arenkiel, B.; Hyldegaard, B. The mechanisms of action of hyperbaric oxygen in restoring host homeostasis during sepsis. *Biomolecules* **2023**, *13*, 1228. [CrossRef]
63. Wei, W.; Ma, N.; Fan, X.; Yu, Q.; Ci, X. The role of Nrf2 in acute kidney injury: Novel molecular mechanisms and therapeutic approaches. *Free Radic. Biol. Med.* **2020**, *158*, 1–12. [CrossRef] [PubMed]
64. Nezu, M.; Souma, T.; Yu, L.; Suzuki, T.; Saigusa, D.; Ito, S.; Suzuki, N.; Yamamoto, M. Transcription factor Nfr2 hyperactivation in early-phase renal ischemia-reperfusion injury prevents tubular damage progression. *Kidney Int.* **2017**, *91*, 381–401. [CrossRef] [PubMed]
65. Soejima, Y.; Ostrowski, R.P.; Manaenko, A.; Fujii, M.; Tang, J.; Zhang, J.H. Hyperbaric oxygen preconditioning attenuates hyperglycemia enhanced hemorrhagic transformation after transient MCAO in rats. *Med. Gas Res.* **2012**, *2*, 9. [CrossRef] [PubMed]
66. Xu, J.; Huang, G.; Zhang, K.; Sun, J.; Xu, T.; Li, R.; Tao, X.; Xu, W. Nrf2 activation in astrocytes contributes to spinal cord ischemic tolerance induced by hyperbaric oxygen preconditioning. *J. Neurotrauma* **2014**, *31*, 1343–1353. [CrossRef]
67. Meng, X.E.; Zhang, Y.; Li, N.; Fan, D.F.; Yang, C.; Li, H.; Guo, D.Z.; Pan, S.Y. Effects of hyperbaric oxygen on the Nrf2 signaling pathway in secondary injury following traumatic brain injury. *Genet. Mol. Res.* **2016**, *15*, 1–7. [CrossRef]
68. Fratantonio, D.; Virgili, F.; Zucchi, A.; Lambrechts, K.; Latronico, T.; Lafere, P.; Germonpre, P.; Balestra, C. Increasing Oxygen Partial Pressures Induce a Distinct Transcriptional Response in Human PBMC: A Pilot Study on the "Normobaric Oxygen Paradox". *Int. J. Mol. Sci.* **2021**, *22*, 458. [CrossRef]
69. Balestra, C.; Mrakic-Sposta, S.; Virgili, F. Oxygen Variations-Insights into Hypoxia, Hyperoxia and Hyperbaric Hyperoxia—Is the Dose the Clue? *Int. J. Mol. Sci.* **2023**, *24*, 13472. [CrossRef]
70. Balestra, C.; Baldelli, S.; Virgili, F.; Salvagno, M.; Mrakic-Sposta, S.; Fratantonio, D. Pulsed hyperoxia acts on plasmatic advanced glycation end products and advanced oxidation protein products and modulates mitochondrial biogenesis in human peripheral blood mononuclear cells: A pilot study on the "Normobaric oxygen paradox". *Int. J. Mol. Sci.* **2024**, *25*, 2394. [CrossRef]
71. Fão, L.; Mota, S.I.; Rego, A.C. Shaping the Nrf2-ARE-related pathways in Alzheimer's and Parkinson's diseases. *Ageing Res. Rev.* **2019**, *54*, 100942. [CrossRef]
72. Haase, V.H.; Hodrea, J.; Balogh, D.B.; Hosszu, A.; Lenart, L.; Besztercei, B.; Koszegi, S.; Sparding, N.; Genovese, F.; Wagner, L.J.; et al. Hypoxia-inducible factors in the kidney. *Am. J. Physiol. Physiol.* **2006**, *291*, F271–F281. [CrossRef] [PubMed]
73. Wenger, R.H.; Stiehl, D.P.; Camenisch, G. Integration of Oxygen Signaling at the Consensus HRE. *Sci. STKE* **2005**, *2005*, re12. [CrossRef]
74. Zuk, A.; Bonventre, J.V. Acute Kidney Injury. *Annu. Rev. Med.* **2016**, *67*, 293–307. [CrossRef]
75. Sendoel, A.; Hengartner, M.O. Apoptotic Cell Death under Hypoxia. *Physiology* **2014**, *29*, 168–176. [CrossRef] [PubMed]
76. Bernhardt, W.M.; Campean, V.C.; Kany, S.; Jurgensen, J.-S.; Weidemann, A.; Warnecke, C.; Arend, M.; Klaus, S.; Gunzler, V.; Amann, K.; et al. Preconditional Activation of Hypoxia-Inducible Factors Ameliorates Ischemic Acute Renal Failure. *J. Am. Soc. Nephrol.* **2006**, *17*, 1970–1978. [CrossRef] [PubMed]
77. Hill, P.; Shukla, D.; Tran, M.G.; Aragones, J.; Cook, H.T.; Carmeliet, P.; Maxwell, P.H. Inhibition of Hypoxia Inducible Factor Hydroxylases Protects Against Renal Ischemia-Reperfusion Injury. *J. Am. Soc. Nephrol.* **2008**, *19*, 39–46. [CrossRef] [PubMed]
78. Weidemann, A.; Bernhardt, W.M.; Klanke, B.; Daniel, C.; Buchholz, B.; Ca, V.; Amann, K.; Warnecke, C.; Wiesener, M.S.; Eckardt, K.U.; et al. HIF Activation Protects From Acute Kidney Injury. *J. Am. Soc. Nephrol.* **2008**, *19*, 486–494. [CrossRef]
79. Kapitsinou, P.P.; Sano, H.; Michael, M.; Kobayashi, H.; Davidoff, O.; Bian, A.; Yao, B.; Zhang, M.-Z.; Harris, R.C.; Duffy, K.J.; et al. Endothelial HIF-2 mediates protection and recovery from ischemic kidney injury. *J. Clin. Investig.* **2014**, *124*, 2396–2409. [CrossRef]

80. Wang, Z.; Schley, G.; Turkoglu, G.; Burzlaff, N.; Amann, K.U.; Willam, C.; Eckardt, K.-U.; Bernhardt, W.M. The protective effect of prolyl-hydroxylase inhibition against renal ischaemia requires application prior to ischaemia but is superior to EPO treatment. *Nephrol. Dial. Transplant.* **2011**, *27*, 929–936. [CrossRef]
81. Kapitsinou, P.P.; Jaffe, J.; Michael, M.; Swan, C.E.; Duffy, K.J.; Erickson-Miller, C.L.; Haase, V.H.; Pastor-Soler, N.M.; Sutton, T.A.; Mang, H.E.; et al. Preischemic targeting of HIF prolyl hydroxylation inhibits fibrosis associated with acute kidney injury. *Am. J. Physiol. Physiol.* **2012**, *302*, F1172–F1179. [CrossRef] [PubMed]
82. Ow, C.P.; Ngo, J.; Ullah, M.M.; Hilliard, L.M.; Evans, R.G. Renal hypoxia in kidney disease: Cause or consequence? *Acta Physiol.* **2018**, *222*, e12999. [CrossRef] [PubMed]
83. Tanaka, T.; Kojima, I.; Ohse, T.; Ingelfinger, J.R.; Adler, S.; Fujita, T.; Nangaku, M. Cobalt promotes angiogenesis via hypoxia-inducible factor and protects tubulointerstitium in the remnant kidney model. *Lab. Investig.* **2005**, *85*, 1292–1307. [CrossRef]
84. Song, Y.R.; You, S.J.; Lee, Y.-M.; Chin, H.J.; Chae, D.-W.; Oh, Y.K.; Joo, K.W.; Han, J.S.; Na, K.Y. Activation of hypoxia-inducible factor attenuates renal injury in rat remnant kidney. *Nephrol. Dial. Transplant.* **2009**, *25*, 77–85. [CrossRef]
85. Ferenbach, D.A.; Bonventre, J.V. Mechanisms of maladaptive repair after AKI leading to accelerated kidney ageing and CKD. *Nat. Rev. Nephrol.* **2015**, *11*, 264–276. [CrossRef] [PubMed]
86. Liu, J.; Wei, Q.; Guo, C.; Dong, G.; Liu, Y.; Tang, C.; Dong, Z. Hypoxia, HIF, and Associated Signaling Networks in Chronic Kidney Disease. *Int. J. Mol. Sci.* **2017**, *18*, 950. [CrossRef] [PubMed]
87. Brkic, P.; Mitrovic, A.; Rakic, M.; Grajic, M.; Jovanovic, T. Hyperbaric oxygen therapy of angiopathic changes in patients with inherited gene imbalance. *Srp. Arh. Celok. Lek.* **2007**, *135*, 669–671. [CrossRef] [PubMed]
88. Weaver, L.K. *Hyperbaric Oxygen Therapy Indications: The Hyperbaric Oxygen Therapy Committee Report*, 13th ed.; Best Publishing Company: North Palm Beach, FL, USA, 2014.
89. Besseling, P.J.; Pieters, T.T.; Nguyen, I.T.N.; de Bree, P.M.; Willekes, N.; Dijk, A.H.; Bovée, D.M.; Hoorn, E.J.; Rookmaaker, M.B.; Gerritsen, K.G.; et al. A plasma creatinine- and urea-based equation to estimate glomerular filtration rate in rats. *Am. J. Physiol. Physiol.* **2021**, *320*, F518–F524. [CrossRef] [PubMed]
90. Benzie, I.F.F.; Strain, J.J. The Ferric Reducing Ability of Plasma (FRAP) as a Measure of "Antioxidant Power": The FRAP Assay. *Anal. Biochem.* **1996**, *239*, 70–76. Available online: http://linkinghub.elsevier.com/retrieve/pii/S0003269796902924 (accessed on 28 March 2024.). [CrossRef] [PubMed]
91. Re, R.; Pellegrini, N.; Proteggente, A.; Pannala, A.; Yang, M.; Rice-Evans, C. Antioxidant activity applying an improved ABTS radical cation decolorization assay. *Free Radic. Biol. Med.* **1999**, *26*, 1231–1237. [CrossRef]
92. Karanovic, D.; Grujic-Milanovic, J.; Miloradovic, Z.; Ivanov, M.; Jovovic, D.; Vajic, U.-J.; Cirovic, S.; Markovic-Lipkovski, J.; Mihailovic-Stanojevic, N. Effects of Losartan, Tempol, and Their Combination On Renal Nitric Oxide Synthases in the Animal Model of Chronic Kidney Disease. *Acta Vet.* **2017**, *67*, 409–425. [CrossRef]

Disclaimer/Publisher's Note: The statements, opinions and data contained in all publications are solely those of the individual author(s) and contributor(s) and not of MDPI and/or the editor(s). MDPI and/or the editor(s) disclaim responsibility for any injury to people or property resulting from any ideas, methods, instructions or products referred to in the content.

MDPI AG
Grosspeteranlage 5
4052 Basel
Switzerland
Tel.: +41 61 683 77 34

International Journal of Molecular Sciences Editorial Office
E-mail: ijms@mdpi.com
www.mdpi.com/journal/ijms

Disclaimer/Publisher's Note: The title and front matter of this reprint are at the discretion of the Guest Editors. The publisher is not responsible for their content or any associated concerns. The statements, opinions and data contained in all individual articles are solely those of the individual Editors and contributors and not of MDPI. MDPI disclaims responsibility for any injury to people or property resulting from any ideas, methods, instructions or products referred to in the content.

www.ingramcontent.com/pod-product-compliance
Lightning Source LLC
Chambersburg PA
CBHW061558210926
51850CB00009B/2146
9783725875368